THE JUAN-CARLOS CRUZ
CALORIE COUNTDOWN
COOKBOOK

THE JUAN-CARLOS CRUZ
CALORIE COUNTDOWN
COOKBOOK

A 5-WEEK EATING STRATEGY FOR SUSTAINABLE WEIGHT LOSS

Juan-Carlos Cruz

Host of Television Food Network's *Calorie Commando* and *Weighing In*

WITH MARTHA ROSE SHULMAN

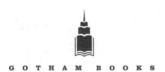

GOTHAM BOOKS

GOTHAM BOOKS
Published by Penguin Group (USA) Inc.
375 Hudson Street, New York, New York 10014, U.S.A.
Penguin Group (Canada), 90 Eglinton Avenue East, Suite 700, Toronto, Ontario M4P 2Y3, Canada
(a division of Pearson Penguin Canada Inc.); Penguin Books Ltd, 80 Strand, London WC2R 0RL,
England; Penguin Ireland, 25 St Stephen's Green, Dublin 2, Ireland (a division of Penguin Books Ltd);
Penguin Group (Australia), 250 Camberwell Road, Camberwell, Victoria 3124, Australia (a division of
Pearson Australia Group Pty Ltd); Penguin Books India Pvt Ltd, 11 Community Centre, Panchsheel
Park, New Delhi – 110 017, India; Penguin Group (NZ), cnr Airborne and Rosedale Roads, Albany,
Auckland 1310, New Zealand (a division of Pearson New Zealand Ltd); Penguin Books (South Africa)
(Pty) Ltd, 24 Sturdee Avenue, Rosebank, Johannesburg 2196, South Africa

Penguin Books Ltd, Registered Offices: 80 Strand, London WC2R 0RL, England

Published by Gotham Books, a division of Penguin Group (USA) Inc.

First printing, January 2007
10 9 8 7 6 5 4 3 2 1

Photo credits:
pp. x, xv, 142: Mark Marriot
p. xiv: Brian Algee
pp. xvii, 45, 50, 57, 59, 60, 62, 63: Robert Campbell
p. 20, 142: Martha Rose Shulman
p. 23: Branimir Kvartuc
pp. 25, 32, 39: Elan Akin
p. 68: Patricia McFarlin
p. 140: Jen Cruz

Insert:
All photographs by Ed Ouellette, with the exception of the photo by Martha Rose Shulman of
Juan-Carlos Cruz holding the tortilla casserole.

Gotham Books and the skyscraper logo are trademarks of Penguin Group (USA) Inc.

LIBRARY OF CONGRESS CATALOGING-IN-PUBLICATION DATA
Cruz, Juan-Carlos.
The Juan-Carlos Cruz calorie countdown : a 5-week eating strategy for sustainable weight loss /
by Juan-Carlos Cruz, with Martha Rose Shulman. — 1st ed.
p. cm.
ISBN-13: 978-1-592-40258-8 (hardcover) 1. Reducing diets. 2. Food—Caloric content.
I. Shulman, Martha Rose. II. Title.
RM222.2.C778 2007
613.2'5—dc22   2006024684

Printed in the United States of America
Set in ITC Century Light

This book is dedicated to the girl I met
in the seventh-grade district choir, my wife, Jennifer.
Thanks for believing in me.

CONTENTS

A few years ago I was what I called a happy fat man. I had a job that I loved and a wife who loved me no matter what shape I was in. Sure, I tried to lose weight from time to time. But to be perfectly honest, my attempts were always halfhearted. The "diet" would always start tomorrow. Sound familiar?

Then one day, just after I'd had one of my typical big, greasy lunches, I felt a stabbing pain on my right side, just under the rib cage. This was not a subtle pain; it felt like someone had stabbed me with a hot ice pick. For the rest of the day I was nearly doubled over

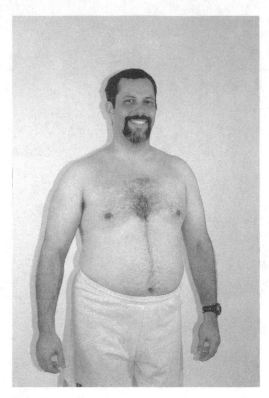

Now *that's* a magnificent gut.

in agony, but I managed to finish off my shift in the bakeshop of the busy hotel where I worked. Then I went home and, being a guy, I didn't do anything about it. It had to happen a few more times before I picked up the phone and made an appointment with my doctor.

I went in for a physical and was told that my gallbladder was the cause of my pain, and that I was most likely trying to pass a stone. While he was at it, my doctor also told me that my blood pressure was through the roof, and that my cholesterol was so high, my blood was thick enough to lubricate a Formula 1 race car. He recommended that I immediately begin taking drugs for both my blood pressure and my cholesterol. I admit I'm scared of most drugs, so I protested. My doctor then told me that if I lost my excess weight, my symptoms would more than likely clear up. And since I felt like my body was actively trying to kill me, those words were all the motivation I needed.

So I did what most red-blooded Americans do. I tried all the fad diets out there—and boy, did I have a lot to choose from. Just look around at the "health and diet" bookshelves at your local bookstore, and you will see diets extolling the virtues of everything from eating only one color for a week or one flavor each day, to cutting out certain food groups, to eating according to your blood type, to eating only raw foods. I tried no-carb diets with some success, but no sooner would I lose some weight than I would gain it right back, and sometimes I'd gain back more than I'd lost. If that's not enough to make you crazy, then I don't now what is. Time and again I found myself saying, "Losing the weight is the easy part. Keeping the weight off is the hard part."

There is a real truth to that. That's why I hate the word *diet*. "Diet" implies a temporary solution. You hear it all the time: "I'm going to go on a diet and lose some weight." Okay, then what? I would go on a diet and lose some weight, but because I couldn't live without carbs for weeks on end, nor could I live without cheese, or meat, or chocolate, I would eventually overcompensate and the weight would come back in spades. If I were going to reach my weight loss goal and stay there, I would need sustainable strategies for getting through the day without feeling deprived.

I would also need to develop strategies for slow, steady weight loss. One of the main reasons people fail in their dieting attempts is because they try to lose too much at one time. It took me a while to become the magnificent fat man that I was, and there was no way that I could lose all that weight quickly and keep it off. I'd been fighting the weight battle for years, but now I saw that if I were going to survive, I needed to win the war, not just a battle. Once I understood this, I began to develop the Calorie Countdown.

My strategies are real-world strategies. They include Pringles®, Taco Bell®, and fast-food hamburgers. Many of you may question this—especially if you are a diet guru who has never been fat (these people drive me crazy; I see them at the gym all the time). But what I'm trying to show you is that you can live in this world and still lose weight, once you have a realistic plan. Yes, it would be nice if you found it easy to "just carry a bag of carrot sticks and drink water all day," as weight-loss professionals often advise. That will work, but if you're at all like me, not for long. Not for a fat person. To this day I still need that piece of chocolate.

The benefits from my weight loss have been amazing. I sleep better, and since I'm not snoring, my wife sleeps better—which makes for a happier household. My energy and endurance are vastly increased. And to those guys out there who are happy fat men like I was, certain body parts perform so much better that you'll feel like you're a teenager again. If I had known about that one benefit, I would have lost weight a long time ago.

Reworking how you think about food is an interesting, sometimes frustrating, but ultimately very rewarding journey. It won't be easy; anyone who says it's easy is lying to you. Can it be done? Absolutely! I was the lab rat for this experiment. Are there still days that I feel fat? Sure. Are there still times when I have to reexamine my own eating program? Yes, I'm only human. But I know that the program works, and that by slowly changing our behaviors, the mind and body follow right along. So give the Calorie Countdown a try, with me as your guide. Thank you for allowing me to come along with you on your journey.

Juan-Carlos Cruz

INTRODUCTION: CONFESSIONS OF A RECOVERING PASTRY CHEF

The word is out. There's a chef teaching low-calorie favorites on the Food Network, and fans are lining up to get on the show. They're coming to New York from as far away as Los Angeles, and they're even paying their own way! That chef is me, Juan-Carlos Cruz, and if you've watched my two shows, *Calorie Commando* and *Weighing In,* you know that I'm a formerly fat chef who will show you how to *keep the taste while you trim your waist.* Dieting just won't work unless you can remember and practice that mantra. As a recovering pastry chef, I ought to know.

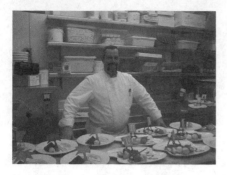

I loved working in that room—every bin behind me was full of chocolate.

For years I ran the pastry kitchen at the elegant Bel Air Hotel, the most exclusive hotel in Los Angeles. I created desserts for the likes of Julia Roberts and Jack Nicholson, Oprah Winfrey and Jim Carrey. My favorite decadent foods surrounded me and beckoned to me at all hours of the day. Chocolate, butter, and sugar were my mealtime, snack-time, and work-time favorites; I regularly indulged in midnight binges at the end of my shift. It wasn't too long before I wouldn't and couldn't wear anything other than my size XXL chef's pants. Those pants eventually went into the garbage, but even when I began to fit into size M, for a long time I continued to wear baggie "fat-boy" chef's pants with the elastic waist.

I was in total denial about this; I'd tell my wife I liked to wear the chef's pants because they were so comfortable. Well, *of course* they were comfortable—*and* I couldn't fit into any of my other, regular pants. I didn't have a mirror in the bedroom. I refused to get on the scale. I didn't want to know. Then I had a health scare, and I needed to know. I needed to weigh in, and *take it off*.

But dieting had never worked for me. I loathed food that tasted like diet food. It went against every professional grain in my supersize chef's body. Whenever I'd gone on a diet, I had denied myself the foods I loved. I'd have some initial success, then I'd blow it, usually in a chocolate-fueled binge. This went on for years; when I was dieting, I probably lost and gained more than a thousand pounds. If I did lose weight, I still held on to the XXL chef's pants, because deep down inside I knew I'd need them again.

DIETING DOESN'T WORK

If fad diets worked, there wouldn't be a new one every year. They don't work for most overweight people, because they're *just too hard to sustain*. If they result in immediate, radical weight loss, the weight loss isn't sustainable, either. If they promise weight loss in the future, they are too tough a test of faith. It's just easier—and certainly more comforting—to eat a burrito and a bowl of ice cream, and then maybe more burritos and bowls of ice cream, to make up for all those burritos and bowls of ice cream that we've been missing.

If I was going to lose my tonnage and keep it off, I was going to have to be able to feel like I wasn't depriving myself while dropping the calories. I finally realized that the only solution would be to transform my favorite dishes into healthier versions that retained the flavors and textures I craved, without so many empty calories and so much fat, and to create new healthy favorites that didn't taste like diet food. I could do this because I'm a chef; I know about food, and how it works. And I know what other people like to eat. I was used to pleasing clients with my pastries. I wanted to continue to please them, and to please myself. My plan worked for me (100 pounds and counting), and I began to share it with others.

And so I became the Calorie Commando. Each challenge—grazing, snacking, identifying trigger foods that could set off binges (for me Numero Uno was chocolate)— required a strategy. Restaurant dining and take-out required strategies. Even going to the movies required a plan. I never gave up an entire food group, or tried to eat all of one type of food. There was no way I was going to give up pasta and bread for the rest of my days. I never gave up cheese—food without cheese, what's the *point*? I didn't try to do without snacking; is a life without chocolate and cookies worth living? My approach was gradual, almost stealthy. I just identified the enemy calories, and little by little, I began to take them out.

My approach worked, and after I'd lost a substantial amount of weight, I threw out my fat clothes. I've incorporated that as a rule in my weight-loss plan. *Throw out your fat clothes*. They're only a license to gain back the weight, and the Calorie Countdown is a program for *permanent, sustainable* weight loss.

THE CALORIE COUNTDOWN

I like to call the theory behind my weight-loss strategy the "chocolate-chip cookie theory." One medium chocolate-chip cookie contains roughly 100 calories. Cutting 100 calories per day will give you a 10-pound weight loss over the course of a year. My chocolate-chip cookie might be your ten potato chips, another 100-calorie package. The trick is to find your own equivalent of chocolate-chip cookies and slowly begin cutting them out of your diet.

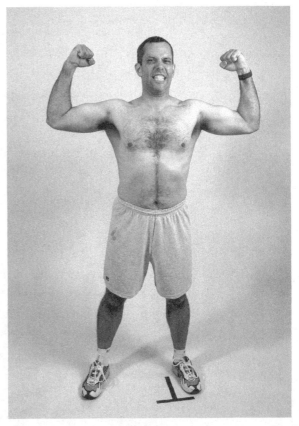

What a difference six months makes.

Using the chocolate-chip cookie theory, you can begin to slowly and gradually increase the number of calories you eliminate from your daily intake. If your eventual weight-loss goal is 10 pounds, then 100 calories a day is all you need to give up, as long as you are willing to give your body time to shed the pounds. The advantage will be that the pounds will stay off. I wanted to lose at least 50 pounds, which meant that eventually I would need to cut 500 calories from my daily intake. So week by week, month by month, I found a selection of "chocolate-chip cookies" in my diet that could be replaced by lower-calorie alternatives.

Extreme deprivation has never been my thing. I allow myself a treat every day, and one decadent dish each weekend. I allow myself a daily cheese fix. When I cook—and this is what I show people how to do in my television shows—I will use a nonfat or low-fat ingredient next to a full-fat one; for example, I might use a low-fat Cheddar side by side with a full-fat goat cheese. The fat and calories savings I make by using the lower-fat ingredient allow me to include some of that full-fat ingredient so that I can preserve the essential flavor and texture of the dish. The idea is to make food that does not taste or feel like diet food.

You can find a lot of "chocolate-chip cookies" in the large portions we Americans are used to eating. Controlling portions will allow you to include some bad-for-you stuff that you love without doing major damage. I have a tricky way of doing this. I'm a charter member of the Clean Plate Club. So I use a smaller plate. Smaller plates make it easier to control how much you eat. This is just one more of the techniques that work when you are trying to lose weight and keep it off.

Exercise is also a crucial part of the Calorie Countdown formula. Weight loss cannot be permanent without it. Our bodies are programmed for survival, and our metabolisms will eventually adjust to lower calorie intakes. That's why people reach plateaus when they diet. Exercise helps the body build muscle mass, and muscle mass requires more calories than fat to maintain, so that your body must constantly burn more energy just to function.

But exercise doesn't mean you have to upend your life, or embarrass yourself in a gym full of fitness buffs. As in calorie reduction, exercise goals will only be attainable if you begin with small changes. When I was 100 pounds heavier than I am today, my beginning goal was just to move, to get myself to the gym. I was ashamed of my body. I had no flexibility, no endurance. Once I'd gotten myself to go to the gym a few times, I went to the next step: fifteen minutes on the treadmill. And so it went. I began riding my bicycle around the block. Then I began biking to work, and everyplace else that I could bike to in Los Angeles. For me it helped to hire a trainer, somebody

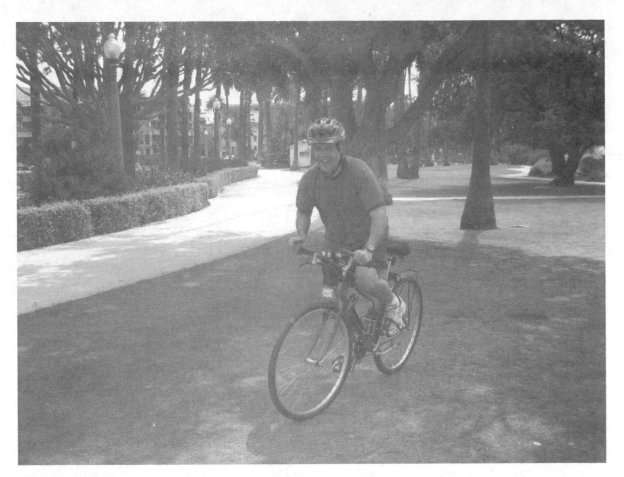

Make being active fun.

who was sympathetic and who could help me figure out how to exercise. I changed my exercise routine every few weeks, whenever I reached a plateau. Little by little, I began to want to have that mirror back in the bedroom.

HOW THE CALORIE COUNTDOWN WORKS

The Calorie Countdown is a five-week program that will introduce you to simple techniques for sustainable weight loss. The crux of my diet is calorie reduction through small changes, gradual weight loss, and maintenance through healthy—but not austere—eating and exercise. The beauty is in its simplicity. There is no complicated science involved. No one food group need be embraced or eschewed. This is a diet that will never go out of fashion. I'm a chef, and I like to eat the same things that most of you like to eat. Check out my recipes and you'll see that you can have your blintzes and brownies and eat them too. You'll have chili con carne and enchiladas. You'll even have cheesesteak. *You'll even have cheese fries!* Check out the menus and you'll see that you'll still be able to grab lunch at a Subway® or a McDonald's®. I've calculated dishes from the real world into this diet. I know what it's like to be fat, and how hard it is to make changes. You won't have to go cold turkey on your favorite foods if you follow my guidelines.

But you will have to become aware of what you eat, and how much. Then you will use the menus on pages 72 to 135 to gradually eliminate calories, 100 at a time, from your diet. You will do this just by cutting out or altering one or two menu items from one week to the next. If you cook, you will have lots of recipes to choose from to meet your caloric guidelines. If you don't cook, you'll use the Menus for the Non-Cook on pages 115 to 135. The food industry has been slow to make healthy changes, but they are beginning to realize that they are killing their customers, and more and more companies are offering healthy alternatives.

WHY THIS DIET WILL WORK FOR YOU

There are a few reasons why this diet will work for you. High up on the list is that it does not involve giving up a whole lot of things you like to eat. Because of my background as a chef in a busy restaurant, I know what people will and will not eat. I know about food. Many diet gurus are doctors. They know something about weight loss, and the impact it has on health. But they don't really know about food—how to make it, and how to make it taste good. My culinary background has taught me what will work when it comes to transforming a dish into something more diet-friendly, and what won't work.

Another reason people have had success with the Calorie Countdown is that it's designed for slow, steady weight loss. My clients from the Food Network show *Weighing In* set realistic goals for a three-month period, and most lost between 12 and 30 pounds. On the low end that's about a pound a week, and that is just fine.

There's another reason why you can trust me with the Calorie Countdown: *I've been there!* I've been fat, I've been a fat chef, I've been a fat pastry chef. I've lost the weight, and gained it back, and lost it again, and gained it back, and finally lost it again for good. I know what it's like to want that candy bar so badly you can hear it talking to you. I know what it's like to feel the humiliation that a fat person feels many times over in the course of a day (did you ever have a person who thought you were cute tell you they wanted to rub your "Buddha belly?") And I also know that when you're in that situation, you'd *rather* eat cookies than go on a diet. It doesn't seem worth it, just to fit into a smaller pair of pants.

But give my weight-loss plan a try. Like my clients, you'll see that the Calorie Countdown works. Begin now, find a daily caloric intake you can live with, and work toward it over the next five weeks. You'll see that when those five weeks are over, you'll have the momentum to continue. One pound a week is all you need to lose. It won't come back if you stick with the program, because this is a weight-loss program that's *sustainable*.

THE JUAN-CARLOS CRUZ
CALORIE COUNTDOWN
COOKBOOK

PART 1

THE

CALORIE

COUNTDOWN

Getting Started

Getting started on a weight-loss plan is always one of the most difficult moments. It's especially difficult if you try to reduce your caloric intake to an extreme. You may lose weight if you do that, but I know from personal experience that weight dropped fast is weight that will come right back—with a vengeance. Then you'll have to repeat that difficult moment again, and again, and *again*. The Calorie Countdown begins sensibly and allows you to move gradually into a sustainable weight-loss program.

HOW FAT IS FAT?

Good question. Do you leave potholes when you run, or make the CD player skip when you dance? Then maybe you have some excess weight. But let's get real. I live on the west side of Los Angeles, where all the beautiful people come to be discovered. So if you walked around my neighborhood, or along Madison Avenue, you would truly get a distorted impression of what real people should look like. You know the old adage that you can never be too skinny or too rich? Well, I disagree, at least with part of that. You *can* be too skinny.

People get so confused with the myriad of methods for determining if they're fat. Some people are, but how do we prove this? Sounds like it should be straightforward—get on the scale, and if it reads 300 pounds you're fat. But how much of that weight is muscle or bones (I love it when people tell me I'm "big-boned")?

Clinically, you are fat if too high a percentage of your body weight is fat tissue. Keeping in mind that we all have different body types and levels of activity, and that bodies change as we age (I don't like this either), a healthy percentage of body fat ranges from 19 to 35 percent in women and 8 to 25 percent in men. As a general rule, athletes have a lower percentage of body fat than most people, and women should be especially careful not to drop below 16 percent. The point, ladies and gentlemen, is not just to be skinny, but to be healthy.

Let's take a quick tour through all the ways of determining body fat. Pick up most books or cruise the Internet and you'll run across the term *body mass index*, or BMI for short. BMI is a very common way of determining if a person is obese, very obese, or—my favorite—morbidly obese. Most of these charts only look at your height versus your weight to determine your BMI. They don't take into account the amount of muscle you have, or the fact that you may have particularly dense bones. BMI charts don't know that you may now be 50 pounds lighter than you were six months ago. So even though these charts are widely used, I find them to be incredibly frustrating. Even at my skinniest the BMI chart told me that I was obese! Well, I had been obese, but that was 100 pounds earlier, and now I didn't jiggle. I worked out daily and had a very healthy diet. I was 16 percent fat and had a resting heart rate of 56 beats per minute. Even though the chart said so, I knew that I wasn't fat, and certainly I wasn't obese. The message here is: Only use the BMI chart as a rough indicator.

One of the coolest ways of determining the amount of excess fat you have is what's known as a *DEXIS® scan*, a kind of digital scan (look it up on Google and you'll see that a lot of nutritionists use it) that can be used to measure the density of your lean tissue, fatty tissue, and bone mass. I had the opportunity to do one of these at the UCLA Center for Human Nutrition. It looks like an MRI machine, but instead of you going into the donut hole, what looks like a crane arm moves slowly up and down your body. The scan takes about 15 minutes (I think—I fell asleep). When it was done, I learned that because I had been carrying around that extra hundred pounds for several years, my bones were actually quite dense and a bit heavier than average. That's what threw off my BMI chart. My body fat ratio according to the scan was 19 percent. Until I had the DEXIS scan, I was in a tailspin over my BMI, when I should have been happy about the fact that I wasn't going to suffer from osteoporosis.

The DEXIS scan is still relatively new, at least for this application, so don't expect your general practitioner to have it. But if you do ever get the opportunity, take it. You will get a printout of your skeletal structure outlined by your soft tissue (the rest of your body). It's a bit freaky to look at but very cool. I have mine on my refrigerator. I took mine when I was about 225 pounds, and wish I had done it when I was 280.

Another frequently used method for determining body fat is called the *skin-fold caliper test*. I had this test at my health club; it was one of the more interesting, and at the same time embarrassing, tests I've done. Using a set of handheld calipers, a professional, such as a nutritionist, physical trainer, or doctor, measures the thickness of folds of skin at strategic parts of the body. Those numbers are then fed into an equation that is used to estimate your overall body fat percentage. If the technician is good this can be very accurate, though the tests can be off by 5 to 10 percent. My body fat ratio came back at 20 percent with this test. I didn't have a follow-up visit because, even though I have a high tolerance for this kind of thing, I found it kind of humiliating. But I can only speak for myself.

At this point your head is swimming, and you're probably saying, "OK, but what do *I* do?" My own favorite method of keeping track of my weight is what's known as the *Bioelectrical Impedance Analysis*, or BIA. What the heck is that? BIA is a method for measuring weight and fat percentage at the same time. While you weigh yourself barefooted, a tiny electrical current runs up one leg and down the other. Every time I work with someone who has never seen one, they want to know if they are going to get shocked by the electrical current. The answer is no, but then, I have never worked with someone with a pacemaker, so I would definitely ask a doctor about that.

When you weigh yourself with a BIA scale you get one measurement for the pounds you weigh, and another measurement for your body fat percentage. Write both of these down and create a chart. As time goes by in the Calorie Countdown, you will notice a fascinating and sometimes confusing thing. The body fat percentage will slowly inch its way down but the weight will stay the same. Good news—you're losing body fat. Then all of a sudden the weight will inch down but the body fat will have gone back up. No, you are not imagining things. What body fat you still have is a higher percentage of your total weight, even though that weight is lower than it was. This can be frustrating, but stick with it; you'll get to where you want to be in a relatively short time.

Several companies make BIA scales. They run about $100, but they're worth the money if you're serious about losing weight, because they really give an accurate measurement of both weight and body fat. There are handheld units but I prefer the all-in-one models that do the whole calculation for you.

Ideally you should work with a doctor. You can discuss this with him or her at your yearly physical. You do get an annual physical, don't you? Maybe you're so embarrassed about your weight that you don't. Well, I too was reluctant to ask my doctor about my caloric needs when I was fat. But my gallbladder made me get over this really fast. Do bear in mind that doctors vary in their approaches to weight loss. If one doctor's advice seems too out there for you, seek a second opinion. And remember, once you have lost some weight and gained muscle mass, your caloric needs will increase again, because your idling speed will be higher. (I'll come back to that later in the book.)

Finally, if you don't want to bother with any of the above, there are plenty of Web sites with useful charts based on sensible methods that take into account the size of your body frame, even if they don't know anything about your muscle mass. If you just want to get started, the charts at www.healthchecksystems.com/height weightchart.htm are useful.

How often should I weigh in?

I confess that I weigh in almost every morning. It can make you crazy to do this, but it helps keep you on the diet. I speak from experience. I found that when I weighed myself once a week, let's say Sunday morning, then on Sunday afternoon, Sunday night, Monday, and well into Tuesday I would not pay really close attention to what I was eating. But I knew by Wednesday that I would be weighing in on Sunday morning, so I would meticulously watch what I ate from Wednesday to Sunday morning. I'm sure that sounds familiar to a lot of you. I've given talks at Weight Watchers groups where almost 100 percent of the folks nod their heads in agreement when I make this point. You really should weigh yourself at least twice a week, and in the beginning, do it every day like I did. It may be compulsive, it may be depressing, but it's worth it.

STEP 1: FINDING YOUR CALORIC GOAL: THE FOOD LOG

Okay, so now you know you need to lose some pounds. The next step is determining how much you should weigh—or want to weigh—and what your caloric intake should be to maintain this weight. Once you have a caloric goal, which will initially only be 100 to 150 calories less per day than you are eating now, you can start making simple cuts.

In order to get to where you're going you have to know where you're starting from. To determine your Calorie Countdown starting point, you have to know how many calories you're consuming on a daily basis to maintain the weight you are now. (This number is known as your *basal metabolic rate*, or BMR, and it should be roughly equivalent to ten times your weight.*) So here's what I'm going to ask you to do: Keep a food journal of everything you eat over a four-day period, one that includes the weekend (most of us eat differently on weekends). Weigh yourself on the first and the last day. You have to be brutally honest with this exercise.

We don't get heavy overnight. For most of us it is a long and sneaky process. I think some of you know what I mean by sneaky. One day we look down and those pants don't quite fit like they used to. The thighs are snug and the waistband leaves that mark on your skin at the end of the day. How did this extra weight sneak up on us?

People gain weight for a lot of different reasons. We eat out of boredom, stress, convenience, time pressure, and yes, there are people who really do have a medical reason for weight gain, such as an underactive thyroid. For myself it was definitely a combination of the above. I am the total stress eater. When I'm stressed out I seek comfort in chocolate-chip cookies, ice cream, and greasy food. Some of my weight gain had to do with economic eating strategies I developed when I was in college. But that 99-cent menu I loved to order at the local fast-food joint turned out to be very expensive in the long run.

Most people I work with are completely unaware of what they're eating. This is what I call *unconscious eating*. In my own case, being a pastry chef in a top hotel kitchen, I was surrounded by some of the best chocolate on the planet, and there were always fresh-baked cookies to be had. Put that on top of working in a stressful environment and it was like pouring gasoline on a fire. I would get to the kitchen at work bright and early every day, pour myself about a quart of OJ and grab a bagel. The orange juice alone came in at about 440 calories, and the bagel added another

---

* This formula for determining your BMR does not take into account your activity level or your muscle mass, both of which would allow for more calories per day.

300 or so. By the end of the day I would not realize that I had eaten from half a dozen to a dozen cookies in one shift, not to mention the goodies that the chefs would send over.

Then one day I got a program for my PDA that tracked caloric intake. I thought it would be very cool to find out how much I was truly taking in. I knew that for this to be accurate I had to be strict: Every time I picked up a cookie I would have to take out my PDA and write it in. Beyond finding out that I was taking in enough fat and sugar for a small army, I was amazed at how many times I was just picking up something and putting it in my mouth without realizing it. That's unconscious eating.

I also consider the excess caloric intake you get when you eat in restaurants and fast-food restaurants unconscious eating. It's so easy and cheap to eat badly that it's no wonder America has a weight problem. You know those "value" supersize meals that you pay a mere 35 cents extra for? Are you aware of the sheer amount of calories, fat, and sugar those meals are packing into your body? If you have not seen the movie *Super Size Me*, go out and rent it. The fast-food joint in the movie no longer has its supersize program, but quite a few others do. The next time you're in a fast-food joint, take a look at that menu and start to think of how much it will cost you to get rid of the weight add-on you get by paying that extra 35 cents. Later on we'll break down choices for eating in fast-food and fine-dining situations. But the first thing we have to do is take a hard look at what we are eating.

When you track what you're eating, you may find that the Calorie Countdown is easier than you thought it would be. One of my clients was used to having two blended coffee drinks every day. She didn't realize that along with these drinks came 600 extra calories. For her to reach her Calorie Countdown goal of a reduction of at least 500 calories a day, all she had to do was find a replacement for those drinks. If you drink sodas on a regular basis, just going from the real thing to the diet version might give you a jump start.

I'm asking you to keep the journal over four days, including a weekend, because most people have a different eating pattern on the weekends. My wife and I always go out for coffee on Saturday and catch up on the week's goings-on. Some of my clients go out for brunch after church. At my church we have donuts and coffee right after the service, and without fail one of the parishioners will call me on being out there with a donut in one hand and coffee in the other. Then I point out that what I have in my hand is half of a glazed donut, and that I sweetened my coffee with Splenda®. In the pre–Calorie Countdown days I would have had the whole donut without a second thought, and certainly not counted this as a meal. Hey, it's once a week, and it's after church. That can't be bad. Once you start adding up all the "it's onlys" you really start packing on the weight.

Here's the chart that I used for my food diary. You'll need a calorie counter, or you can get food diary software to help you track your food and calories (see Appendix for resources). You can download this from my Web site, caloriecountdown.net, then load it into your PDA like I did, so it's always with you. Isn't technology great?

CALORIE COUNTDOWN FOOD LOG

	DAY 1	CALORIES	DAY 2	CALORIES
5:00 AM–9:00 AM	**Breakfast**		**Breakfast**	
SUBTOTAL				
9:00 AM–12:00 PM	**Midmorning Snack**		**Midmorning Snack**	
SUBTOTAL				
12:00 PM–3:00 PM	**Lunch**		**Lunch**	
SUBTOTAL				
3:00 PM–6:00 PM	**Afternoon Snack**		**Afternoon Snack**	
SUBTOTAL				
6:00 PM–10:00 PM	**Dinner**		**Dinner**	
SUBTOTAL				
TOTAL CALORIES				

CALORIE COUNTDOWN FOOD LOG

	DAY 3	CALORIES	DAY 4	CALORIES
5:00 AM–9:00 AM	Breakfast		Breakfast	
SUBTOTAL				
9:00 AM–12:00 PM	Midmorning Snack		Midmorning Snack	
SUBTOTAL				
12:00 PM–3:00 PM	Lunch		Lunch	
SUBTOTAL				
3:00 PM–6:00 PM	Afternoon Snack		Afternoon Snack	
SUBTOTAL				
6:00 PM–10:00 PM	Dinner		Dinner	
SUBTOTAL				
TOTAL CALORIES				

Now here's an example of a food log that a 29-year-old overweight man did for me. You can see why he was overweight when you observe the number of calories he was consuming:

DAY 1	CALORIES	DAY 2	CALORIES
Breakfast		**Breakfast**	
½ cup Quaker® Oats and Honey granola	225	1 cup instant oatmeal	151
½ cup whole milk	80	1 cup coffee with sugar	15
1 cup coffee with sugar	15	½ cup whole milk	160
1 cup chocolate milk	226		
	546		**326**
Midmorning Snack		**Midmorning Snack**	
Large mocha	490	Large mocha	490
1 bagel	430	1 bagel	430
	920		**920**
Lunch		**Lunch**	
Roast beef sandwich	450	2 carne asada tacos	500
2 chocolate-chip cookies	220	1 steak quesadilla	550
1 (12-oz) Coke®	145	1 (12-oz) Coke	145
	815		**1,195**
Afternoon Snack		**Afternoon Snack**	
Venti® Frappuccino®	310	Venti Frappuccino	310
½ cup cashews	393	Pecan diamond	490
	703		**800**
Dinner		**Dinner**	
3 slices pepperoni pizza	797	Caesar salad	395
3 bread sticks	345	Beef lasagne	824
2 beers	300	2 beers	300
	1,442		**1,519**
TOTALS	**4,426**		**4,760**

DAY 3		DAY 4	
	CALORIES		**CALORIES**
Breakfast		**Breakfast**	
Biscuits and gravy	280	Pancakes with butter and syrup	520
1 cup whole milk	160	Caramel mocha	282
	440		**802**
Midmorning Snack		**Midmorning Snack**	
Large mocha	490	Large mocha	490
1 bagel	430	Granola bar	188
	920		**678**
Lunch		**Lunch**	
Spicy chicken sandwich	430	Steak and cheese sandwich	700
Large fries	530	1 (7-oz) bag potato chips	1,051
1 (12-oz) Coke	145	1 (12-oz) Coke	145
	1,105		**1,896**
Afternoon Snack		**Afternoon Snack**	
1 (12-oz) Coke	145	Venti Frappuccino	310
2 shortbread cookies	200	Cranberry-walnut pound cake	390
	345		**700**
Dinner		**Dinner**	
Large beef nachos	1,420	2 cups beef stew	444
1 beer	150	Dinner roll with butter	200
		1 glass red wine	104
		1 cup ice cream	356
	1,570		**1,104**
TOTALS	**4,380**		**5,180**

Sneaky Snack Attack

Does this sound familiar? "I don't eat that much, so why am I not losing any weight?" Or, "I'm careful about what I eat but I'm still gaining weight." I hear that on a daily basis, and I must admit that I have been guilty of the thought myself. But after keeping a food diary, you'll find out the awful truth: There's a lot of snacking that goes on, and 90 percent of the time you aren't even aware of it.

Almost everybody snacks. Those who don't usually snack don't have a weight problem. With me it's chocolate and cookies. For my lovely wife it's potato chips. She won't touch my chocolate, and I seldom get into her potato chips. I know from painful experience that if I go a few days without snacks I'll end up having an eating binge that will undo all the benefits of my previous self-denial efforts. I can see you nodding your head in agreement.

To retain both my sanity and my weight loss I had to factor my snacks into my eating plan, and they had to be snacks that gave me pleasure. Open up most diet plan books and you'll see advice that recommends snacking on carrot sticks or celery sticks, or something like that. That really is good advice, but I know myself, and I know what I'm going to do and not do. Carrying around carrot and celery sticks is not something I'm going to do. I had to be realistic, so I began looking for alternatives that would fulfill my need for snacking and my particular desires, and yet not increase my waistline.

I realized that I had to do this after a couple of false starts. It all came to a head the day I emptied my house of everything that was bad for me. I felt good about it until that night, when I found myself ransacking the shelves in my kitchen, looking for a forgotten piece of chocolate from a holiday baking project. It was almost 11 o'clock in the evening, and the overpriced yuppie mart around the corner was about to close. I was in full binge form, so I put on my sneakers, walked down to the market, marched myself over to a bin of individually wrapped chocolate truffles, and plunged my hand into them. With my handful of truffles I made my way to the checkout stand with only minutes to go before they closed the register. I was all ready to pay when the clerk behind the counter said, "Hey, Juan, that weight-loss plan is really starting to work."

Now I was faced with a dilemma: Do I wolf down the handful of truffles or do I put them all back and sulk my way home? I stood there for a few seconds that felt like minutes and thought about it. I turned around and put all but one truffle back. I don't think the cash register drawer had even closed by the time I was enjoying that hazelnut milk chocolate truffle. I can honestly say it was ecstasy. The clerk behind the counter then said, "So, that's your secret! You just get one piece of chocolate a day but really enjoy it!" Most guys will recognize what I mean when I say that I answered,

"Yeah, I meant to do that! That's my secret!" But from then on I would make a daily late-afternoon pilgrimage to the yuppie mart, exchange pleasantries, and enjoy my decadent treat.

I share that story not because I want you to eat chocolate to lose weight (that would be nice, wouldn't it) but to illustrate the importance of planning snacks. And not to slam the health benefits of carrot sticks and celery sticks with peanut butter, but we all live in a fast-paced convenience food world. So my eating plans include snacks that are already portioned out. For example, I know that my chocolate truffle is about 70 calories, and that my Dove® Promises® chocolate bar is 42 calories. I have one client who can't get through the day without cheese, and by cheese I mean real cheese. So for her snacks she has two Laughing Cow® Babybel® cheeses with Melba toast. The cheeses are 70 calories apiece; so she gets her cheese fix from a snack that is well under 200 calories.

I was on the treadmill at the gym the other day discussing this very topic with one of my nutritionist friends. She wasn't very impressed by the idea of chocolate bars and cheese snacks, and argued that they weren't very healthy foods. She may be right, strictly speaking. But my main concern is to get you to eat fewer calories. Once you become aware of what you're eating and how much, you can work your way up to healthy snacking.

My general rule is that if I allot about 100 to 200 calories per snack, I won't feel deprived. My own snacking occurs in the late afternoon and sometimes just before bedtime, so that's when I plan my snacks. According to many of the food logs I've looked at, that's when a lot of people want to treat themselves to something. What follows are a few of my favorite snack recommendations. By no means does this list end here; if you want to go the carrot and celery route, so much the better. I like to portion out my snacks into 100-calorie plastic bags, or 4-ounce bags, depending on the food. You can either weigh or measure out the food. Luckily many companies are cluing in to this trend, and I for one love it!

Sneaky Snack List

For the chocolate lover (that's me: I must have chocolate!!!):

- Lindt Lindor chocolate truffle; my favorite is the peanut butter (73 calories each)

- Dove dark chocolate or milk chocolate Promises bar (42 calories each)

- Fat Free Fudgsicle® bar (71 calories)

- Brownie (page 281; 92 calories)
- Chocolate-Chip Cookie (page 285; 68 calories)

For the cheese lover:

- Laughing Cow Babybel (70 calories each)
- Individually packaged string cheese (80 calories each)

100-calorie packages

- Nabisco® and Pringles® are making lower-calorie snacking easy, and I hope others will follow their lead. Nabisco makes a line of snacks that come in prepackaged 100-calorie bags, and I love them! They include mini versions of Oreo® Thin Crisps, graham crackers, Wheat Thins®, Peanut Butter Cookie Crisps, and more. You grab a bag and throw it in your purse, brief-case, backpack, or glove compartment and you know you have a snack that is exactly 100 calories. In addition to the Nabisco products, Pringles has also started making 100-calorie packages. Okay, I know we're looking at potato chips. But what I'm stressing here is portion control, not just nutri-tion. So if having a fix of 100 calories' worth of Pringles keeps you from go-ing on a 3,000-calorie bender, you'll still be ahead of the game!!

For the frozen desserts lover:

- Frozen fruit and juice bars (75 calories)
- Tofutti Cuties® (120 calories)
- I've even seen very small individual servings of premium ice cream that are about 100 calories.

Miscellaneous and always good:

- Dannon® Light 'n Fit™ 6-ounce yogurts (80 calories) with 1 banana (105 calories)
- 12 almonds (85 calories)
- ½ cup Kashi™ cereal or raisin bran with ½ cup 1% milk (128 to 148 calories)
- ½ cup 1% cottage cheese (82 calories)
- Barbecued Popcorn (page 271; 3 cups = 72 calories) or light microwave popcorn

- The second half of your lunch

- Campbell's® Microwavable Soup bowls

- Kashi GOLEAN® Waffles (85 calories each)

- Jamba Juice® choices from their "Enlightened" line

- ½ high-fiber English muffin with 1 tablespoon low-fat cream cheese (110 calories)

And of course, you can't go wrong with fresh fruit. Don't pay attention to the people who tell you that they're full of carbs. If you like fruit, go for it.

- 1 medium banana (105 calories)

- 1 medium apple (80 calories)

- 1 cup grapes (110 calories)

- 1 cup strawberries (50 calories)

- 1 orange (45 to 86 calories, depending on the size)

- 1 peach (37 calories)

- 1 pear (96 calories)

- 1 cup blueberries (41 calories)

- 1 cup cantaloupe (60 calories)

- 1 cup watermelon (46 calories)

STEP 2: REDUCING THE CALORIES: LET THE CALORIE COUNTDOWN BEGIN!

After four brutal days, you are now done keeping the eating journal. You've looked at your journal and know how many calories you're really taking in. You've looked at a few charts and identified what you think, more or less, your target weight should be. Multiply your target weight by 10 and subtract that from the number of calories you now know you are consuming on a daily basis. That will tell you roughly how many calories you need to cut from your diet.

Don't despair! The Calorie Countdown takes a gradual approach to cutting calories, and there are lots and lots of recipes for yummy, gooey dishes in this book. Also, once you begin your exercise program and increase your muscle mass, you'll be able to consume more calories and still lose weight.

Here is what you need to do with the information in your food log:

1. Identify your unconscious eating. Where is the snacking? How much high-calorie food are you actually consuming? Are you a grazer or a meal eater (or both)?

2. Identify the caloric input that you don't control. If you don't cook for yourself and rely on restaurants and take-out for most of your caloric needs, it can be the portion size alone that is resulting in your eating more calories than your body can use.

3. Figure out how to modify the above by:

   - Reducing the number of times you put food into your mouth each day

   - Creating a meal plan that works for you (see my "Five-Meal Day" menus, pages 29–31)

   - Finding substitutes for some of the foods you do put into your mouth (see all the recipes in this book)

   - Reducing portion size

STEP 3: INCREASING YOUR MUSCLE MASS: GETTING MOVING

Exercise is a crucial part of the Calorie Countdown formula. Weight loss cannot be permanent without it. Our bodies are programmed for survival, and our metabolisms will eventually adjust to lower calorie intakes. That's why people reach plateaus when they diet. *When you eat something, you're making a commitment to the universe to use it or store it.* Without exercise, the body will eventually store it, because it thinks that famine is just around the corner.

But as the mother in *Absolutely Fabulous* said to her daughter in response to admonitions to eat less and exercise more, *"If it was that easy, darling, everyone would do it."* Here too the strategy is to begin slowly. When I was 100 pounds heavier than I am today, my beginning goal was just to move, to get myself to the gym. I was ashamed of my body. I had no flexibility, no endurance. Once I'd gotten myself to go to the gym a few times, I went to the next step: fifteen minutes on the treadmill. And so it went. I began riding my bicycle around the block. Then I began biking to work, and everyplace else that I could bike to in Los Angeles. For me it helped to hire a trainer, somebody who was sympathetic and who could help me figure out how to exercise. I changed my exercise routine every few weeks, whenever I reached a plateau. Little by little, I began to want to have that mirror back in the bedroom. I threw out my fat clothes and bought some nice duds; I'm still working toward fitting into one, tighter pair of pants.

As in calorie reduction, exercise goals will only be attainable if you begin with small changes. First, get moving. Walk a little bit one day; then walk a little more. *The best exercise for you is the exercise that you will do.* This can just as easily be salsa dancing or yoga as weight training or jogging. Ideally, your exercise options should eventually include some form of weight-bearing exercise, so that your body produces more muscle mass. Muscle mass requires more energy to maintain than fat. It gives your body a bigger engine to work with; it increases your body's idling speed. That's one of the reasons you'll keep off the weight you lose on my Calorie Countdown eating plan. But first, just begin to do *something*. When you begin to feel and to see results, you'll be motivated to do a little more. Eventually, exercise—*the one you like to do*—will be part of your life.

THE CALORIE COUNTDOWN KITCHEN

Here are some of the dieting weapons I have in my kitchen.

Equipment

- Nonstick cookware. Invest in some heavy-duty nonstick cookware. A 12-inch pan and a 10-inch pan are most useful. Nonstick omelet pans are also essential for making omelets without added fat.

- A 12 × 15-inch sheet pan or cookie sheet, with a rack that fits in it. You'll be using this a lot to oven-fry (I call it *air-frying*) foods.

- Wood or urethane utensils for the nonstick cookware

- A good chef's knife and paring knife, and a steel for honing. Vegetables, ginger, and garlic add bulk, flavor, and texture to many of my dishes, and to prepare them easily you need a sharp knife. A dull knife is much more dangerous than a sharp one, because dull knives slip off the food.

- Hand blender. This is like the samurai sword of the healthy cook. It makes it very easy to puree soups.

- Regular blender. You'll be making lots of Calorie Countdown shakes.

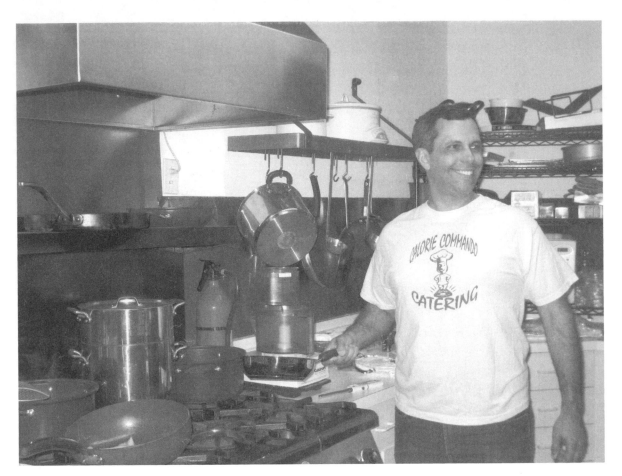

Welcome to the Commando Lab.

- Microwave oven

- Toaster oven

- Barbecue

- George Foreman® grill or a similar grill for easy kitchen grilling

- Food processor

- Lots of disposable plastic food containers. This makes batch cooking of a large meal and then dividing the meal out for the rest of the week very practical. I buy lots of containers of the same size so I don't have to fish around for the appropriate lid.

- Small plastic zipper bags for packing snacks

QUICK TIP

This sounds like a no-brainer, but always go shopping on a full stomach. There will be less of a temptation to pick up bad treats and snacks that call out to you as you walk down the aisle.

Foods

- Oil sprays:

  - Canola oil

  - Olive oil

  - Garlic-flavored oil

  - Butter-flavored

  (Note on sprays: I tried using one of those pump sprayers that you fill yourself, with disastrous results. The oil clogged the nozzle and I ended up throwing it in the trash in frustration.)

- Canola oil

- Olive oil

- Balsamic vinegar

- Seasoned rice wine vinegar

- Nonfat low-sugar yogurt (I freeze this for a quick snack)

- Fat Free Fudgsicles (at 71 calories, these are a great way to get your chocolate fix and not blow your calorie budget)

- Splenda®

- Splenda Sugar Blend for Baking

- Almonds: Premeasure them by the quarter cup into plastic zipper bags and keep them in the freezer for quick snacks.

- Individual Dove Promises bars. OK, now you think I'm nuts, but I often have one Dove Bar late in the day to fix my chocolate craving. The small bars are great for portion control—but the trick is to not eat the whole bag.

- Lots of spice blends. If I had to pick one thing to improve healthy cooking (and unhealthy, too, for that matter) I would get a rack of various spice blends, like jerk seasoning, barbecue rub, five-spice, etc. I have dozens in my pantry and find new ones every time I go to the market. They make it easy to infuse food with lots of nonfat flavor without having to work like crazy.

> **QUICK TIP**
>
> Always read the ingredient list when buying packaged foods. If the ingredient list has the word *hydrogenated* in it, then stay away from it. When it comes to calories, fat is fat, but when it comes to the effect on your body, the type of fat really matters. Hydrogenated fats will slap your arteries shut so fast your ears will pound with the sound of your heart trying to pump the sludge that once was blood.

- Garlic chili sauce. You can find this in the ethnic foods section of the super-market, with the Asian ingredients.

- Teriyaki sauce

- Hoisin sauce

- Oyster sauce

- Low-sodium soy sauce

- Babybel cheeses. I carry one in my pocket and get my cheese fix once a day with this finite amount of cheese.

- Reduced-fat peanut butter

- Low-fat cream cheese

- Light butter

- Water-packed canned tuna

- Dannon Light 'n Fit yogurts

- Lots of Lean Cuisine® and similar frozen dinners

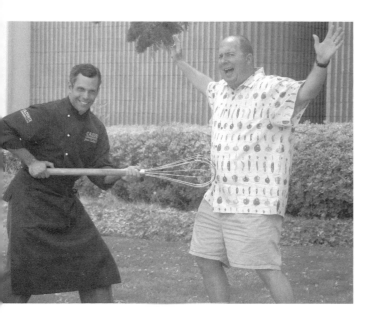

Week Minus 1 and Counting

Here are the things you need to do first, before you even begin to live by the menus starting on page 72 and cook all of the wonderful food in this book.

1. Write down the date, your starting weight, height, and age.

2. Write down the weight you would like to be.

3. Multiply your present weight by 10 to get a rough idea of the number of calories you are presently consuming to maintain this weight (this is known as your basal metabolic rate, or BMR).

4. Multiply your ideal weight by 10 to get a rough idea of the number of calories you should be consuming.

5. Create a four-day food log that includes a weekend to see what your caloric intake really is. Add the four days' totals together, then divide by 4 to get your average daily caloric intake.

6. Subtract the answer to Step 4 from the average daily caloric intake indicated in Step 5. This should be the number of calories you need to cut from your daily intake. You have five weeks to reach this goal.*

*If the goal is more than 500 calories, take one week for every 100 calories above 500. The Calorie Countdown eating plans range from 1,200 calories a day to 2,500.

Copy this chart, or download it from my Web site, www.caloriecountdown.net, and stick it on your refrigerator.

CALORIE COUNTDOWN WORKSHEET

WEEK MINUS 1 AND COUNTING

Name: _____ Age: _____ Height: _____

Date: _____ Weight: _____

(a) Weight × 10: _____(approximate BMR)

(b) Ideal Weight: _____

(c) Ideal Weight × 10: _____ (approximate ideal BMR)

(d) Food Log Calories/Day: _____

(e) Subtract (d − c): _____ (the number of calories to cut)

Now you are ready for Week 1 of the diet.

Remember, this is a gradual diet. Our goal is *sustainable weight loss*.

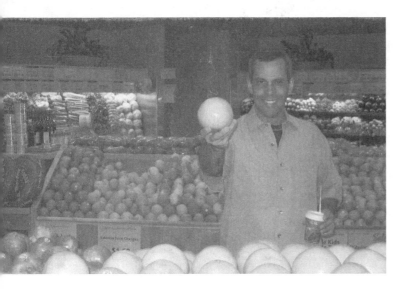

Week 1

100 to 150 calories

Strategies

- Count Down. Look at your food log from last week. Find 100 calories that you can eliminate: 100 calories can be found in a cookie; a piece of bread; a cup of orange juice; a glass of wine; a beer; half a bagel; a soda; a flavored yogurt.

- Truly become aware of *what* you are eating. Be brutally honest.

- Become aware of *why* you are eating. Are you eating because you're hungry? Or because somebody else is? Are you eating because you're stressed or depressed?

- Throw out all the crappy junk food in your pantry. Don't think about it, just do it.

- Start eating five times a day: breakfast, snack, lunch, snack, dinner.

- Go shopping for a gym. Find something that's comfortable for you. Don't go someplace that's intimidating.

- Take diet sodas for a test drive. I've been drinking diet sodas for about 6 years, and some will always taste nasty to me. I happen to like Diet Dr Pepper® and diet cherry Coke (I have a real sweet tooth). Find something that you like.

- If you drink whole milk, switch to 2% milk.

- Stop going to big-box stores. The problem with these stores is that you buy hundreds of the same item, and if it's in your home, you're going to eat it. They also tend to sell the least healthy, most heavily processed foods.

- Weigh yourself every day at the same time. It may seem frustrating at first but it's the best method for preventing backsliding.

FOODS TO AVOID (TRIGGER FOODS)	SUBSTITUTIONS
Soda	Diet soda
Sports drinks	Noncaloric flavored water
Orange juice from concentrate	4 ounces fresh orange juice
Full-fat coffee drinks	Lighter (nonfat), smaller coffee drinks
Blended coffee drinks (e.g., Frappuccino)	Small, light blended coffee drinks

FAST OR CHAIN FOODS TO AVOID	SUBSTITUTIONS
Baja Fresh® Burrito Ultimo® (1,010 to 1,120 calories)	Baja Fresh "Baja Style" Tacos (280 to 310 calories)
California Pizza Kitchen® Classic Caesar salad (1,453 calories)	California Pizza Kitchen ½ Original Barbecue Chicken pizza (600 calories)
Koo-Koo-Roo® California Burrito (810 calories)	Koo-Koo-Roo BBQ Chicken Salad (365 calories)

THE PANTRY RAID

Taking a good and brutal look into our pantries and refrigerators can be both entertaining and horrifying. It is an expedition into the realm of our guilty pleasures, where the dreaded snack foods reside. Some snack foods fall into a category called *trigger foods*, and they can be deadly. These are the foods that don't seem to have any built-in mechanisms for letting you know when you've had enough. Nutritionists coined the term "trigger foods" because they trigger binge eating.

In my own case, I have to be very careful about chocolate. Chocolate and I have a very strange relationship. I can't have it around the house, or I'll eat it all. But if I don't have a small piece of chocolate every day I'll miss it so much that I'll overcompensate and I'll go on a bender. Yes, even after all these years I have to find ways to control my cravings. I am, after all, a recovering pastry chef. And as I said before, my wife, on the other hand, couldn't care less about chocolate. But put her in a room with salty, crunchy junk like potato chips and she's done for.

Admitting that I was powerless in the face of chocolate was the first step to my recovery. Recognizing *why* I sometimes ate uncontrollably was a second step. We binge for different reasons. Sometimes they're purely emotional. I for one am a stress eater. When I'm stressed, chocolate makes me feel good. Others eat out of boredom, anxiety, even joy. I had one client who told me, "I eat when I'm feeling depressed; and I eat when I'm feeling very happy."

Given that we don't always have control over our emotions and the binge eating that certain foods provoke, there is one thing we can do to regain the upper hand: *Get rid of the trigger foods*—open up our pantries and, to put it bluntly, *start dumping the crap*.

This may be easy for me to say now, but believe me, I know it can be hard. I grew up in a family that did not waste food, so the thought of going into my pantry and actually throwing out something that was perfectly good was horrifying. It went against every fiber of my being. I will also admit to a fair amount of cheapness (we shall call it frugality): If I paid for that box of high-fat, high-carb scalloped potatoes, I'd be damned if I was going to just throw it out. At one point I figured I would just prepare everything I had in there and eat it. Bad plan. It led to weight gain, and it cost me a lot more to get rid of the weight than it would have to throw out the convenience food.

Okay, where do we start? First, go get the trash can. You might be tempted, if you're like me and you have trouble throwing food away, to get some boxes and fill them with items you can take to your church or local food bank. The problem I had with this approach was that I procrastinated for a couple of weeks, so the boxes just sat there and teased me. When I actually got the trash can and threw the foods away, I had a triumphant feeling of victory: I was taking control of the foods that once controlled me.

Now, go straight to your pantry and open up the cupboards. Take a look around, and you'll be amazed at what you find. Every time I do this with a client, it's like going on an archaeological dig. We find packaged foods and convenience foods they didn't even know were there. How do you choose what to chuck? First rule: If you've forgotten it's in there, throw it out. Second rule: If it's dusty, throw it out. Third and most important rule: *If it has no nutritional value, throw it out.*

LET ME GET THIS STRAIGHT:
YOU WANT ME TO EAT MORE????? (THE FIVE-MEAL DAY)

I love this question! I usually get it after I've told someone they should be eating five times per day. Most of us grow up eating three times per day: breakfast, lunch, and dinner—breakfast being a light meal, lunch medium, and dinner the main meal of the day. Never mind that in an ideal dieter's world we would start big and end small. This is what we have to work with.

If you really think about it, breakfast, lunch, and dinner are just the meals we *call* meals, and plan for if we plan our eating at all. In actual fact, most of us snack throughout the day and don't count that snacking as really eating. Why not change the way we look at our snacking, and actually plan five meals a day?

If you go to the bookstore and look at a bunch of diet books, you'll see explanations ranging all over the map as to why this eating strategy works. Some books will tell you that it keeps your insulin levels constant, some give explanations that I can't follow at all. I do know this: If you eat every few hours, you won't allow your body to become hungry. And by not allowing your body to become hungry you are less likely to snack unconsciously. Unconscious snacking is the main reason people put on weight and don't even realize it until they can't get into their favorite pair of pants.

When you look over the weekly menus on pages 72 to 135, you will notice that I include a snack every morning and every afternoon. Planning that snack is vitally important! The midmorning snack, which I call *second breakfast* and my wife calls *elevenses*, is sometimes the hardest one to figure out. Most of us don't even realize that we are having a second breakfast, but if you think about that midmorning coffee break at Starbucks and the muffin that you order with your coffee, and consider how many calories are in that muffin (more than 400), you realize that you are in the middle of a minefield. You would do better having an actual second breakfast. No, I don't mean a large helping of steak and eggs and bacon with orange juice and coffee. But it's not unusual for me to have a second bowl of cereal or piece of fruit with some yogurt in the midmorning. If I'm really on the run I throw one of those Kashi GOLEAN Waffles in the toaster, or half a whole-wheat English muffin, and eat it with some reduced-calorie peanut butter. My wife takes Campbell's Microwavable Soup bowls to work and heats them up for snacks. Sometimes I'll make a half a sandwich using left-over chicken salad from the day before. Or I'll just grab a string cheese and an apple. The important thing is that I know I'm going to have that small meal, and I have lots of options.

It would be easy for me to say "just have a bag of carrot sticks," and that would be very good advice. But if you are anything like me, you need a little bit of the bad stuff every day. That is why you see Dove Promises bars and chocolate truffles in the menus. Cravings are tough to ignore, and if we ignore them completely they will find a way to sabotage us. I find that I crave the bad stuff in the afternoon, and I always al-low myself that cappuccino and a bit of chocolate if that's what I want. But the cap-puccino is nonfat, and the chocolate, whether it's a Dove bar or a truffle, comes in at under 100 calories.

Another thing you can do for your afternoon snack is finish your lunch. You'll see that in the section of this book on strategies for restaurants (page 40), I recom-mend that you ask the waiter for a to-go box when you order your meal. Since the portions in most restaurants are oversized, one of the most effective ways for you to control your portions is to transfer part of your restaurant meal into the to-go box be-fore you begin eating. If you do this at lunch, take the box back home or to the office and open it again in the afternoon when you want to eat something. That will defi-nitely keep you from snacking until dinnertime.

Of course, it's best to have as healthy a snack as possible, the most obvious be-ing a piece of fruit, some nonfat yogurt, or some crudités. And that's where I would like you to end up. But meanwhile, don't be shocked that I've written in Ritz® 100-Calorie Snack Packs throughout the menus. They might not be the healthiest snacks, but at least you know that they're exactly 100 calories, and by planning your meals this way, you won't be unwittingly loading your body with more calories than it can use.

Sample Five-Meal Days
(see pages 72–135 for complete calorie counts)

1,600 to 1,700 calories

BREAKFAST

2 poached eggs
2 slices whole-wheat toast
½ cup orange juice

MIDMORNING SNACK

1 banana

6-oz Dannon Light 'n Fit yogurt

LUNCH

Subway 6-inch Veggie Delite® Sandwich

Iced tea

AFTERNOON SNACK

1 peanut-butter cookie

1 cup 1% milk

DINNER

Eggplant Parmesan (page 237)

Green salad with Creamy Italian Dressing (page 180)

1 (4-oz) glass red wine

½ cup fruit sherbet

1,500 to 1,600 calories

BREAKFAST

Kashi GOLEAN Hot Cereal

½ cup blueberries

1 cup 1% milk

MIDMORNING SNACK

1 cup grapes

6-oz Dannon Light 'n Fit yogurt

LUNCH

Roasted Bell Pepper and Lentil Salad (page 172)

Mineral water or diet soda

AFTERNOON SNACK

100-Calorie Snack Pack

1 nonfat cappuccino

DINNER

Gazpacho (page 156)

Crab and Avocado Quesadillas (page 221)

Steamed asparagus

Banana Cream Pie (page 278)

1,250 to 1,400 calories

BREAKFAST

½ cup scrambled Egg Beaters®

½ high-fiber English muffin

½ cup orange juice

MIDMORNING SNACK

½ cup Kashi Mighty Bites™ Honey Crunch cereal

½ cup nonfat milk

LUNCH

Boston Market® Tortilla Soup with Toppings

1 slice whole-wheat bread

Boston Market Seasonal Fruit Salad

Iced tea

AFTERNOON SNACK

1 apple

1 Nabisco 100-Calorie Snack Pack

1 nonfat cappuccino

DINNER

Air-Fried Pork Chops (page 184)

Steamed broccoli

Green salad with fat-free dressing

1 (4-oz) glass red wine

1 peach

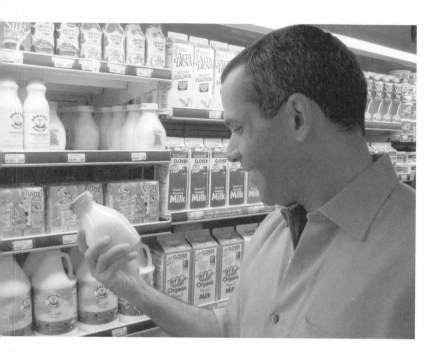

Week 2

150 to 200 calories

Strategies

■ Count Down. Use the menus starting on page 72. Find your calorie range and go to the set of menus with a calorie range that is 100 to 150 calories less than the week before.

■ Sign up at a gym. You shopped for one last week. Now sign up.

■ Test drive a personal trainer if you can afford it. This could be at the gym, through the Y, or somebody who comes to your home. It's his or her job to help you attain your goal, not to criticize you or judge you. If he does, fire him on the spot. Be careful, this becomes an intimate relationship quickly. Entire sitcom episodes have been devoted to the relationships that develop between people and their trainers. The message is that it's often harder to fire your trainer than it is to break up with your lover.

■ Be sure to eat breakfast! This is critically important. Start your day with a cereal that has at least 3 grams of fiber, something like oatmeal or Kashi GOLEAN cereal. See further suggestions below.

■ Go to the market and purchase new seasonings and spices, including spice blends.

- Switch to 1% milk if you're drinking 2% milk.

- Learn to eat slowly. You eat less if you eat slowly.

- Eat in one place in your home, to avoid unconscious eating.

- Buy lots of small containers for portioning out food.

- Beware of salads bearing noodles. Especially crispy noodles!

FOODS TO AVOID (TRIGGER FOODS)	SUBSTITUTIONS
Potato chips and crunchy snack foods	Air-fried tortilla chips (page 195)
Dips	Salsa
Sugar and honey	Splenda
Mashed potatoes	Whole grains
Butter for cooking	Pan spray
Muffins	Cereal

FAST OR CHAIN FOODS TO AVOID	SUBSTITUTIONS
Subway Double Bacon & Cheese on Deli Roll (460 calories)	Subway Honey Mustard Ham and Egg on Deli Roll (270 calories)
Subway 6-inch Chicken & Bacon Ranch Sandwich (530 calories)	Subway 6-inch Turkey Breast & Ham Sandwich (290 calories)
Saladworks® Mandarin Chicken Salad (589 calories)	Saladworks Newport Salad (184 calories)
Chili's® Awesome Blossom® (2,710 calories!)	Chili's Fajitas (330 calories)

STARTING THE DAY OFF RIGHT

I hate to channel my mother, your mother, my first-grade teacher, your school nurse, and every nutritionist I've ever met. But here I go!!

Breakfast is the most important meal of the day.

All right, I said it. I got it out of my system. But a truer statement has never been made. It cracks me up when I hear people say, "If I just don't eat anything until lunch I can eat more," only to find when they look at their food diary, that they've consumed all kinds of excess calories. Study after study has proven that people who don't eat a good breakfast end up consuming more calories throughout the day. Why? Because they're hungry!!

But what you eat and how much you eat for breakfast is what matters. Most breakfasts are either really sugar-laden or fat-laden. The large yuppie coffee drink and muffin that you stop for on your way to work (and I'm guilty of this too; believe me, I am not passing judgment) do not constitute a healthy breakfast. Let's face it, muffins are just cake! Even the ones that say "low-fat" are full of sugar. And don't be fooled by bran muffins; your average muffin will have between 450 and 600 calories. You can get your fiber without laying the foundation for another layer of fat. Here is a simple equation:

muffins = cake = tummy rolls

Don't be conned by other "nonfat" or "reduced-calorie" baked goods. That is a marketing scam. I was getting a reduced-calorie chocolate twist at my local coffee store until I went to their Web page and found that this so-called reduced-calorie twist was 450 calories. My question is, Reduced from what? The same goes for bagels, which rose to fame during the nonfat craze of the early nineties. I love bagels! But a large plain bagel weighs in at about 320 calories. Try half a multigrain bagel with reduced-calorie peanut butter or light cream cheese, and you'll still come in at around 200 calories.

I live in the same fast-paced world that you live in, and I know that most days you just don't have the time to make breakfast from scratch. I wish you did because the Blueberry Ricotta Pancake recipe on page 145 is something else. But you need to begin your day with something that's going to give you enough energy to make it through to a midmorning snack (or "second breakfast"). Most popular breakfast cereals are no better than muffins. The problem with having a sugary cereal is that your body metabolizes the sugar quickly, leaving you feeling hungry in a very short time. Luckily there are some good alternatives to having Cocoa Puffs® for breakfast.

After working with a few nutritionists, I kept seeing the same breakfast cereal, called Kashi GOLEAN, coming out on their eating plans. I—of course—made the obvious deduction that this cereal must taste like twigs and bark. I had begun to diet, and was eating instant oatmeal for breakfast, and even though that was better than the quart of orange juice and large bagel I had been eating before, it still had a lot of sugar. I was beginning to plateau and was not happy about it, so one day in the supermarket I said, "What the heck, let's give this Kashi stuff a try." And to my amazement, I found that the stuff was pretty good! It also had a good balance of carbohydrates and protein. The carbohydrates came in the form of fiber, and when you're trying to lose weight, fiber is a friend; it makes you feel full longer.

I tried the cereal with a little nonfat yogurt and some blueberries, and it rocked. Kashi also puts out several flavors of oatmeal, hot cereal, high-fiber, high-protein waffles, and breakfast pilafs that are pretty good. You'll definitely see these products in my eating plans.

Oatmeal is one of my other favorite breakfast products. I would be lying if I said I never had the instant packet types. But when I'm paying particular attention to my weight I stay away from the instant stuff and take the extra two minutes to make my oatmeal in the microwave with a little nonfat milk. Of course, oatmeal needs brown sugar, and Splenda is putting out a good product that fits the bill.

CALORIE COUNTDOWN BREAKFASTS

1 cup oatmeal (147 calories)
1 cup 1% milk (105 calories)
1 medium banana (105 calories)

1 cup Total® Raisin Bran (150 calories)
1 cup 1% milk (105 calories)
1 medium banana (105 calories)

1 small whole-wheat bagel (110 calories)
1 T fruit preserves or jam
1 cup 1% milk (105 calories)
½ cup fresh fruit (melon, berries, pineapple, citrus) (50–60 calories)

½ cup All-Bran® cereal (80 calories)
1 cup 1% milk (105 calories)
1 cup fresh grapefruit juice (96 calories)

1 cup Fiber One® Bran Cereal (120 calories)
½ cup 1% milk (53 calories)

1 cup low-fat fruit yogurt (160 calories)
½ cup fresh orange juice (56 calories)

½ high-fiber English muffin (75 calories)
1 T reduced-fat peanut butter (95 calories)
1 cup 1% milk (105 calories)

1 high-fiber English muffin (150 calories)
1 T low-fat cream cheese (35 calories)
1 cup 1% milk (105 calories)

1 cup strawberries (50 calories)

2 T sugar-free maple-flavored syrup (50 calories)

1 cup 1% milk (105 calories)

½ cup scrambled Egg Beaters (60 calories)

½ high-fiber raisin English muffin (75 calories)

1 cup 1% milk (105 calories)

½ cup fresh orange juice (56 calories)

1 cup Kashi Organic Promise® Autumn Wheat™ cereal (190 calories)

½ cup 1% milk (53 calories)

1 medium banana (105 calories)

1 cup Kashi GOLEAN cereal (190 calories)

½ cup 1% milk (105 calories)

1 medium banana (105 calories)

1 packet Kashi GOLEAN Hearty Honey & Cinnamon Hot Cereal (150 calories)

½ cup blueberries (41 calories)

½ cup 1% milk (53 calories)

2 Kashi GOLEAN Waffles (170 calories)

1 T I Can't Believe It's Not Butter!® Squeeze (60 calories)

2 T sugar-free maple-flavored syrup (50 calories)

½ cup fresh orange juice (56 calories)

1 packet Kashi GOLEAN Creamy Truly Vanilla Hot Cereal (150 calories)

1 medium banana (105 calories)

½ cup fresh orange juice (56 calories)

GOOD CARBS VERSUS BAD CARBS

Contrary to popular opinion, not all carbohydrates are bad. The body needs carbs to run properly. When your blood sugar gets low, you get cranky. Blood sugar comes from carbohydrates. The trick is to consume the type of carbohydrates that takes a long time to metabolize, so that your blood sugar doesn't spike and drop. This is what makes you feel energetic for a minute, and hungry and low very soon afterward.

I like to compare quick-burning carbohydrates to vaporized gasoline and slow-burning carbs to coal. If you take a pound of gasoline and a pound of coal and light them both, the vaporized gasoline will burn up completely in a flash, whereas the coal will burn slowly. When you consume lots of simple, quick-burning carbohydrates and your body doesn't metabolize them all as energy, the ones that are left over are metabolized as, guess what, fat. Slower-burning carbs will be more likely to be slowly burned as energy.

Quick-burning carbohydrates are also known as *simple carbohydrates*, and they include sugar and white flour, which means cake, cookies, muffins, white bread, sugary cereals, and some pasta. Most snack foods, like potato chips and French fries, are simple carbs, and so are things we think of as healthy, like granola bars and even many meal replacement bars. Meal replacement bars may have some protein, but some of them also have the caloric and nutritional equivalent of brownies. Full-sugar frozen yogurt and ice cream are also loaded with simple carbohydrates.

Carbohydrates that burn more slowly are called *complex carbohydrates*, and include whole grains—that means whole-grain breads (like multigrain, oatmeal, and whole-wheat pumpernickel), whole-grain pastas, and vegetables. Vegetables are great sources of complex carbohydrates. Fruit has lots of natural sugar, but it also has lots of fiber, and the more fiber a food has, the slower it takes your body to burn it; fruit is a good carbohydrate.

FAT VERSUS FAT

Even though fat calories are the hardest calories to burn, you can't just cut out all fats from your diet and expect to lose weight. The body needs fat to metabolize fat-soluble vitamins, and for other important functions as well. It's true that a low-fat diet is much healthier than any other type of diet, but low-fat doesn't mean no-fat. Which is a good thing, since a world without fat wouldn't be much fun.

When it comes to calories, fat is fat, but when it comes to what it does inside your body, not all fats are created equal, and some are downright evil. Enemy Number One: hydrogenated or partially hydrogenated fats. Unfortunately this ingredient is in darn near all commercial baked goods, not to mention chips of all kinds, French fries, and every other type of fried food you love to order at fast-food chains. It would take several paragraphs to explain what it does to the body, but trust me, it's bad and it makes weight loss very difficult.

So what is this hydrogenated fat anyway? You've seen it and tasted it, and can recognize it as Crisco® or " shortening," as well as most margarine spreads. But it's hidden in most baked goods, loved by the food industry because of its shelf life and

QUICK TIP

Be careful of flavored milk, even if it's made with 2% milk; 2% milk can still have a significant number of calories.

ability to retain moisture. So turn that muffin over and read the ingredient list. The higher it is on the list, the more there is of it inside the muffin.

What about other fats? Here's an easy rule: *If it's solid at room temperature, try to avoid it.* Butter is solid at room temperature. Margarine and lard (don't laugh, lots of people use it) are, too. The tasty fat that runs out of your roast beef is solid by the time you get to doing the dishes. Fats that come from animals are not the good fats. Whole milk and even 2% milk are very high in those fats. So is cheese. And chicken skin is really bad. In the Calorie Countdown you'll be cooking with skinless chicken and light turkey, and you'll be using low-fat dairy products, although every once in a while there will be some real cheese and real butter. Life without cheese is not worth living, as far as I'm concerned.

The good fats—the ones that actually help your body metabolize fats—are found in olive oil, canola oil, Enova™ oil, and avocados. I try to eat half an avocado on most days. They have just the right type of fat for your body. Nuts are also good sources of good fats—think almonds, pecans, macadamia nuts, and peanuts. But you still have to watch the amount you eat: no more than one-quarter cup per day. I buy nuts in bulk and measure them out into plastic snack bags, a quarter-cup per bag. I keep them in the freezer and grab them for healthy snacks. Which is what I want you to do, too.

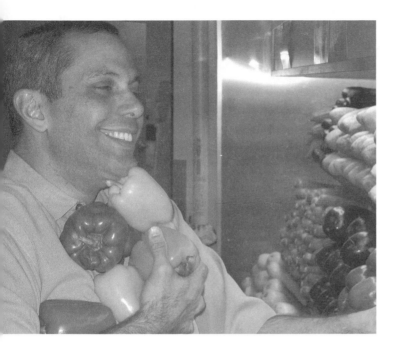

Week 3

200 to 300 calories

Strategies

■ Count Down. Use the menus starting on page 72. Find your calorie range and go to the set of menus with a calorie range that is 100 to 150 calories less than the week before.

■ Drink an 8-ounce glass of water with each meal. Carry a water bottle and drink all day. You'll clean out your kidneys and lose some weight in the process.

■ Switch to nonfat milk.

■ Take lunch to work two days of the week.

■ Keep healthy snacks at work.

■ Go out and get some decent nonstick pans. You don't have to spend a fortune, but don't get the cheapest ones either—they're too thin. You'll save so many calories by not having to use fat while cooking that it makes it worth the investment.

■ Have a strategic plan for restaurants. Plan ahead for restaurant meals. If they have a Web site, look at the menu. Ask them to fax the menu to you if they don't. Focus on light proteins: broiled and grilled foods, with sauces on the side. Remember—a Caesar salad can have over 1,000 calories!

FOODS TO AVOID (TRIGGER FOODS)	SUBSTITUTIONS
French fries	Air Fries (page 250)
Energy bars as snacks	Sneaky snacks (see page 15)
Full-fat and 2% milk	Nonfat and 1% milk
Half-and-half	1% or 2% milk
Bagels	Small whole-wheat or half bagels

FAST OR CHAIN FOODS TO AVOID	SUBSTITUTIONS
Quiznos® Signature Classic with Dressing (1,084 calories)	Quiznos Sierra Smoked Turkey with Raspberry Chipotle Sauce (350 calories)
Boston Market Pastry Top Chicken Pot Pie (750 calories)	Boston Market Chicken Tortilla Soup and Caesar Side Salad (380)
McDonald's Big Mac® and small fries (790 calories)	McDonald's Cheeseburger, no fries (310 calories)

I DON'T WANT TO BE A PRISONER! LET'S GO OUT TO DINNER!: STRATEGIES FOR RESTAURANTS

I hate the thought of being a prisoner in my own home, not being able to go out to eat because I'm trying to lose weight. Dining out for me is one of life's great sensual pleasures. But remember, it's up to you and you alone to look out for yourself when you venture out into the world of restaurants. I know that sounds hard-core, but it's true. Dining out can still be a sensual experience if you follow my guidelines.

I spent two wonderful years at the California Culinary Academy learning how to cook. I only spent a week during those two years studying nutrition, and that had nothing to do with healthy cooking, but with how nutrition works. When a chef puts together his meals, all he's interested in is making sure you have a wonderful experience, not necessarily a healthy one.

For the most part Americans are impressed more with value than with healthy. Just look at the portion sizes you get in most restaurants. I mean who needs a pasta bowl the size of your head? To keep myself sane, I allow myself one meal a week where I can have anything I want, but I don't go overboard with the portions. So if I want barbecue with white bread, I get barbecue with white bread. But I ask for a to-go box when I make my order, put half of the food into the box for later, and I enjoy every bit of my meal.

So it's Saturday night and your friends or family want to go out. What do you do? The first thing you should have done is gotten to know the restaurants in your area and what the best choices might be. I have a collection of menus from all of my neighborhood restaurants, and have gone through and looked for the healthiest alternatives. I've even been known to call a restaurant up and ask them to fax over a menu.

Let's say it's too late for that. You're hungry, you're from out of town, and you're looking for a place to eat. Luckily, most restaurants will accommodate a request for a healthier version of a dish. Don't be afraid to ask! I was a waiter for a lot longer than I care to remember, and what I wanted as a waiter was to make good tips. I made those tips by making sure my guests were happy. It actually made me crazy if the guest made a comment about the dish after he'd finished the meal. If he had made a request earlier I could have done something about it.

Here are some general guidelines for dining out:

- Make reservations. The less time you have to wait for a table, the less ravenous you will become. If you are absolutely starving by the time you sit down you will not be able to implement the next suggestion.

- Send back the free bread at the beginning of the meal. And don't you dare dive into that basket of deep-fried tortilla chips. I like to call those "deep-fried triangles of death." If you must have bread, have it brought with the meal.

- Don't order the Caesar salad. Trust me, it was my job to make the Caesar dressing at one hotel I worked at, and it's all high-calorie fat! If you want proof, go to www.CalorieKing.com and punch in "Caesar Salad."

- Beware of most main-dish salads. These salads are often piled high with cheese, bacon, olives, and in the case of taco salads, ground beef.

- Stay away from cream soups.

- Don't even think about shoestring fries or curly fries! If you must have fries on that rare special occasion, then order the steak fries. They have less surface area to a soak up grease.

- Don't butter that bread!! Don't get me wrong, I love butter. But there have been several studies that say that people who dip their bread in olive oil tend to eat fewer calories in the long run. And at least olive oil is a good fat.

- Order each course one at a time. How many times have you been out to dinner and had an appetizer, then a soup, then wondered how you're going to get the main course down because you're already full?

- Ask about splitting an order. Some places will charge an extra fee for this, but for me the fee is worth it.

- Split your order into a to-go box. Ask if the kitchen can do that. So you spend an extra three dollars—you'll get an extra meal out of it without blowing your calorie budget.

- If the kitchen will not split the meal for you, then do it yourself. Ask for a to-go box when the meal comes.

- Instead of pasta or potatoes for the side, have all vegetables, steamed and lightly finished with some butter (every restaurant I've worked in finishes the vegetables in butter no matter what. Just know that for future reference.)

- Don't be shy about asking how a dish is prepared. Sometimes the menu won't make it obvious when something is fried, or deep-fried, or even if it's finished with a cream sauce.

- Always go for broiled, grilled, baked, braised, and of course poached. When you go out for breakfast, poached eggs are your best option.

- Order from the kids' menu; the portions are smaller. I have had arguments with waiters about this. I tell them to go ahead and charge me whatever they need to charge me. I just want the smaller portion. Sometimes waiters can be from Mars, and they just don't understand.

- Halfway through your meal, ask yourself if you're still hungry. If you are not, then by all means stop!!

- Order an appetizer and a side salad as your whole dinner. I do this so often that sometimes I don't even read the rest of the menu.

- Order fruit or sorbet for dessert.

- If you're done eating, don't pick at your plate. Take your napkin and place it right on top.

- If you must have a decadent chocolate or other dessert, order one for the table and a whole bunch of forks to split it.

As I'm always saying, the Calorie Countdown is all about choices, and luckily some of the major chains out there are offering some pretty good ones. Here are some examples. For more ideas, see the Menus for the Non-Cook, starting on page 115, and check the Web sites of your favorite restaurants.

- Applebee's®: Weight Watchers menu

- Hard Rock® Cafe: Smoked Turkey Sandwich or Grilled Chinese Chicken Salad

- Olive Garden®: Shrimp Primavera or Pasta e Fagioli

- Ruby Tucsday®: Smart Eating℠ menu

- Outback Steakhouse®: Victoria's Filet® or Shrimp Griller

- Chili's: Guiltless Grill® menu

If you're seeing a pattern of lean proteins, then you are on to me. Just remember, there are hidden dangers in every cuisine. But there are also many healthy choices.

FAST-FOOD STRATEGIES

Let me tell you this up front: I love fast food! A few years ago I had the pleasure of being on a panel of chefs being interviewed by a major magazine, and I was asked what restaurants I frequented most often. My response was Taco Bell®. There was a bit of laughter, and then I explained that on most nights chefs get off work after midnight, and who else is open at that time of night but fast-food joints? Most of the other chefs admitted to a reliance on convenience food on the way home from work. Hey! We cook all day, we're hungry and want to get home, and we just want something quick and easy.

It just blows my mind how cheap fast food is these days. No wonder America has become obese, especially low-income America. Walk into any chain and you'll find that for about two dollars you can come out with a good 1,500-calorie meal. "Good" here does not refer to quality, just quantity.

But there are healthier meals out there, even in fast-food restaurants. Flip through some of the menus on pages 72 to 135 and you'll notice that I have included some places that you may be surprised to see in the Calorie Countdown. Sure, I admit that eating at McDonald's every day is not a good idea; see the movie *Super Size Me* and you'll see what I mean. But if you are craving a hamburger, a regular cheeseburger at McDonald's is not a bad caloric buy at 310 calories. Choose that over the Big Mac (530 calories) and you're saving over 200 calories. Subway sandwiches have also made quite an impact with their "6 Grams of Fat or Less" choices, and Taco Bell now has a lower-calorie "Fresco Style" line.

I may have mentioned this before, but I am a caffeine fanatic. I've tried to go cold turkey, but at least once a week I allow myself a blended coffee drink from Starbucks. However, even at Starbucks you can make healthier choices. Compare a large blended drink with whipped cream to a small light version without, and you'll see that you can save yourself up to 400 calories. Again, the message here is: *Plan*.

Here are some good choices at fast-food joints:

- Schlotzsky's Deli℠ Dijon Grilled Chicken sandwich with the fresh fruit salad
- Subway 6-inch sandwiches with 6 grams of fat or less
- Subway Turkey Breast Wrap
- McDonald's Grilled Chicken California Cobb Salad
- McDonald's Chicken McGrill® with no mayo
- Wendy's® small Chili
- Taco Bell "Fresco Style" items
- Panda Express® Chicken with String Beans
- Panda Express Beef with Broccoli
- Pizza Hut® Fit N' Delicious™ menu

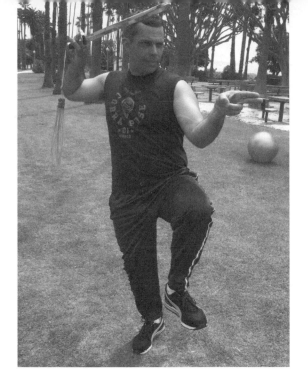

Week 4

300 to 400 calories

Strategies

- Count Down. Use the menus starting on page 72. Find your calorie range and go to the set of menus with a calorie range that is 100 to 150 calories less than the week before.

- Review your eating from the past three weeks. What changes have you made? Which ones were the most difficult? What changes do you want to make?

- Reward yourself with a nonfood treat. You deserve it. This is important, because so many times, rewards revolve around food. Think of all the times you've gone out to eat to celebrate something. Finding a nonfood way to congratulate yourself is good for your waistline. Buy some clothes or a piece of jewelry.

- Try a new exercise, something you've never done. Be creative and brave. Try dancing! You never know what you'll like.

- Get into the habit of reading labels. Beware of labels that say "low-fat." It doesn't mean it's low in calories. Same goes for "low-carb."

- Stay away from free food.

FOODS TO AVOID (TRIGGER FOODS)	SUBSTITUTIONS
Free snacks in bars and restaurants, free food in general	Well-chosen appetizers or meals
Full-fat ice cream	Low-fat or nonfat ice cream
White bread	Whole-wheat high-fiber bread
Baked potatoes with toppings	Baked potatoes with salsa and low-fat cheese
Full-fat salad dressings	Nonfat dressings

FAST OR CHAIN FOODS TO AVOID	SUBSTITUTIONS
Baja Fresh Fajitas (almost all over 1,000 calories)	Baja Ensalada with Charbroiled Steak and Salsa (465 calories)
Taco Bell Grilled Stuft Steak Burrito (680 calories)	Taco Bell Fresco Style Steak Burrito Supreme® (350 calories)
Jamba Juice Smoothies	Jamba Juice Enlightened Smoothies

STRATEGIES FOR THE HEALTHY FAMILY

Today kids are fatter than they have ever been. Many suffer from type 2 diabetes, a disease that in the past afflicted only older, sedentary adults. A recent study suggests that the present generation will be the first generation to have a shorter life expectancy than their parents; and it's all related to obesity caused by a sedentary lifestyle. These findings really scare me.

Many parents don't understand that their own lifestyle will determine the lifestyle of their kids, which in turn will impact their health. This was made all too clear to me one day about a year ago, when I was making my rounds at Children's Hospital Los Angeles. I volunteer there with my dog Maggie, in the animal-assisted therapy program.

Ninety-nine percent of the time when I'm in my volunteer uniform, no one recognizes me from my television shows. And my dog is so cute that no one notices me anyway. But on that day the mother of the child whom my dog was visiting knew who I was, and she went on about how she loved my show (I always love to hear that; to this day I get a kick out of being recognized). Both the mother and the daughter were, for lack of a better term, obese. Not just a little, but a lot. We talked about diets and weight loss while my dog played with the little girl.

A few minutes into the conversation another family member arrived with lunch from the McDonald's in the lobby, and it was like a scene from the movie *Super Size Me*. They had every bad thing that McDonald's has to offer. I started to collect Maggie so that they could enjoy their lunch, when the conversation turned to their daughter's type 2 diabetes, which was why she was in the hospital. They told me that no one else in the family had diabetes, and that it was mystery to them how their daughter got it. At this point I began to feel like I was in an episode of *The Twilight Zone*.

Now remember, I'm there with the animal-assisted therapy program, so it was not my place to say anything. When we receive our training for this program we are discouraged from even asking questions about why the child is in the hospital. But when I left the room I nearly burst into tears. They had obviously watched many shows on weight loss and the health effects of obesity, but had never taken any of it to heart. My dog and I have volunteered at Children's Hospital for more than three years and have seen many heartwarming and heartbreaking cases. But that encounter still haunts me. It's one of the reasons I'm inspired to do what I do, to teach people to become aware of what they're eating.

Bringing up a healthy family must be the hardest task on this planet. I once attended a lecture on family dynamics, and the family structure was compared to one of those hanging mobile sculptures, where everything was in perfect balance. Anything that helped to keep that balance and make it easier to get through the day was a good thing. Unfortunately, keeping that balance has led to some unintended consequences. I totally understand when a parent says, "I can only get things done when Johnny's playing video games," or the one I used to hear around my house when I was growing up: "The television is our babysitter." Which explains why I know every television theme song from the 1970s.

But to raise a healthy family, you may have to shake things up. That delicately balanced mobile may go through some rough times. It's easier in the long run, though, to instill healthy habits in a young person than to try to retrain them after they have developed bad habits and a weight problem. And avoiding the inevitable health problems that result from being overweight will ultimately make life easier for the entire family.

So what's a family to do?

The best thing is to live the message. Kids see what their parents do and pattern that behavior. If you skip breakfast, it's likely that your kid will think that skipping breakfast is normal. If you are always snacking, then your kids will do the same. On the other hand, if you see that your kids are becoming too fat and try to control their eating while not changing your own habits, you will fail. If everyone in the house gets a Drumstick® for dessert except for little Benny, then little Benny is going to develop some sneaky ways of getting that treat.

No one ever said that bringing up healthy, well-balanced children would be easy. And I'm sure that when all you hear is them whining about how it's not fair that so-and-so gets ice cream on a regular basis and they don't, it would be easier to give in. But let's raise kids to be healthy, active, and well-adjusted adults.

Tips for Living the Message

- Limit sedentary behavior, like watching television, playing video games, and, of course, surfing the Internet.

- If they must play video games, by all means go out and get Dance Dance Revolution. Even try it yourself! Your kids may laugh at you, but it's one heck of a workout.

- Never use food as a reward. How many times have you said, "If you're good, you'll get candy," or "If you get a good grade, we'll take you out for a nice dinner"? I used to get a banana split every time I won a sporting event.

- Get rid of all, and I do mean *all,* unhealthy snacks in the house.

- Have plenty of healthy snacks on hand. These include fresh fruit, graham crackers, low-fat vanilla wafers, nonfat yogurt with fruit, reduced-fat natural peanut butter with whole-wheat crackers, fat-free pudding, fruit juice bars, and my favorite, fat-free Fudgsicles.

- If you want your kids to eat fruit, then they had better see you eating fruit.

- Never make exercise a punishment.

- Schedule family outings that involve physical activity, like bike rides, hikes, and Sundays at the local pool or beach.

- Get outside and play games with your kids; play tag and hide-and-seek with the little ones; shoot baskets, play baseball, soccer, or football with the bigger ones.

- Eat breakfast every day.

- Don't even think about having full-sugar soft drinks in the house.

- Never criticize your child about his or her weight.

- Start with small servings. Let your child ask for more if he or she is still hungry. Use smaller plates.

- 100% juice is 100 percent sugar. It may sound healthy, but fruit juices are a sugar delivery system. This is particularly important when it comes to babies. If you want to give them juice, dilute it by half with water. Many babies are overweight because they are drinking too much juice, leading to a lifelong addiction to sugar.

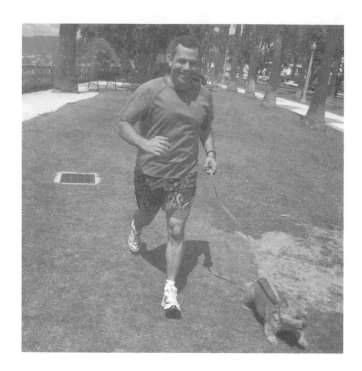

Week 5

500 calories: GOAL!

Strategies:

- Count Down. Use the menus starting on page 72. Find your calorie range and go to the set of menus with a calorie range that is 100 to 150 calories less than the week before.

- The hardest weeks are Week 1 and Week 5. Week 1 because it's difficult to make changes, Week 5 because you may become discouraged and bored. You've done really well on some things, but you're human. Don't beat yourself up about not doing some things "right." Look at the things you've done right, and continue to do them. Strive to change the things you haven't. Remember that we are trying to win a war here, not just a battle, and that by the time you have reduced your daily caloric intake by 500 calories, you've accomplished a great deal. The changes you've made are ones that you can sustain, and you will continue to lose weight at about 1 pound a week. You may experience plateaus as your body continuously adjusts to its new muscle mass and caloric needs, but don't be discouraged by them. They are normal and they aren't forever.

- Be prepared for friends and family not supporting you. This may sound odd, but friends and family are not always 100 percent supportive after you've been on a lifestyle change for a while, so don't expect them to be. Usually it's unconscious on their part, but they can sabotage you. When I had been losing weight for some time and I'd go out with friends, often they'd say, "Are you still on that diet?" and inevitably what would follow would be something like, "Oh have some nachos and another beer, this one time won't hurt!" Or you may go to visit your parents, and your mother will make lots of your childhood favorite desserts. She may act hurt if you refuse, but don't let her kill you with love! My response to these situations is "I'm not on a diet. This is my lifestyle. Respect it."

- Avoid and be conscious of situations that promote overeating, like a birthday party at the office or at school, or a cocktail party with a buffet. Stay away from the buffet table at the cocktail party and avoid sitting down near a bowl of chips.

- Try not to eat for comfort or to relieve stress. Think of substitutions, the same strategy you use for food. For me, walking my dog is a big stress reliever, and it gets me out of the house and gets me some exercise at the same time.

- *Be flexible!!!* None of this is written in stone. These are guidelines.

- This is something to do in the weeks to come: Throw out your fat clothes! You've crossed the Rubicon. You're not going back.

FOODS TO AVOID (TRIGGER FOODS)	SUBSTITUTIONS
Nachos	Calorie Countdown Nachos (page 163)
Regular beer	Light beer
Wine coolers	Wine spritzers made with sparkling water
Regular bacon	Turkey bacon, Canadian bacon
Butter	I Can't Believe It's Not Butter!

FAST OR CHAIN FOODS TO AVOID	SUBSTITUTIONS
Applebee's Southwest Philly Rollup with Salsa (1,605 calories)	Applebee's Teriyaki Steak 'N Shrimp Skewers (370 calories)
Arby's® Chicken Breast Fillet (500 calories)	Arby's regular Roast Beef sandwich (320 calories)
Sizzler® Hamburger (625 calories)	Sizzler 6-oz Dakota Ranch Steak (315 calories)

THE DARK NIGHT OF THE SOUL: DEALING WITH PLATEAUS

The dark night of the soul, that sounds like a heavy title. But you will undoubtedly find yourself there when you hit your first plateau, about five or six weeks into the Calorie Countdown.

When I got serious about losing weight, I started working out regularly, and thought I monitored my food intake carefully. I was determined to lose that gut as quickly as I could. All was going well until I hit a six-week-long plateau. Six weeks! I weighed myself every day and that scale did not move an inch. This was making me crazy. I did what any determined dieter would do. I ate less and worked out more. That darn needle on the scale still did not move!

Out of desperation I made an appointment with a nutritionist. She counted up my calories and what I was eating, compared that with how much I was working out, and came to the remarkable conclusion that I was not eating enough and I was working out too much! I'm sure I looked at her like she had lobsters coming out of her ears. She had me cut down my workout schedule from five days a week to three days a week, and add an avocado a day to my strict eating regime. She instructed me to eat half the avocado early in the day and the other half of the avocado later in the day. This advice sounded completely insane to me. How could cutting back on my training and adding a cup of fat to my diet help? But since I had already paid for her time and, cheap as I am, I was not about to ignore advice that I had paid for, I did what she said.

Within about a week the needle on the scale began to move in the direction I wanted it to. To say that I was amazed is no understatement. You could have knocked me over with a feather!

I had been making two of the most common mistakes in my effort to reshape my body; well, really three: 1) I wasn't eating enough; 2) I was working out too hard; and, most importantly, 3) I was not being patient with my body. Patience is the most important attribute to have when you set out to lose weight and become fit. I did not get fat overnight, and I was not about to get in shape overnight either.

Plateaus . . . we all have them. I guarantee that you will have this experience. And I guarantee that it will frustrate you. And it won't frustrate you in a minor way; it will make you crazy. You will question your commitment, and whether this weight-loss program is worth it. I know what I'm talking about! Some of you may recognize the term "the dark night of the soul," which comes out of spirituality and religious practice. It refers to those times in our lives when we question our beliefs, when we feel alone and cut off. When I was up in the middle of the night, frustrated and ready to dive into that pint of Ben & Jerry's®, that was a dark night of the soul.

Plateaus can occur at any time in a diet. As I learned from my nutritionist, the major causes can be—ironically enough—not eating enough and exercising too much. The reason why undereating can cause them is because the body is such a magnificently designed machine. The more I learn about it the more I am amazed by it. It has one major goal, and that is survival. To survive, the body thinks it has to store energy for later use. It hasn't quite caught up with the times, so it doesn't know that we don't use most of the energy we consume in calories on a daily basis, out plowing the back 40, or even walking to the corner grocery store. What we don't use up, we store. We call that stored energy fat.

Sometimes we need to play games with the body so that it doesn't operate so efficiently in survival mode. When you're dieting like mad, eating only carrot sticks and drinking only water, your body senses that there's a famine, and its survival mechanisms take over. Instead of releasing some of its fat reserves, the body says "Heck no!!! I'm not giving anything up—can't you see there is a famine out there?" And the needle on the scale stays put.

Another, even more dangerous thing can occur with serious undereating. The body will continue to conserve fat when it thinks there's a famine out there, but it needs to consume something for energy, so it will consume muscle tissue. Some of you might be saying, "That's okay, I don't want to be all muscle-bound anyway." But stop for a moment—what you may not realize is that the heart is muscle tissue too! You might be able to live without biceps, but you're not going to get too far without a heart.

That's why I take the approach to dieting that I take, only cutting a few hundred calories at a time and allowing the body to adjust to each reduction. The body will not sense deprivation if you withdraw calories gradually. It won't stop burning its fat stores, at least for a while.

But even on the Calorie Countdown you are bound to experience plateaus. It's how you handle them that will be the deciding factor in your success or failure with the program. Knowing what you now know about the body, do you just go out and start eating more? Yes and no. What you need to do is make some gentle changes in your eating patterns for a few weeks. Where are you in the Calorie Countdown? Try adding some healthy fats, like the avocado I added to mine, or some olive oil, and see what happens. Your body will be forced to readjust. This will also give you an excuse to try new things. Don't go crazy though; your body doesn't need Ben & Jerry's to know there isn't a famine going on.

The other most common culprit when it comes to plateaus is doing the same workout day after day. I've been living this "healthy lifestyle" for some time now, and

I've noticed something at the gym. Week after week, month after month, and yes, even year after year I see the same people doing the exact same exercises, and their bodies don't change. They may be in great cardiovascular shape, but their bodies have learned how to become very efficient at what they're doing. If you do something long enough, the body becomes accustomed to doing it efficiently, and will use less and less energy for the same activity.

Take a walk around any gym and I'm sure you will see the same thing. When I started watching some top-notch athletes (there are plenty in my neighborhood, as it's full of actors whose living depends on looking fabulous and being in the best shape possible) I noticed that they are constantly changing their workout. One day they're on the treadmill, the next day they're doing a spinning class, and the next day they're in a core workout class.

I learned this lesson firsthand when a friend talked me into joining his aerobics class, the last time I experienced a plateau. I've always enjoyed doing martial arts. It's a "guy thing," and I do it for my cardio. I also weight train and consider myself to be in pretty good shape. The aerobics class was geared for athletes, with a stair component. Now keep in mind that I've been working out consistently for the last five years and do martial arts several times a week. I thought this class would be a cakewalk, especially when I realized I was the only guy in a roomful of starlets in training. But I have to say, the class kicked my behind! I thought I was going to die!! The day before this I had been in a boxing ring holding my own against a very big guy, and now I was gasping for air in a roomful of beautiful young women! What the heck was going on?

The answer is quite simple. My body had become accustomed to the rhythms of sparring, but was totally shocked by this aerobics class. Since this class uses weights, I replaced some of my weight training with the aerobics class, and boy, did I break through my plateau. Another benefit has been that since I've been doing this class and challenging my cardiovascular endurance, my martial arts skills have improved considerably.

Sometimes we think we're experiencing a plateau, but it isn't a plateau at all. Your weight may not be going down because your body's muscle mass is increasing, and muscle weighs more than fat. I've experienced this a few times. I'm eating right, getting the proper amount of exercise, but my weight isn't going down. Then I have to remember that the number on the scale is not the only indication of how I'm doing. Thanks to my trusty scale (the one I talked about on page 5 that measures body fat percentage), I can see that even though my weight hasn't budged, my body fat percentage has gone down. At the same time I notice that my clothes are fitting much better (how your clothes fit is usually a much better indicator of your progress than the needle on the scale.) This is when taking a really big deep breath and relaxing comes in very handy. My wife would call it taking a chill pill.

So, let's recap. This is how you should deal with plateaus:

- Reevaluate what you are eating, and make sure you are eating enough. You don't want the body to think that it's experiencing a famine.

- Reevaluate your workout regime, and change things up. You don't necessarily have to go all out and run a marathon, but if you've been spending all your time on the exercise bike at the gym, try an entirely different activity. To prevent my workouts from becoming stale I now change my routine every two to four months. That sometimes even includes my trainer. This has given me the excuse to try salsa and hip-hop dance classes. I've never been that good a dancer, but I'm going to lose some weight trying to become one.

- The most important thing of all: Be patient with yourself! You didn't get fat overnight, and the weight is not going to go away overnight, either.

Your Exercise Program

In my fantasy house I have a full gym, with all the cardio equipment I like, a weight training area, all the core training equipment I could dream of, a martial arts/yoga area, and one of those really cool endless pools that has a current of water that you swim against, like the swimmer's version of a treadmill. But all that won't fit into my condo.

Is exercise really necessary to lose weight? Only if you want to keep it off. And since this diet is all about sustainable weight loss, that means that the answer to this question is a resounding YES. And let's face it, exercise also makes it easier to lose weight. A 1-pound glob of fat is equivalent to 3,500 calories of stored energy. To lose 1 pound a week, you have to create a 500-calorie deficit every day. In addition to doing all of the things I've been urging you to do in this book—losing the cookies, eating smaller meals more often, changing over to diet sodas, controlling your snacking—you can chisel off some of that weight with exercise.

The reason exercise is so important is because it changes your body's resting metabolism. Resting metabolism is the amount of energy (read calories) your body needs to burn, even when you're sleeping, in order for you to stay alive. In simple guy terms (this analogy worked for me), it's the idling speed of your body's motor. If you're sitting in traffic with the motor running, your car needs gas. The bigger the engine, the more gas it needs. When you exercise, you build more muscle mass, and muscle mass requires more energy to maintain than fat, even when you're sitting still. You've created a bigger motor. Weight training in particular builds a bigger motor, but all exercise helps your body both lose fat and trade some for muscle.

LATE-NIGHT TELEVISION IS THE ANSWER! (JUST KIDDING)

So what exercise should you do? If you watch a lot of late-night television, you'll see a lot of gizmos and gadgets that claim to make exercise and weight loss easy, painless, and quick. What 99 percent of these products do, very efficiently I might add, is lighten your wallet. I truly wish that the gizmos and gadgets were as magical as their infomercials claim they are. But if any one of them were truly a magic bullet, there wouldn't be a new weight-loss gimmick every time you turned on late-night TV.

Runners will tell you that running is best, because it burns the most calories in the shortest amount of time. You can run on a

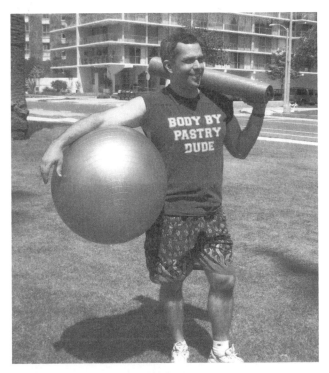

You don't need a gym to get a good workout.

treadmill in the gym or on one at home, or you can run outside on a track or in your local park or through your neighborhood (running outdoors burns more calories than running indoors on a treadmill). But I hate running, I truly hate it. I find it boring and it makes my knees hurt. If you love it, you're lucky, go for it. But I'll only do it if I'm getting in shape for a particular event. Running is not an exercise that I will do consistently, and that, as I've said repeatedly, is what I want you to find.

Look around and you'll see that the options are endless. There's yoga and Pilates, weight training and aerobics, water aerobics and swimming, biking, treadmills and exercise bikes, elliptical trainers and spinning. When I started trying to get into shape I did a lot of research into what was best. I wanted to burn as much fat as I could in the shortest amount of time. I must admit I even purchased a few of those exercise machines and tapes advertised on late-night television. My in-home gym soon became a dust-covered sculpture whose main task was to hold the dry cleaning. To this day I have some VHS exercise tapes still in their shrink wrap. Learn from my experience: Don't go out and purchase expensive equipment before you know whether you're going to use it. Take out a trial membership at a gym and see what you like to do.

After "Do I need to exercise to lose weight?" the next most frequently asked exercise-related question I get is "Which is better, weight training or aerobic training?" The truth is, if you want to lose weight and look really good, a combination of the two is best. Many women ask me if they'll end up looking muscle-bound if they do weight training. But you won't; you'll look like a body builder only if you set out to look like a body builder.

BABY STEPS

If you're starting completely from Square One, and by that I mean you're sitting on the sofa with a bag of Cheetos® reading this, and you've never exercised, and you don't have the financial means to join a gym or hire a trainer, get up and start walking. You can begin the weight training later, but let's get you moving first. Okay, I know, I live in sunny Southern California and where you are it's snowing. But even here in Southern California we can have bad weather. My parents go to the mall on blazing hot summer days and do their laps there.

The two pieces of equipment I would recommend, not just for beginners but for anybody who is serious about exercising, are: 1) a pedometer, and 2) something to listen to music on. First, the pedometer. This is a little device, about the size of a very small pager, that counts your steps. It tells you how much time you've spent walking, and how far you've walked. They're inexpensive, and a great way to gauge your physical activity. I've never been able to set the stride right on mine, so it keeps telling me I've gone about half as far as I think I have. But if it says I've taken 10,000 steps, I believe it. Pedometers also sometimes have calorie meters, but I pay no attention to those.

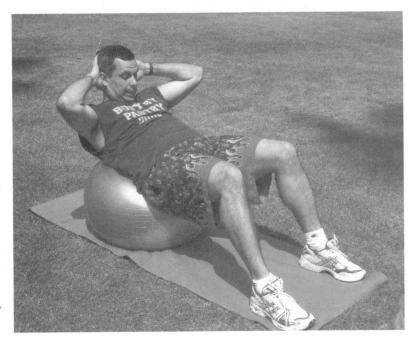

There's a six-pack in there somewhere.

The second piece of equipment is equally important, because it will prevent you from becoming bored when you exercise. It can be a Walkman®, an iPod, a CD player, or an MP3 player of some sort, even a radio. You don't have to spend a fortune. CD players are getting cheaper all the time; I saw one this morning going for $10 in my local drugstore. What to listen to is purely up to you. Personally I like to listen to books on tape. I download them off the Internet and I know I'll have a good five hours' worth of listening. I only listen to them while I'm doing my cardio exercise, which is especially motivating if it's an exciting book. If you're not able to download, you can go to the library and pick up books on CD. See, you can't get away with the budget excuse here.

Some gyms provide individual television sets for each piece of cardio equipment. You plug in headphones and choose your station. Some will have six televisions on a wall, and you tune your radio to the station of the TV you want to watch. I must admit I enjoy watching the reruns of my favorite TV shows on the individual televisions on the cardio equipment at my gym. There are times I extend my workout just so I can see the last ten minutes of a show.

QUICK TIP

Make sure to have a pre-workout snack of about 250 calories, such as a bowl of cereal or container of yogurt.

TODDLER STEPS

Let's say you're not starting from Square One, and you're willing and able to spend some money. Should you buy some equipment for the home, or join a gym? This really depends on you. In my own experience, I didn't have the discipline to work out on my own at home, and I also didn't really know how to use my equipment. Finally I do-

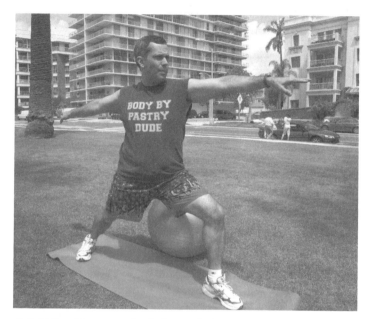

At first I thought yoga was for sissies, but it kicked my butt!

nated it to a worthy charity and joined a gym. But if you're able to commit to working out at home, and are more likely to do it than to go to a gym, by all means invest in some high-quality aerobics equipment. These will fall into three different categories: the treadmill, the elliptical trainer, and the bicycle. Forget about the abdominal machines advertised on late-night infomercials.

If you're going to invest in a home treadmill, don't waste your money on a cheap one; be prepared to spend at least $1,000. It should feel solid and durable. Many of the good ones fold up and save space. I prefer elliptical trainers, the ones with pedals that go up and around, because they give me a very good workout and they're much easier on my knees and back. They do take up more space than a treadmill, because they don't fold up, but the higher-end ones have some very cool features, like built-in exercise programs that vary speed and incline, and digital readouts. Some even remember your previous workout data. As for weight training, it's hard to beat some of the all-in-one machines by Bowflex®. They don't take up much room, and you can do 101 exercises on them. They're not cheap, but they're great.

If joining a gym is the right answer for you, you should know that not all gyms are created equal. Some are really fancy and expensive, others are more basic. But you can get just as effective a workout at the YMCA as you can at the Sports Club LA, where Hollywood's rich and famous go.

I suggest taking a tour of the neighborhood and seeing what is available. Make sure that you are comfortable in the gym, because if you're not, you won't go. I've had a few different memberships in the last five years, mostly because of my work situations, and I can tell you that gym atmospheres vary greatly. One gym I went to was frequented by the kids from UCLA; I hope this doesn't make me sound too old, but cool as it was to be with the kids, the music was just too darn loud. I also went to a gym that I would call a muscle-head gym; bodybuilders used this gym, and even though I found most of the bodybuilders to be perfectly charming, I felt a bit out of place. One place I loved, even though it wasn't the right fit for me, resembled a 1940s boxing gym, with no mirrors, heavy punching bags, and medicine balls. It even had a card table for playing poker after your workout! Finally I found a gym not far from my home that caters to professionals. They keep the equipment clean and in good repair, and play music I can relate to. So shop around.

When you're shopping around, try out all of the classes offered by the gym. I've tried Latin dance classes, aerobics classes, mat Pilates and yoga classes, spinning, and even kickboxing. Sometimes I feel like I look silly, but I get a heck of a workout.

As a totally out-of-shape fat man, the only thing worse than not going to the gym for me was going to the gym and not accomplishing anything. I had no idea how to use the equipment. So I purchased a series of ten sessions with a trainer, and by doing this I accomplished two things: First, I created accountability for at least ten visits to the gym. If I didn't show up, I lost the money. Second, I had somebody to show me how to use every piece of equipment in the gym properly. Since I was working on a budget, I told my new trainer that I could only afford the ten sessions, and wanted him to show me how to use all of the equipment properly, and set up a program that I could follow for the next few months, until I could afford another ten sessions. This was the best thing I could have done; I learned to use the machines properly, ensuring workouts that were efficient and much less likely to cause me injury. This was truly the beginning of my exercise career.

It really helps, especially in the beginning, if you create some kind of accountability for exercising. For me, paying for those training sessions in advance got me to the gym. Some people do this by working out with a partner or friend, or with a group. I had a workout partner for a while who wouldn't go to the gym unless I went.

FUEL FOR THE TREADMILL

This information might motivate you to change your eating habits when you go to fast-food joints. Small changes at the counter can mean huge time savings in the gym.

Just for fun, let's see how long it takes to burn off the calories in certain foods, beginning with that apocryphal chocolate-chip cookie. How long will it take to burn off the cookie's 120 calories?

The average 150-pound woman working out on a treadmill or elliptical trainer burns about 100 calories per mile, or 7 calories per minute. So it will take her a little more than 17 minutes to burn off the chocolate-chip cookie. For every 420 calories she'll have to work out for an hour. If she eats a 580-calorie Big Mac she'll be on that treadmill for an hour and thirteen minutes.

In recent years a women's gym franchise called Curves® has popularized a new gym concept that I absolutely love. These gyms have a limited number of machines set out in a particular workout order. You begin on one machine, and after a set amount of time move on to the next one. The workout is not exactly tailor-made for one individual, but it gives everybody a varied routine. Most large gyms are now including this workout somewhere on the premises.

What about workouts like Pilates or yoga? Both of these are wonderful for building strength and flexibility. But make sure that you add in an aerobics component, like running, elliptical training, fast walking, aerobics classes, or swimming.

THE DREADED PLATEAU

This happens to everyone. And I do mean *everyone*. We all reach a point where we plateau: No matter what we do, we aren't losing weight. Research has shown, and I myself could have been the guinea pig for this study, that if you continue doing the same exercise month after month, year after year, the body will become very efficient

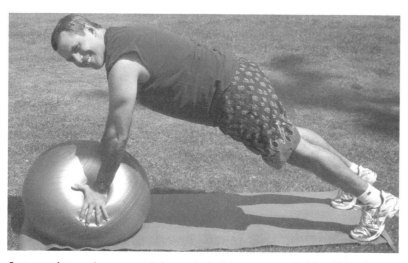

Core exercises work every muscle in your body. I dare you to try holding this position for more than a minute!

at doing the exercise, and eventually it won't require as much fuel to accomplish it. That's one of the reasons I like belonging to a big gym: There is so much available that I can change my exercise routine every two to four months, no matter how strong I'm feeling. Recently I went from weight training three mornings per week to doing one of those aerobics classes that uses steps, a medicine ball, and light hand weights. They call this class "Core and More" at my gym, but it goes by different names at different places. I thought I was in pretty good shape when I went to that class, but that trainer kicked my behind. I'll do this workout for another three months, then I'll change to an intense flow yoga class. After that, who knows? The point is, I won't get stuck in a rut. And you won't plateau either if you change your routine regularly.

WHAT ABOUT JUNIOR?

I know this is a book for adults, but childhood obesity is a huge problem and a huge subject that is getting a lot of attention. I truly believe that we lead by example, and once we begin to move, we've got to get our kids moving, the way kids should.

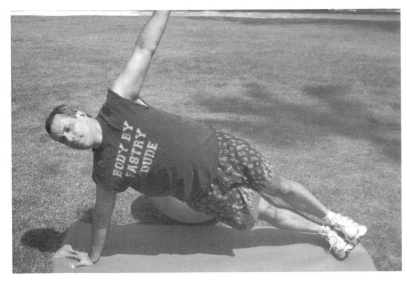

Yoga in the park—how California can you get?!

Encourage activities such as bicycle riding and roller-skating. I confess that in my former life I used to spend hours playing video games. My hand-eye coordination was pretty good, but my gut was pretty impressive, too. I recently had the opportunity to play Dance Dance Revolution 2 on PlayStation®2 with some kids. I must say it was one heck of a workout! If you've never seen this, it's a dance game where you have to do dance movements by stepping on the control pad

to the beat of the game. The developers are working on more products, and I hope they come out with a martial arts version. I can just see telling Junior that he can't play Star Wars™ until he reaches a new high score on Dance Dance Revolution. Meanwhile, you could always impose a rule that for every half hour on the PlayStation he has to spend thirty minutes doing some kind of physical play.

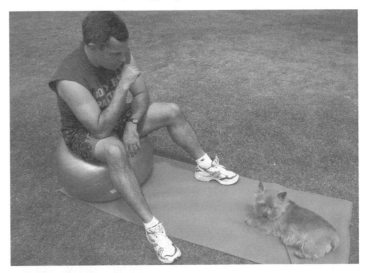

Don't overdo it, make sure to take rests (and make sure your workout partner is a good listener).

PART 2

THE
CALORIE
COUNTDOWN
MENUS

Introduction to the Menus

Counting calories can be a big bore, so big that it prevents some people from dieting. So I've counted the calories for you and created eighteen weeks' worth of menus, each week with a caloric value that is 100 to 200 calories lower than the week before. The weekly menus range from 2,400 calories per day to under 1,200. I've provided you with this wide range because you're all going to be starting from a different place. My own ultimate goal was 1,900 calories a day, so my Calorie Countdown began at 2,400 (well, actually I was consuming amounts more similar to the ones in the food log

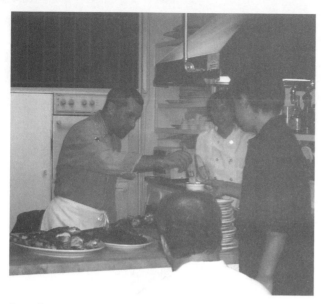
Spreading the good news: Calorie Countdown food is as hearty and tasty as it looks.

on page 12, so I'd actually been losing weight for a while by the time I got to the 2,400-calorie starting point). You may be starting from 1,800 calories a day, with a 1,300 calorie a day goal. So you would begin by using the menus in the 1,650 to 1,800 calorie week on page 115.

So that you can really understand my "chocolate-chip cookie theory"—that notion I keep going back to about making choices and substitutions in your diet so you still get treats and sweets and other things you like to eat while reducing caloric intake—I've made every two sets of menus *identical* except for one or two items, and laid them out side by side on the page. For example, in my 1,900 to 1,650 Calorie Countdown Menus for the week beginning on page 86, the menus on the left side of the page represent a daily caloric intake of 1,800 to 1,900 calories. Those on the right represent a daily caloric intake of 1,650 to 1,800 calories. But they're essentially the same menus, except you've lost at least 100 calories because of one small change. Look at the meals on Day 1: All you did from one week to the next was give up one piece of bread at lunch and one Dove Promises bar in the afternoon (you still got to eat one), and you saved 152 calories. On Day 2 you got your lunch at Quiznos, and the first week you had a Turkey Ranch & Swiss sandwich, which cost you 691 calories. The second week you ordered a small Sierra Smoked Turkey with Raspberry Chipotle Sauce at Quiznos and saved 341 calories! This is such a good savings that you could, if you wanted to, add a 100-calorie chocolate-chip cookie to your menu. You also lost calories by choosing nonfat milk over 1% milk for your afternoon snack. There are notes after each daily set of menus telling you just where you lost the calories.

Because there are nutritional analyses for all of my recipes, you can make your own substitutions by finding dishes with similar caloric values if you'd rather have something else for a meal. And since I know you're not going to bring your lunch to work every day, I've included fast-food places and restaurants that post their nutritional values online, so that you can make your own choices here too.

In fact, you'll find six separate Calorie Countdown Menus for the Non-Cook on

pages 115 to 135, because I know that you don't all cook. In fact, most of you probably don't cook; that's one of the main reasons you got fat! Well, I don't cook at home
very often either, and I'm a chef! Open my freezer and you'll find a lot of frozen meals.
But they're Lean Cuisine or Weight Watchers brands, so I can keep track of my calories. Open the cupboard and it's full of Campbell's Microwavable Soups. We eat them
for lunch and my wife takes them to work for snacks. I've done the research for you,
so you can keep going to the Subway chain or whatever, but you need to know what
to order to stay within your calorie range.

Doctors and nutritionists, and maybe you, may look at these menus and wonder
why a diet guy is recommending that you have your afternoon snack at Starbucks®
with a cappuccino and a Dove chocolate bar, instead of eating vegetables and a
healthy dip. And why am I recommending a Wendy's hamburger for lunch? My answer is that I live in the real world, and people who need to lose weight live in the
real world. I didn't have to leave this world to lose weight, and neither do you. You
just have to become aware of what you're eating. If you choose to make healthier
choices than the ones I'm presenting in the menus, that's terrific—you're ahead of
the game. But if you love Starbucks and convenience food, you'll find it very difficult
to sustain a weight loss plan that doesn't take this into account. Everyone can do the
Calorie Countdown, and you don't have to give up your Subway sandwich or your afternoon cappuccino to do it. What should keep coming back to you as you eat your
way through these menus is that *the Calorie Countdown is all about choices.*

Recap: How to Use the Menus

1. Go to the Calorie Countdown Weekly Menus section that has the caloric
   value you are starting from. These are your menus for Week 1. If you wish,
   you can substitute foods and dishes with similar caloric values for those on
   the menu. Use a pocket calorie counter, an online source, and the nutritional values for the recipes on pages 143 to 303 to help you with your
   choices. Note that there are also Six Weekly Menus for the Non-Cook. Use
   them if you fall into this group.

2. For each subsequent week, use the next Calorie Countdown set of menus,
   until you reach your goal of a weekly reduction of 500 calories (you'll find
   that it will actually be more like 500 to 600 calories). Note that every two
   Countdown Menus for the week are identical, except for one or two items
   that you will omit or change.

3. When you have achieved an overall reduction in your diet of 500 to 600 calories a week, you should stick with that caloric intake for several weeks. Then, if you want to keep reducing, you can continue to use these menus to reduce calories. But for the weight loss to be sustainable, you need to give your body time to adjust to the regimen. You can download a Calorie Countdown spreadsheet from my Web site, www.CalorieCountdown.net, if you want to continue to create your own menus.

As you work your way through the Calorie Countdown, *make sure that you also follow the advice in Part 1 of this book.*

Weekly Menus from 2,400 Calories to 1,200 Calories a Day

2,400 to 2,250 Calorie Countdown

DAY 1: 2,400 calories

	CALORIES
Breakfast	
2 eggs	160
2 slices bacon	86
2 slices toast	220
1 cup orange juice	112
	578
Midmorning Snack	
Starbucks blueberry muffin	380
1 Grande Latte®	260
	640
Lunch	
Chile-Cheese Rice Burritos (page 192)	225
Sweetened iced tea	100
	325
Afternoon Snack	
Power Crunch Peanut Butter Creme Bar	185
	185
Dinner	
Pita Steak Sandwich with Dill Sauce (page 151)	341
Broccoli with Garlic Chili Sauce (page 254)	48
Green salad with Creamy Italian Dressing (page 180)	100
1 (6-oz) glass red wine	145
Fat Free Fudgsicle®	71
	705
TOTALS	**2,433**

DAY 1: 2,250 to 2,300 calories

	CALORIES
Breakfast	
1 egg	80
2 slices bacon	86
1 slice toast	110
1 cup orange juice	112
	388
Midmorning Snack	
Starbucks blueberry muffin	380
1 Grande Latte	260
	640
Lunch	
Chile-Cheese Rice Burritos (page 192)	225
Sweetened iced tea	100
	325
Afternoon Snack	
Power Crunch Peanut Butter Creme Bar	185
	185
Dinner	
Pita Steak Sandwich with Dill Sauce (page 151)	341
Broccoli with Garlic Chili Sauce (page 254)	48
Green salad with Creamy Italian Dressing (page 180)	100
1 (6-oz) glass red wine	145
Fat Free Fudgsicle®	71
	705
	2,243

Your Calorie Countdown Choices: You lost 190 calories at breakfast, just by having 1 egg instead of 2 and 1 slice of toast instead of 2.

DAY 2: 2,400 calories

	CALORIES
Breakfast	
¾ cup raisin bran	150
1 cup 1% milk	105
1 medium banana	105
1 Tall cappuccino	150
	510
Midmorning Snack	
1 cup grapes	100
1 cup fruit-flavored low-fat yogurt	252
1 Tall nonfat cappuccino	75
	427
Lunch	
Deli roast beef sandwich (small)	414
Mineral water	0
2 Oatmeal-Craisin Cookies (page 291)	98
	512
Afternoon Snack	
2 Dove Promises bars	84
	84
Dinner	
Air-Fried Pork Chops (page 184)	321
½ cup rice	103
Stir-Fried Asparagus and Peppers (page 264)	49
1 (12-oz) beer	150
Chocolate Angel Food Cake with Strawberries (page 282)	136
	759
TOTALS	**2,292**

DAY 2: 2,250 to 2,300 calories

	CALORIES
Breakfast	
¾ cup raisin bran	150
1 cup 1% milk	105
1 medium banana	105
1 Tall cappuccino	150
	510
Midmorning Snack	
1 cup grapes	100
6-oz Dannon Light 'n Fit Nonfat Strawberry Yogurt	60
1 Tall nonfat cappuccino	75
	235
Lunch	
Deli roast beef sandwich (small)	414
Mineral water	0
2 Oatmeal-Craisin Cookies (page 291)	98
	512
Afternoon Snack	
2 Dove Promises bars	84
	84
Dinner	
Air-Fried Pork Chops (page 184)	321
½ cup rice	103
Stir-Fried Asparagus and Peppers (page 264)	49
1 (12-oz) beer	150
Chocolate Angel Food Cake with Strawberries (page 282)	136
	759
TOTALS	**2,100**

Your Calorie Countdown Choices: By switching from a 1-cup serving of low-fat fruit yogurt to a 6-ounce serving of Dannon Light 'n Fit nonfat yogurt, you lost 192 calories.

DAY 3: 2,400 calories

	CALORIES
Breakfast	
1 plain bagel	360
2 T light cream cheese	70
1 cup orange juice	112
1 Tall cappuccino	150
	692
Midmorning Snack	
¾ cup raisin bran	150
½ cup 1% milk	53
	203
Lunch	
Baja Fresh Veggie & Cheese Bare Burrito™	580
Diet soda	0
	580
Afternoon Snack	
Chocolate Angel Food Cake with Strawberries (page 282)	136
1 Tall nonfat cappuccino	75
	211
Dinner	
Broccoli-Halibut Stir-Fry (page 220)	221
½ cup rice	103
Apple-Pear Slaw (page 168)	72
1 (6-oz) glass white wine	145
Pound Cake (page 297)	216
	757
TOTALS	**2,443**

DAY 3: 2,250 to 2,300 calories

	CALORIES
Breakfast	
1 plain bagel	360
2 T light cream cheese	70
1 cup orange juice	112
1 Tall nonfat cappuccino	75
	617
Midmorning Snack	
¾ cup raisin bran	150
½ cup 1% milk	53
	203
Lunch	
Baja Fresh Charbroiled Chicken Tacos	560
Diet soda	0
	560
Afternoon Snack	
1 apple	80
1 Tall nonfat cappuccino	75
	155
Dinner	
Broccoli-Halibut Stir-Fry (page 220)	221
½ cup rice	103
Apple-Pear Slaw (page 168)	72
1 (6-oz) glass white wine	145
Pound Cake (page 297)	216
	757
TOTALS	**2,292**

Your Calorie Countdown Choices: You lost 20 calories by having 2 Charbroiled Chicken Tacos instead of the Veggie & Cheese Burrito at lunch. You lost another 56 calories by choosing an apple instead of angel food cake for your afternoon snack. You said good-bye to another 75 by swapping out a regular cappuccino for a nonfat cappuccino at breakfast.

DAY 4: 2,400 calories

	CALORIES
Breakfast	
1 cup Kashi GOLEAN cereal	190
½ cup 1% milk	53
1 banana	105
1 Tall cappuccino	150
	498
Midmorning Snack	
1 large bagel	360
1 Grande Light Caramel Frappuccino, no whip	180
	540
Lunch	
Garden Turkey Burger (page 196)	267
Potato Salad (page 171)	110
	377
Afternoon Snack	
Post-Workout Shake (page 275)	200
	200
Dinner	
Creamy Four-Cheese Macaroni with Broccoli (page 233)	408
Air-Fried Okra (page 252)	84
Green salad with vinaigrette	120
1 (6-oz) glass red wine	145
Roasted Pineapple (page 301)	82
	839
TOTALS	**2,454**

DAY 4: 2,250 to 2,300 calories

	CALORIES
Breakfast	
1 cup Kashi GOLEAN cereal	190
½ cup 1% milk	53
1 banana	105
1 Tall cappuccino	150
	498
Midmorning Snack	
1 large bagel	360
1 Grande Light Caramel Frappuccino, no whip	180
	540
Lunch	
Garden Turkey Burger (page 196)	267
Green salad with fat-free ranch dressing	31
	298
Afternoon Snack	
13.6-oz Jamba Juice Enlightened Berry Fulfilling™ smoothie	160
	160
Dinner	
Creamy Four-Cheese Macaroni with Broccoli (page 233)	408
Air-Fried Okra (page 252)	84
Green salad with vinaigrette	120
1 (6-oz) glass red wine	145
Roasted Pineapple (page 301)	82
	839
	2,335

Your Calorie Countdown Choices: By choosing a green salad instead of potato salad for your lunch, you dropped 79 calories. You saved another 40 in the afternoon by substituting an Enlightened Jamba Juice for the Post-Workout Shake.

DAY 5: 2,400 calories

	CALORIES
Breakfast	
½ cup Fruit & Fibre® Cereal	105
½ cup 1% milk	53
1 banana	105
1 cup orange juice	112
1 Tall cappuccino	150
	525
Midmorning Snack	
2 string cheeses	160
1 apple	80
	240
Lunch	
BLT (3 strips bacon, 1 T mayo)	421
Iced tea	0
	421
Afternoon Snack	
1 Grande Light Caramel Frappuccino, no whip	180
12 almonds	85
	265
Dinner	
Oven-Fried Chicken Breasts (page 202)	175
Mashed Potatoes with Horseradish (page 261)	275
½ cup steamed green beans	22
Green salad with vinaigrette	120
1 (6-oz) glass red wine	145
Chocolate Tofu Cheesecake (page 286)	185
	922
TOTALS	**2,373**

DAY 5: 2,250 to 2,300 calories

	CALORIES
Breakfast	
½ cup Fruit & Fibre Cereal	105
½ cup 1% milk	53
1 banana	105
½ cup orange juice	56
1 Tall cappuccino	150
	469
Midmorning Snack	
2 string cheeses	160
1 apple	80
	240
Lunch	
BLT (3 strips bacon, 1 T mayo)	421
Iced tea	0
	421
Afternoon Snack	
1 Tall Light Frappuccino, no whip	113
12 almonds	85
	198
Dinner	
Oven-Fried Chicken Breasts (page 202)	175
Mashed Potatoes with Horseradish (page 261)	275
½ cup steamed green beans	22
Green salad with vinaigrette	120
1 (6-oz) glass red wine	145
Chocolate Tofu Cheesecake (page 286)	185
	922
	2,250

Your Calorie Countdown Choices: You traded a Grande Light Caramel Frappuccino for a Tall Frappuccino in the afternoon and lost 67 calories. You gave up another 56 calories by drinking 4 ounces of orange juice instead of 8 ounces for breakfast.

DAY 6: 2,400 calories

	CALORIES
Breakfast	
2-egg cheese omelet	360
1 cup orange juice	112
1 English muffin	150
1 T butter	100
1 Tall cappuccino	150
	872
Midmorning Snack	
1 banana	105
Diet Snapple® (noncaloric)	0
	105
Lunch	
Tuna Salad (page 178)	143
1 cup 1% milk	105
1 slice whole-wheat bread	110
	358
Afternoon Snack	
Pringles 100-Calorie Pack	100
1 (12-oz) light beer	110
1 apple	80
	290
Dinner	
Open-Faced Chili Dog (page 150)	314
Air Fries (page 250)	92
Mixed Salad Greens with Balsamic Vinaigrette (page 169)	89
1 (12-oz) regular beer	150
Roasted Ginger Papaya (page 300)	146
	791
TOTALS	**2,416**

DAY 6: 2,250 to 2,300 calories

	CALORIES
Breakfast	
2-egg cheese omelet	360
½ cup orange juice	56
1 English muffin	150
1 T butter	100
1 Tall cappuccino	150
	816
Midmorning Snack	
1 banana	105
Diet Snapple (noncaloric)	0
	105
Lunch	
Tuna Salad (page 178)	143
1 cup 1% milk	105
	248
Afternoon Snack	
Pringles 100-Calorie Pack	100
1 (12-oz) light beer	110
1 apple	80
	290
Dinner	
Open-Faced Chili Dog (page 150)	314
Air Fries (page 250)	92
Mixed Salad Greens with Balsamic Vinaigrette (page 169)	89
1 (12-oz) regular beer	150
Roasted Ginger Papaya (page 300)	146
	791
TOTALS	**2,250**

Your Calorie Countdown Choices: You lost 110 calories by eliminating 1 slice of bread at lunch and another 56 with 4 ounces less orange juice at breakfast.

DAY 7: 2,400 calories

	CALORIES
Breakfast	
3 Kashi GOLEAN Waffles	255
1 T butter	100
2 T light syrup	50
½ cup orange juice	56
1 Tall cappuccino	150
1 banana	105
	716
Midmorning Snack	
2 Babybels	140
5 pieces Melba toast	60
Mineral water	0
	200
Lunch	
Campbell's Chunky™ Sirloin Burger with Country Vegetables soup	160
1 slice whole-wheat bread	110
Iced tea	0
1 orange	86
1 Oatmeal-Craisin Cookie (page 291)	49
	405
Afternoon Snack	
3 cups Barbecued Popcorn (page 271)	120
1 (12-oz) light beer	110
	230
Dinner	
Chicken Asopa (page 187)	288
Sourdough roll	150
Green salad with vinaigrette	120
1 (6-oz) glass white wine	145
Zinfandel-Poached Pears (page 303)	191
	895
TOTALS	**2,445**

DAY 7: 2,250 to 2,300 calories

	CALORIES
Breakfast	
2 Kashi GOLEAN Waffles	170
1 T I Can't Believe It's Not Butter!®	60
2 T light syrup	50
½ cup orange juice	56
1 Tall cappuccino	150
1 banana	105
	591
Midmorning Snack	
2 Babybels	140
5 pieces Melba toast	60
Mineral water	0
	200
Lunch	
Campbell's Chunky Sirloin Burger with Country Vegetables Soup	160
1 slice whole-wheat bread	110
Iced tea	0
1 orange	86
1 Oatmeal-Craisin Cookie (page 291)	49
	405
Afternoon Snack	
3 cups Barbecued Popcorn (page 271)	120
1 (12-oz) light beer	110
	230
Dinner	
Chicken Asopa (page 187)	288
Sourdough roll	150
Green salad with vinaigrette	120
1 (6-oz) glass white wine	145
Zinfandel-Poached Pears (page 303)	191
	895
TOTALS	**2,320**

Your Calorie Countdown Choices: You lost 125 calories by just giving up 1 waffle and using a butter substitute at breakfast.

2,200 to 1,900 Calorie Countdown

DAY 1: 2,100 to 2,200 calories

	CALORIES
Breakfast	
1 small whole-wheat bagel	110
1 T light cream cheese	70
1 boiled egg	80
½ cup orange juice	56
1 Tall cappuccino	150
	466
Midmorning Snack	
1 banana	105
6-oz Dannon Light 'n Fit yogurt	60
	165
Lunch	
Koo-Koo-Roo Chinese Chicken Salad (no dressing)	550
Iced tea	0
	550
Afternoon Snack	
Post-Workout Shake (page 275)	200
	200
Dinner	
Calzones (page 231)	403
Green salad with fat-free ranch dressing	31
1 (6-oz) glass red wine	145
¾ cup Dreyer's/Edy's Fat Free Black Cherry Vanilla Swirl Frozen Yogurt	135
	714
TOTALS	**2,095**

DAY 1: 1,900 to 2,100 calories

	CALORIES
Breakfast	
1 small whole-wheat bagel	110
1 T light cream cheese	70
1 boiled egg	80
½ cup orange juice	56
1 Tall cappuccino	150
	466
Midmorning Snack	
1 banana	105
6-oz Dannon Light 'n Fit yogurt	60
	165
Lunch	
Koo-Koo-Roo BBQ Chicken Salad (no dressing)	365
Iced tea	0
	365
Afternoon Snack	
Post-Workout Shake (page 275)	200
	200
Dinner	
Calzones (page 231)	403
Green Salad with fat-free ranch dressing	31
1 (6-oz) glass red wine	145
¾ cup Dreyer's/Edy's Fat Free Black Cherry Vanilla Swirl Frozen Yogurt	135
	714
TOTALS	**1,910**

Your Calorie Countdown Choices: By switching from Koo-Koo-Roo Chinese Chicken Salad at 550 calories to their BBQ Chicken Salad at 365 calories you lost 185 calories. Next time go for their Chicken Caesar at 288 calories.

DAY 2: 2,100 to 2,200 calories

	CALORIES
Breakfast	
1 cup oatmeal	147
½ cup 1% milk	53
½ apple, grated	40
1 tsp honey	21
1 Tall cappuccino	150
	411
Midmorning Snack	
½ cup 2% cottage cheese	102
12 almonds	85
1 Tall nonfat cappuccino	75
	262
Lunch	
Cali Cheesesteak (page 147)	344
Diet soda	0
	344
Afternoon Snack	
1 banana	105
1 T peanut butter	94
	199
Dinner	
Spicy Orange Chicken Lo Mein (page 200)	508
Green salad with fat-free ranch dressing	31
1 (12-oz) regular beer	150
Zinfandel-Poached Pears (page 303)	191
	880
TOTALS	**2,096**

DAY 2: 1,900 to 2,100 calories

	CALORIES
Breakfast	
1 cup oatmeal	147
½ cup 1% milk	53
½ apple, grated	40
1 tsp honey	21
1 Tall nonfat cappuccino	75
	336
Midmorning Snack	
½ cup nonfat cottage cheese	62
12 almonds	85
1 Tall nonfat cappuccino	75
	222
Lunch	
Cali Cheesesteak (page 147)	344
Diet soda	0
	344
Afternoon Snack	
1 banana	105
1 T peanut butter	94
	199
Dinner	
Spicy Orange Chicken Lo Mein (page 200)	508
Green salad with fat-free ranch dressing	31
1 (12-oz) light beer	110
Zinfandel-Poached Pears (page 303)	191
	840
	1,941

Your Calorie Countdown Choices: By switching from a regular beer (150 calories) to a light beer at dinner you lost 40 calories. By switching to a nonfat cappuccino at breakfast you lost another 75. You lost another 40 at midmorning snack by going from 2% to nonfat cottage cheese.

DAY 3: 2,100 to 2,200 calories

	CALORIES
Breakfast	
1 packet Kashi GOLEAN Hot Cereal™	150
1 cup orange juice	112
1 Tall cappuccino	150
	412
Midmorning Snack	
Granola bar	140
1 cup 1% milk	105
	245
Lunch	
Kalamata Halibut (page 226)	238
Green salad with vinaigrette	120
	358
Afternoon Snack	
Fat Free Fudgsicle	71
1 Tall cappuccino	150
	221
Dinner	
Garlic-Roasted Tenderloin (page 198)	447
½ cup steamed potatoes	68
½ cup steamed broccoli	22
1 (6-oz) glass red wine	145
Zinfandel-Poached Pears (page 303)	191
	873
TOTALS	**2,109**

DAY 3: 1,900 to 2,100 calories

	CALORIES
Breakfast	
1 packet Kashi GOLEAN Hot Cereal	150
1 cup orange juice	112
1 Tall cappuccino	150
	412
Midmorning Snack	
1 banana	105
1 cup 1% milk	105
	210
Lunch	
Kalamata Halibut (page 226)	238
Green salad with Creamy Italian Dressing (page 180)	100
	338
Afternoon Snack	
Fat Free Fudgsicle	71
1 Tall nonfat cappuccino	75
	146
Dinner	
Garlic-Roasted Tenderloin (page 198)	447
Mashed Cauliflower (page 260)	65
½ cup steamed broccoli	22
1 (6-oz) glass red wine	145
Zinfandel-Poached Pears (page 303)	191
	870
	1,976

Your Calorie Countdown Choices: You saved 35 calories by swapping a banana for a granola bar. You saved 20 calories at lunch by choosing Creamy Italian Dressing instead of vinaigrette. You saved another 75 calories by swapping out a regular cappuccino for a nonfat one in the afternoon.

DAY 4: 2,100 to 2,200 calories

	CALORIES
Breakfast	
1 cup Kashi GOLEAN Cereal	190
½ cup 1% milk	53
½ cup blueberries	41
1 Tall cappuccino	150
	434
Midmorning Snack	
GOLEAN Crunchy! Chocolate Peanut Bar	180
1 cup 1% milk	105
	285
Lunch	
Tuna Salad (page 178)	143
1 slice whole-wheat bread	110
	253
Afternoon Snack	
1 peach	37
1 cup grapes	100
	137
Dinner	
Chili con Carne (page 195)	378
2 corn tortillas	100
2 Quick String Cheese Quesadillas (page 152)	260
Green salad with oil and vinegar	120
1 (12-oz) light beer	110
4-oz Häagen-Dazs® Orchard Peach fat-free sorbet	130
	1,098
TOTALS	**2,207**

DAY 4: 1,900 to 2,100 calories

	CALORIES
Breakfast	
1 cup Kashi GOLEAN cereal	190
½ cup 1% milk	53
½ cup blueberries	41
1 Tall cappuccino	150
	434
Midmorning Snack	
Granola bar	140
1 cup 1% milk	105
	245
Lunch	
Tuna Salad (page 178)	143
1 slice whole-wheat bread	110
	253
Afternoon Snack	
1 peach	37
1 cup grapes	100
	137
Dinner	
Chili con Carne (page 195)	378
2 corn tortillas	100
2 Quick String Cheese Quesadillas (page 152)	130 130
Green salad with oil and vinegar	120
1 (12-oz) light beer	110
4-oz Häagen-Dazs Orchard Peach fat-free sorbet	130
	968
TOTALS	**2,037**

Your Calorie Countdown Choices: By losing 1 Quick String Cheese Quesadilla at dinner, you got a 130-calorie reduction. You still had a hearty meal. You lost another 40 calories in the morning by choosing a granola bar over the GOLEAN Crunchy! Chocolate Peanut Bar.

DAY 5: 2,100 to 2,200 calories

	CALORIES
Breakfast	
2 Kashi GOLEAN Waffles	170
1 T I Can't Believe It's Not Butter!	60
2 T light syrup	50
½ cup orange juice	56
1 Tall cappuccino	150
	486
Midmorning Snack	
1 apple	80
1 string cheese	80
24 almonds	170
	330
Lunch	
Subway 6-inch Cold Cut Combo sandwich	410
Iced tea	0
	410
Afternoon Snack	
2 Oatmeal-Craisin Cookies (page 291)	98
1 Tall cappuccino	150
	248
Dinner	
Spicy Seared Scallops (page 229)	187
½ cup steamed rice	103
6 spears steamed asparagus with	27
1 tsp sesame oil	40
1 (6-oz) glass white wine	145
Pound Cake (page 297)	216
	718
TOTALS	**2,192**

DAY 5: 1,900 to 2,100 calories

	CALORIES
Breakfast	
2 Kashi GOLEAN Waffles	170
1 T I Can't Believe It's Not Butter!	60
2 T light syrup	50
½ cup orange juice	56
1 Tall cappuccino	150
	486
Midmorning Snack	
1 apple	80
1 string cheese	80
24 almonds	170
	330
Lunch	
Subway 6-inch Turkey Breast & Ham sandwich	290
Iced tea	0
	290
Afternoon Snack	
2 Oatmeal-Craisin Cookies (page 291)	98
1 Tall cappuccino	150
	248
Dinner	
Spicy Seared Scallops (page 229)	187
½ cup steamed rice	103
6 spears steamed asparagus with	27
1 tsp sesame oil	40
1 (6-oz) glass white wine	145
Pound Cake (page 297)	216
	718
TOTALS	**2,072**

Your Calorie Countdown Choices: You lost 120 calories by choosing a Subway Turkey Breast & Ham sandwich at 290 calories instead of the Cold Cut Combo at 410 calories.

DAY 6: 2,100 to 2,200 calories

	CALORIES
Breakfast	
2 scrambled eggs	260
2 tablespoons salsa	9
1 English muffin	150
½ grapefruit	41
1 Tall cappuccino	150
	610
Midmorning Snack	
¾ cup raisin bran	150
½ cup 1% milk	53
	203
Lunch	
Saladworks Chicken Caesar Salad	423
Iced tea	0
	423
Afternoon Snack	
1 banana	105
1 Tall Frappuccino	113
	218
Dinner	
Feta-Artichoke Lasagne (page 239)	190
Arugula & Tomato Salad (page 170)	123
1 (6-oz) glass red wine	145
Chocolate Cake with Chocolate Frosting (page 284)	191
	649
TOTALS	**2,103**

DAY 6: 1,900 to 2,100 calories

	CALORIES
Breakfast	
2 scrambled eggs	260
2 tablespoons salsa	9
1 English muffin	150
½ grapefruit	41
1 Tall cappuccino	150
	610
Midmorning Snack	
¾ cup raisin bran	150
½ cup 1% milk	53
	203
Lunch	
Saladworks Newport Salad	184
Iced tea	0
1 slice whole-wheat bread	110
	294
Afternoon Snack	
1 banana	105
1 Tall Frappuccino	113
	218
Dinner	
Feta-Artichoke Lasagna (page 239)	190
Arugula & Tomato Salad (page 170)	123
1 (6-oz) glass red wine	145
Chocolate Cake with Chocolate Frosting (page 284)	191
	649
TOTALS	**1,974**

Your Calorie Countdown Choices: You lost 239 calories just by choosing the Saladworks Newport Salad instead of the Chicken Caesar. The Newport Salad is just as big, but at less than half the caloric cost. So you got to add some bread.

DAY 7: 2,100 to 2,200 calories

	CALORIES
Breakfast	
1 packet Kashi GOLEAN Hot Cereal	150
1 banana	105
½ cup orange juice	56
1 Tall cappuccino	150
	461
Midmorning Snack	
1 Tall Frappuccino	113
	113
Lunch	
Black Forest Ham and White Bean Panini (page 148)	356
Mineral water	0
	356
Afternoon Snack	
2 Peanut Butter–Banana Cookies (page 293)	252
1 cup 1% milk	105
	357
Dinner	
Chicken Asopa (page 187)	340
½ cup sautéed zucchini	54
Green salad with vinaigrette	120
1 (12-oz) regular beer	150
Roasted Ginger Papaya (page 300)	146
	810
TOTALS	**2,097**

DAY 7: 1,900 to 2,100 calories

	CALORIES
Breakfast	
1 packet Kashi GOLEAN Hot Cereal	150
1 banana	105
½ cup orange juice	56
1 Tall cappuccino	150
	461
Midmorning Snack	
1 Tall nonfat cappuccino	75
	75
Lunch	
Black Forest Ham and White Bean Panini (page 148)	356
Mineral water	0
	356
Afternoon Snack	
Fat Free Fudgsicle	71
1 cup 1% milk	105
	176
Dinner	
Chicken Asopa (page 187)	340
½ cup sautéed zucchini	54
Green salad with vinaigrette	120
1 (12-oz) regular beer	150
Roasted Ginger Papaya (page 300)	146
	810
	1,878

Your Calorie Countdown Choices: In the afternoon you traded the Peanut Butter–Banana Cookies for the Fudgsicle and saved 181 calories in the bargain. You lost another 38 by choosing a nonfat cappuccino instead of a Tall Frappuccino for your midmorning snack.

1,900 to 1,650 Calorie Countdown

DAY 1: **1,800 to 1,900 calories**	CALORIES	DAY 1: **1,650 to 1,800 calories**	CALORIES
Breakfast		**Breakfast**	
1 cup Kashi Organic Promise Strawberry Fields™ cereal	120	1 cup Kashi Organic Promise Strawberry Fields cereal	120
½ cup 1% milk	53	½ cup 1% milk	53
1 banana	105	1 banana	105
Coffee or tea with 1% milk and Splenda	12	Coffee or tea with 1% milk and Splenda	12
	290		**290**
Midmorning Snack		**Midmorning Snack**	
½ Strawberry–Toasted Pecan Chicken Salad sandwich (page 174)	115	½ Strawberry–Toasted Pecan Chicken Salad sandwich (page 174)	115
1 cup nonfat milk	91	1 cup nonfat milk	91
	206		**206**
Lunch		**Lunch**	
Roasted Bell Pepper and Lentil Salad (page 172)	294	Roasted Bell Pepper and Lentil Salad (page 172)	294
Diet Snapple (noncaloric)		Diet Snapple (noncaloric)	
2 slices whole-wheat bread	220	1 slice whole-wheat bread	110
	514		**404**
Afternoon Snack		**Afternoon Snack**	
2 Dove Promises bars	84	1 Dove Promises bar	42
1 Tall nonfat cappuccino	75	1 Tall nonfat cappuccino	75
	159		**117**
Dinner		**Dinner**	
Braised Shrimp (page 219)	246	Braised Shrimp (page 219)	246
½ cup steamed rice	103	½ cup steamed rice	103
Green salad with vinaigrette	120	Green salad with vinaigrette	120
Banana Cream Pie (page 278)	197	Banana Cream Pie (page 278)	197
Mineral water	0	Mineral water	0
	666		**666**
TOTALS	**1,835**		**1,683**

Your Calorie Countdown Choices: By giving up 1 slice of bread at lunch you lost 110 calories. You lost another 42 calories by having 1 Dove Promises bar instead of 2 for your afternoon snack.

DAY 2: 1,800 to 1,900 calories

	CALORIES
Breakfast	
¾ cup raisin bran	150
6-oz Dannon Light 'n Fit vanilla yogurt	60
1 banana	105
Coffee or tea with 1% milk and Splenda	12
	327
Midmorning Snack	
1 string cheese	80
12 almonds	85
	165
Lunch	
Quiznos Turkey Ranch & Swiss sandwich	691
Iced tea	0
	691
Afternoon Snack	
100-Calorie Snack Pack	100
1 cup 1% milk	105
	205
Dinner	
Spaghetti Squash Spaghetti and Meatballs (page 244)	306
½ cup steamed broccoli	22
Mixed Salad Greens with Balsamic Vinaigrette (page 169)	89
1 cup cantaloupe	54
	471
TOTALS	**1,859**

DAY 2: 1,650 to 1,800 calories

	CALORIES
Breakfast	
¾ cup raisin bran	150
6-oz Dannon Light 'n Fit vanilla yogurt	60
1 banana	105
Coffee or tea with 1% milk and Splenda	12
	327
Midmorning Snack	
1 string cheese	80
12 almonds	85
	165
Lunch	
Quiznos Small Sierra Smoked Turkey with Raspberry Chipotle Sauce	350
Iced tea	0
	350
Afternoon Snack	
100-Calorie Snack Pack	100
1 cup nonfat milk	91
	191
Dinner	
Spaghetti Squash Spaghetti and Meatballs (page 244)	306
½ cup steamed broccoli	22
Green salad with vinaigrette	120
1 cup cantaloupe	54
1 Chocolate-Chip Cookie (page 285)	68
	570
	1,603

Your Calorie Countdown Choices: You substituted a Quiznos Small Sierra Smoked Turkey with Raspberry Chipotle Sauce sandwich for the Quiznos Turkey Ranch & Swiss sandwich and saved 341 calories, so you got to add some vinaigrette and a Chocolate-Chip Cookie to your menu! You also lost calories by choosing nonfat milk over 1% milk for your afternoon snack.

DAY 3: 1,800 to 1,900 calories

	CALORIES
Breakfast	
1 English muffin	150
1 T I Can't Believe It's Not Butter!	60
1 soft-boiled egg	80
½ grapefruit	53
Coffee or tea with 1% milk and Splenda	12
	355
Midmorning Snack	
6-oz Dannon Light 'n Fit nonfat yogurt	60
1 Tall nonfat cappuccino	75
	135
Lunch	
6.5-oz bowl Boston Market Chicken Tortilla Soup with Toppings	170
Boston Market Caesar Side Salad	300
	470
Afternoon Snack	
1 Babybel	70
5 Melba toasts	60
	130
Dinner	
Chile-Cheese Rice Burritos (page 283)	310
Green salad with Creamy Italian Dressing (page 180)	100
1 cup black beans	210
1 (12-oz) light beer	110
Fat Free Fudgsicle	71
	801
TOTALS	**1,891**

DAY 3: 1,650 to 1,800 calories

	CALORIES
Breakfast	
1 English muffin	150
1 T I Can't Believe It's Not Butter!	60
1 soft-boiled egg	80
½ grapefruit	53
Coffee or tea with 1% milk & Splenda	12
	355
Midmorning Snack	
6-oz Dannon Light 'n Fit nonfat yogurt	60
1 Tall nonfat cappuccino	75
	135
Lunch	
6.5-oz bowl Boston Market Chicken Tortilla Soup (no toppings)	80
Boston Market Caesar Side Salad	300
	380
Afternoon Snack	
1 Babybel	70
5 Melba toasts	60
	130
Dinner	
Chile-Cheese Rice Burritos (page 283)	310
Green salad with fat-free ranch dressing	31
1 cup black beans	210
1 (12-oz) light beer	110
Fat Free Fudgsicle	71
	732
	1,732

Your Calorie Countdown Choices: You got the tortilla soup without the toppings at Boston Market and saved 90 calories. At dinner you switched from vinaigrette to fat-free dressing and saved another 69.

DAY 4: 1,800 to 1,900 calories

	CALORIES
Breakfast	
1 cup oatmeal	150
1 cup 1% milk	105
½ grated apple	40
½ cup orange juice	56
Coffee or tea with 1% milk and Splenda	12
	363
Midmorning Snack	
Almonds and Yogurt Snack (page 276)	194
	194
Lunch	
Herb Turkey Wrap (page 147)	262
Green salad with vinaigrette	120
Iced tea	0
	382
Afternoon Snack	
1 banana	105
12 almonds	85
1 Tall nonfat cappuccino	75
	265
Dinner	
Broccoli-Halibut Stir-Fry (page 220)	221
½ cup steamed rice	103
Green salad with vinaigrette	120
1 (6-oz) glass white wine	145
Roasted Pineapple (page 301)	82
	671
TOTALS	**1,875**

DAY 4: 1,650 to 1,800 calories

	CALORIES
Breakfast	
1 cup oatmeal	150
1 cup nonfat milk	91
½ grated apple	40
½ cup orange juice	56
Coffee or tea with 1% milk and Splenda	12
	349
Midmorning Snack	
2 Babybels	140
	140
Lunch	
Herb Turkey Wrap (page 147)	262
Crudités with Creamy Italian Dressing (page 180)	100
Iced tea	0
	362
Afternoon Snack	
1 banana	105
12 almonds	85
1 Tall nonfat cappuccino	75
	265
Dinner	
Broccoli-Halibut Stir-Fry (page 220)	221
½ cup steamed rice	103
Mixed Salad Greens with Balsamic Vinaigrette (page 169)	89
1 (6-oz) glass white wine	145
Roasted Pineapple (page 301)	82
	640
	1,756

Your Calorie Countdown Choices: By substituting 2 Babybel cheeses for the Almonds and Yogurt Snack you lost 54 calories. You lost another 14 by switching to nonfat milk at breakfast, and at lunch you chose Creamy Italian Dressing instead of vinaigrette for another 20-calorie savings. At dinner you traded vinaigrette for Balsamic Vinaigrette and saved another 31 calories.

	CALORIES		CALORIES
Breakfast		**Breakfast**	
1 small whole-wheat bagel	110	1 small whole-wheat bagel	110
2 T low-fat cream cheese	70	2 T low-fat cream cheese	70
½ cup orange juice	56	½ cup orange juice	56
Coffee or tea with 1% milk and Splenda	12	Coffee or tea with 1% milk and Splenda	12
	248		**248**
Midmorning Snack		**Midmorning Snack**	
Nabisco Honey Maid® Cinnamon Thin Crisps Snack Pack	100	Nabisco Honey Maid Cinnamon Thin Crisps Snack Pack	100
1 cup nonfat milk	91	1 cup nonfat milk	91
	191		**191**
Lunch		**Lunch**	
Open-Faced Chili Dog (page 150)	314	Open-Faced Chili Dog (page 150)	314
Iced tea	0	Iced tea	0
	314		**314**
Afternoon Snack		**Afternoon Snack**	
1 cup grapes	100	1 cup grapes	100
	100		**100**
Dinner		**Dinner**	
Eggplant Parmesan (page 237)	246	Eggplant Parmesan (page 237)	246
½ cup steamed green beans	22	½ cup steamed green beans	22
2 slices French bread	150		
Green salad with vinaigrette	120	Green salad with vinaigrette	120
1 (6-oz) glass red wine	145	1 (6-oz) glass red wine	145
Tiramisu (page 302)	350	Tiramisu (page 302)	350
	1,033		**883**
TOTALS	**1,886**		**1,736**

Your Calorie Countdown Choices: All you did here was eliminate the French bread from your dinner for a 150-calorie savings.

DAY 6: 1,800 to 1,900 calories

	CALORIES
Breakfast	
2 Kashi GOLEAN Blueberry Waffles	170
1 T I Can't Believe It's Not Butter!	60
2 T light syrup	50
Coffee or tea with 1% milk and Splenda	12
	292
Midmorning Snack	
1 Tall Frappuccino	113
	113
Lunch	
Tuna Salad sandwich on rye (page 178)	343
1 cup nonfat milk	91
	434
Afternoon Snack	
1 cup cantaloupe	53
6-oz Dannon Light 'n Fit yogurt	60
	113
Dinner	
Garlic-Roasted Tenderloin (page 198)	447
Mashed Potatoes with Horseradish (page 261)	275
6 spears steamed asparagus	18
Green salad with fat-free dressing	31
Chocolate Angel Food Cake with Strawberries (page 282)	136
	907
TOTALS	**1,859**

DAY 6: 1,650 to 1,800 calories

	CALORIES
Breakfast	
2 Kashi GOLEAN Blueberry Waffles	170
1 T I Can't Believe It's Not Butter!	60
2 T light syrup	50
Coffee or tea with 1% milk and Splenda	12
	292
Midmorning Snack	
1 Tall Frappuccino	113
	113
Lunch	
Tuna Salad (page 178)	143
1 cup nonfat milk	91
	234
Afternoon Snack	
1 cup cantaloupe	53
6-oz Dannon Light 'n Fit yogurt	60
	113
Dinner	
Garlic-Roasted Tenderloin (page 198)	447
Mashed Potatoes with Horseradish (page 261)	275
6 spears steamed asparagus	18
Green salad with fat-free dressing	31
Chocolate Angel Food Cake with Strawberries (page 282)	136
	907
	1,659

Your Calorie Countdown Choices: Instead of a Tuna Salad sandwich for lunch you had a Tuna Salad without bread and saved 200 calories.

DAY 7: 1,800 to 1,900 calories

	CALORIES
Breakfast	
1 Egg Beaters Southwestern omelet	60
2 slices whole-wheat toast	220
1 T I Can't Believe It's Not Butter!	60
1 Tall nonfat cappuccino	75
½ cup orange juice	56
	471
Midmorning Snack	
6-oz Dannon Light 'n Fit yogurt	60
1 banana	105
	165
Lunch	
Club Salad (page 175)	271
1 slice whole-wheat bread	110
Mineral water	0
	381
Afternoon Snack	
½ cup grapes	50
1 Babybel	70
1 Tall nonfat cappuccino	75
	195
Dinner	
Oven-Fried Chicken Breasts (page 202)	175
Mango-Coconut Salsa (page 166)	57
Toasted Almond Green Beans (page 266)	89
½ cup roasted sweet potato	79
Low-fat fruit ice	202
	602
TOTALS	**1,814**

DAY 7: 1,650 to 1,800 calories

	CALORIES
Breakfast	
1 Egg Beaters Southwestern omelet	60
1 slice whole-wheat toast	110
1 T I Can't Believe It's Not Butter!	60
1 Tall nonfat cappuccino	75
½ cup orange juice	56
	361
Midmorning Snack	
6-oz Dannon Light 'n Fit yogurt	60
1 banana	105
	165
Lunch	
Club Salad (page 175)	271
1 slice whole-wheat bread	110
Mineral water	0
	381
Afternoon Snack	
½ cup grapes	50
1 Babybel	70
1 Tall nonfat cappuccino	75
	195
Dinner	
Oven-Fried Chicken Breasts (page 202)	175
Mango-Coconut Salsa (page 166)	57
Toasted Almond Green Beans (page 266)	89
½ cup roasted sweet potato	79
Low-fat fruit ice	202
	602
	1,704

Your Calorie Countdown Choices: You dropped 110 calories just by dropping 1 slice of bread at breakfast.

1,700 to 1,500 CALORIE COUNTDOWN

DAY 1: 1,600 to 1,700 calories

	CALORIES
Breakfast	
1 cup Kashi GOLEAN cereal	190
½ cup 1% milk	53
1 medium banana	105
Coffee or tea with 1% milk and Splenda	12
	360
Midmorning Snack	
100-Calorie Snack Pack	100
Noncaloric flavored water	
	100
Lunch	
Baja Fresh Grilled Mahi Mahi Taco	300
Diet soda or mineral water	
1 Chocolate-Chip Cookie (page 285)	68
	368
Afternoon Snack	
2 Dove Promises bars	84
1 Tall nonfat cappuccino	75
	159
Dinner	
Turkey Meatloaf (page 217)	236
6 spears steamed asparagus	18
1 tsp Molly McButter®	5
Green salad with fat-free ranch dressing	31
Maple-Roasted Butternut Squash (page 259)	159
Roasted Ginger Papaya (page 300)	146
	595
TOTALS	**1,582**

DAY 1: 1,500 to 1,600 calories

	CALORIES
Breakfast	
1 cup Kashi GOLEAN cereal	190
½ cup 1% milk	53
1 medium banana	105
Coffee or tea with 1% milk and Splenda	12
	360
Midmorning Snack	
100-Calorie Snack Pack	100
Noncaloric flavored water	0
	100
Lunch	
Baja Fresh Grilled Mahi Mahi Taco	300
Diet soda or mineral water	
1 Chocolate-Chip Cookie (page 285)	68
	368
Afternoon Snack	
2 Dove Promises bars	84
1 Tall nonfat cappuccino	75
	159
Dinner	
Turkey Meatloaf (page 217)	236
6 spears steamed asparagus	18
1 tsp Molly McButter	5
Green salad with fat-free ranch dressing	31
Roasted Ginger Papaya (page 300)	146
	436
	1,423

Your Calorie Countdown Choices: You lost 159 calories by eliminating the Maple-Roasted Butternut Squash from your dinner.

DAY 2: 1,600 to 1,700 calories

	CALORIES
Breakfast	
2 poached eggs	160
2 slices whole-wheat toast	220
½ cup orange juice	56
Coffee or tea with 1% milk and Splenda	12
	448
Midmorning Snack	
1 banana	105
6-oz Dannon Light 'n Fit yogurt	60
	165
Lunch	
Subway 6-inch Veggie Delite Sandwich	230
Iced tea	0
	230
Afternoon Snack	
1 Peanut Butter–Banana Cookie (page 293)	126
1 cup 1% milk	105
	231
Dinner	
Eggplant Parmesan (page 237)	246
Green salad with Creamy Italian Dressing (page 180)	100
1 (6-oz) glass red wine	145
½ cup fruit sherbet	125
	616
TOTALS	**1,690**

DAY 2: 1,500 to 1,600 calories

	CALORIES
Breakfast	
Egg Beaters Southwestern omelet	60
2 slices whole-wheat toast	220
½ cup orange juice	56
Coffee or tea with 1% milk and Splenda	12
	348
Midmorning Snack	
1 banana	105
6-oz Danon Light 'n Fit yogurt	60
	165
Lunch	
Subway 6-inch Veggie Delite Sandwich	230
Iced tea	0
	230
Afternoon Snack	
1 Peanut Butter–Banana Cookie (page 293)	126
1 cup nonfat milk	91
	217
Dinner	
Eggplant Parmesan (page 237)	246
Green salad with Creamy Italian Dressing (page 180)	100
1 (6-oz) glass red wine	145
½ cup fruit sherbet	125
	616
	1,576

Your Calorie Countdown Choices: For breakfast you saved yourself 100 calories by substituting an Egg Beaters Southwestern omelet for the 2 poached eggs. If you choose to have 1 slice of toast instead of 2 you'll cut out another 110 calories. You also lost 14 calories in the afternoon by choosing nonfat milk over 1% milk.

DAY 3: 1,600 to 1,700 calories

	CALORIES
Breakfast	
2 Kashi GOLEAN Waffles	170
1 T I Can't Believe It's Not Butter!	60
2 T light syrup	50
½ cup orange juice	56
Coffee or tea with 1% milk and Splenda	12
	348
Midmorning Snack	
1 Babybel	70
½ high-fiber English muffin	75
	145
Lunch	
Koo-Koo-Roo Rotisserie Chicken breast and wing	355
Green salad with vinaigrette	120
	475
Afternoon Snack	
2 cups Barbecued Popcorn (page 271)	80
1 cup V8 juice	50
	130
Dinner	
Ginger Packet Salmon (page 225)	195
½ cup quinoa	120
Cucumber-Dill Salad (page 177)	41
Light Pear Crisp (page 288)	211
	567
TOTALS	**1,665**

DAY 3: 1,500 to 1,600 calories

	CALORIES
Breakfast	
2 Kashi GOLEAN Waffles	170
1 T I Can't Believe It's Not Butter!	60
2 T light syrup	50
½ cup orange juice	56
Coffee or tea with 1% milk and Splenda	12
	348
Midmorning Snack	
1 Babybel	70
½ high-fiber English muffin	75
	145
Lunch	
Koo-Koo-Roo Rotisserie Chicken breast and wing	355
Green salad with fat-free dressing	31
	386
Afternoon Snack	
2 cups Barbecued Popcorn (page 271)	80
1 cup V8 juice	50
	130
Dinner	
Ginger Packet Salmon (page 225)	195
½ cup quinoa	120
Cucumber-Dill Salad (page 177)	41
Roasted Ginger Papaya (page 300)	146
	502
	1,511

Your Calorie Countdown Choices: You lost 89 calories at lunch by switching to fat-free dressing. You dropped another 65 calories by choosing Roasted Ginger Papaya instead of Light Pear Crisp for dinner.

DAY 4: 1,600 to 1,700 calories

	CALORIES
Breakfast	
1 packet Kashi GOLEAN Hot Cereal	150
½ cup 1% milk and Splenda	53
½ cup orange juice	56
Coffee or tea with 1% milk and Splenda	12
	271
Midmorning Snack	
¾ cup nonfat cottage cheese	120
12 almonds	85
	205
Lunch	
Herb Turkey Wrap (page 149)	262
Mineral water or diet soda	0
1 Oatmeal-Craisin Cookie (page 291)	49
	311
Afternoon Snack	
1 apple	80
1 string cheese	80
	160
Dinner	
Garlic-Roasted Tenderloin (page 198)	447
Zucchini Latkes (page 268)	66
½ cup steamed green beans	22
1 (6-oz) glass red wine	145
Fat Free Fudgsicle	71
	751
TOTALS	**1,698**

DAY 4: 1,500 to 1,600 calories

	CALORIES
Breakfast	
1 packet Kashi GOLEAN Hot Cereal	150
½ cup nonfat milk and Splenda	46
½ cup orange juice	56
Coffee or tea with 1% milk and Splenda	12
	264
Midmorning Snack	
½ cup nonfat cottage cheese	80
½ cup diced fresh pineapple	37
	117
Lunch	
Herb Turkey Wrap (page 149)	262
Mineral water or diet soda	0
	262
Afternoon Snack	
1 apple	80
1 string cheese	80
	160
Dinner	
Garlic-Roasted Tenderloin (page 198)	447
Zucchini Latkes (page 268)	66
½ cup steamed green beans	22
1 (6-oz) glass red wine	145
Fat Free Fudgsicle	71
	751
	1,554

Your Calorie Countdown Choices: You saved 88 calories by substituting fresh pineapple for almonds at your midmorning snack, and reducing the cottage cheese amount by ¼ cup. You saved another 49 calories at lunch by forgoing the cookie, and you saved another 7 at breakfast by choosing nonfat milk.

DAY 5: 1,600 to 1,700 calories

	CALORIES
Breakfast	
1 packet Kashi GOLEAN Hot Cereal	150
½ cup blueberries	41
1 cup 1% milk	105
Coffee or tea with 1% milk and Splenda	12
	308
Midmorning Snack	
1 cup grapes	100
6-oz Dannon Light 'n Fit yogurt	60
	160
Lunch	
Roasted Bell Pepper and Lentil Salad (page 172)	294
Mineral water or diet soda	0
1 slice whole-wheat bread	110
	404
Afternoon Snack	
100-Calorie Snack Pack	100
1 Tall nonfat cappuccino	75
	175
Dinner	
Crab and Avocado Quesadillas (page 221)	263
6 spears steamed asparagus	18
Gazpacho (page 156)	87
Banana Cream Pie (page 278)	197
	565
TOTALS	**1,612**

DAY 5: 1,500 to 1,600 calories

	CALORIES
Breakfast	
1 packet Kashi GOLEAN Hot Cereal	150
½ cup blueberries	41
1 cup 1% milk	105
Coffee or tea with 1% milk and Splenda	12
	308
Midmorning Snack	
1 cup grapes	100
6-oz Dannon Light 'n Fit yogurt	60
	160
Lunch	
Roasted Bell Pepper and Lentil Salad (page 172)	294
Mineral water or diet soda	0
	294
Afternoon Snack	
100-Calorie Snack Pack	100
1 Tall nonfat cappuccino	75
	175
Dinner	
Crab and Avocado Quesadillas (page 221)	263
6 spears steamed asparagus	18
Gazpacho (page 156)	87
Banana Cream Pie (page 278)	197
	565
	1,502

Your Calorie Countdown Choices: All you did was take away 1 slice of bread from your lunch and you lost 110 calories.

DAY 6: 1,600 to 1,700 calories

	CALORIES
Breakfast	
Breakfast Taco (page 144)	231
½ cup orange juice	56
Coffee or tea with 1% milk and Splenda	12
	299
Midmorning Snack	
½ cup fruit salad	100
½ cup nonfat cottage cheese	80
	180
Lunch	
Strawberry–Toasted Pecan Chicken Salad (page 174)	230
1 slice whole-wheat bread	110
Iced tea	0
	340
Afternoon Snack	
2 Lindt chocolate truffles	146
1 Tall nonfat cappuccino	75
	221
Dinner	
Wild Mushroom Manicotti (page 248)	193
Green salad with Creamy Italian Dressing (page 180)	100
1 (6-oz) glass red wine	145
Zinfandel-Poached Pears (page 303)	191
	629
TOTALS	**1,669**

DAY 6: 1,500 to 1,600 calories

	CALORIES
Breakfast	
Breakfast Taco (page 144)	231
½ cup orange juice	56
Coffee or tea with 1% milk and Splenda	12
	299
Midmorning Snack	
½ cup fruit salad	100
½ cup nonfat cottage cheese	80
	180
Lunch	
Strawberry–Toasted Pecan Chicken Salad (page 174)	230
1 slice whole-wheat bread	110
Iced tea	0
	340
Afternoon Snack	
2 Lindt chocolate truffles	146
1 Tall nonfat cappuccino	75
	221
Dinner	
Wild Mushroom Manicotti (page 248)	193
Green salad with Creamy Italian Dressing (page 180)	100
Zinfandel-Poached Pears (page 303)	191
	484
TOTALS	**1,524**

Your Calorie Countdown Choices: You lost 145 calories by eliminating the wine from your dinner. If you want to keep the wine you can cut out the bread at lunch, or the afternoon chocolate.

DAY 7: 1,600 to 1,700 calories

	CALORIES
Breakfast	
Blueberry Ricotta Pancakes (page 145)	277
1 T I Can't Believe It's Not Butter!	60
½ cup orange juice	56
Coffee or tea with 1% milk and Splenda	12
	405
Midmorning Snack	
Small blended coffee drink	113
	113
Lunch	
Tuna Salad (page 178)	143
Iced tea	0
1 slice whole-wheat bread	110
	253
Afternoon Snack	
Pringles 100-Calorie Pack	100
Diet soda	0
	100
Dinner	
Air-Fried Pork Chops (page 184)	321
Air Fries (page 250)	92
Rapid Ratatouille (page 263)	59
Green salad with fat-free ranch dressing	31
Tiramisu (page 302)	310
	813
TOTALS	**1,684**

DAY 7: 1,500 to 1,600 calories

	CALORIES
Breakfast	
Blueberry Ricotta Pancakes (page 145)	277
1 T I Can't Believe It's Not Butter!	60
½ cup orange juice	56
Coffee or tea with 1% milk and Splenda	12
	405
Midmorning Snack	
Small blended coffee drink	113
	113
Lunch	
Tuna Salad (page 178)	143
Iced tea	0
	143
Afternoon Snack	
Pringles 100-Calorie Pack	100
Diet soda	0
	100
Dinner	
Air-Fried Pork Chops (page 184)	321
Air Fries (page 250)	92
Rapid Ratatouille (page 263)	59
Green Salad with fat-free ranch dressing	31
Tiramisu (page 302)	310
	813
	1,574

Your Calorie Countdown Choices: You dropped 110 calories by eliminating the bread at lunch.

1,500 to 1,250 Calorie Countdown

DAY 1: **1,400 to 1,500 calories**	CALORIES	DAY 1: **1,250 to 1,400 calories**	CALORIES
Breakfast		**Breakfast**	
1 small whole-wheat bagel	154	1 small whole-wheat bagel	154
1 T low-fat cream cheese	35	1 T low-fat cream cheese	35
½ cup orange juice	56	½ cup orange juice	56
1 boiled egg	80	1 boiled egg	80
Coffee or tea with 1% milk and Splenda	12	Coffee or tea with 1% milk and Splenda	12
	337		**337**
Midmorning Snack		**Midmorning Snack**	
1 banana	105	1 banana	105
6-oz Dannon Light 'n Fit yogurt	60	6-oz Dannon Light 'n Fit yogurt	60
	165		**165**
Lunch		**Lunch**	
Shrimp Cocktail (page 155)	134	Shrimp Cocktail (page 155)	134
1 slice whole-wheat bread	110	1 slice whole-wheat bread	110
Iced tea	0	Iced tea	0
	244		**244**
Afternoon Snack		**Afternoon Snack**	
1 Dove Promises bar	42	1 Dove Promises bar	42
1 Tall nonfat cappuccino	75	1 Tall nonfat cappuccino	75
	117		**117**
Dinner		**Dinner**	
Quick Shoyu Chicken (page 206)	162	Quick Shoyu Chicken (page 206)	162
½ cup steamed rice	103	½ cup steamed rice	103
½ cup steamed green beans	22	½ cup steamed green beans	22
1 (6-oz) glass white wine	145	1 (6-oz) glass white wine	145
Light Pear Crisp (page 288)	211	Brownie (page 281)	92
	643		**524**
TOTALS	**1,506**		**1,387**

Your Calorie Countdown Choices: At dinner, ironically, my Brownie gave you 119 calories less than my Light Pear Crisp.

DAY 2: 1,400 to 1,500 calories

	CALORIES
Breakfast	
1 packet Kashi GOLEAN Hot Cereal	150
½ cup blueberries	41
½ cup 1% milk	53
Coffee or tea with 1% milk and Splenda	12
	256
Midmorning Snack	
1 string cheese	80
12 almonds	85
	165
Lunch	
Panda Express Chicken with String Beans	160
½ cup steamed rice	103
Green tea	0
	263
Afternoon Snack	
Ritz 100-Calorie Snack Mix	100
1 Tall nonfat cappuccino	75
	175
Dinner	
Ginger Packet Salmon (page 225)	195
½ cup quinoa	128
Green salad with fat-free dressing	31
1 (6-oz) glass red wine	145
Roasted Pineapple (page 301)	82
	581
TOTALS	**1,440**

DAY 2: 1,250 to 1,400 calories

	CALORIES
Breakfast	
1 packet Kashi GOLEAN Hot Cereal	150
½ cup blueberries	41
½ cup 1% milk	53
Coffee or tea with 1% milk and Splenda	12
	256
Midmorning Snack	
1 string cheese	80
12 almonds	85
	165
Lunch	
Panda Express Chicken with String Beans	160
½ cup steamed rice	103
Green tea	0
	263
Afternoon Snack	
Ritz 100-Calorie Snack Mix	100
1 Tall nonfat cappuccino	75
	175
Dinner	
Ginger Packet Salmon (page 225)	195
½ cup quinoa	128
Green salad with fat-free dressing	31
Mineral water	0
Roasted Pineapple (page 301)	82
	436
TOTALS	**1,295**

Your Calorie Countdown Choices: You had mineral water instead of wine with your dinner and lost 145 calories. That was the only change you made.

DAY 3: 1,400 to 1,500 calories

	CALORIES
Breakfast	
1 cup Kashi GOLEAN cereal	190
½ cup 1% milk	53
1 banana	105
Coffee or tea with 1% milk and Splenda	12
	360
Midmorning Snack	
6-oz Dannon Light 'n Fit yogurt	60
1 Tall nonfat cappuccino	75
	135
Lunch	
Campbell's Chunky Microwavable Beef with Country Vegetables Soup	150
1 slice whole-wheat bread	110
Diet soda	0
	260
Afternoon Snack	
2 Lindt chocolate truffles	146
Coffee with 1% milk and Splenda	12
	158
Dinner	
Portobello Mushroom–Phyllo Packets (page 243)	221
Rapid Ratatouille (page 263)	59
1 (6-oz) glass red wine	145
Roasted Ginger Papaya (page 300)	146
	571
TOTALS	**1,484**

DAY 3: 1,250 to 1,400 calories

	CALORIES
Breakfast	
1 cup Kashi GOLEAN cereal	190
½ cup nonfat milk	46
1 banana	105
Coffee or tea with 1% milk and Splenda	12
	353
Midmorning Snack	
6-oz Dannon Light 'n Fit yogurt	60
1 Tall nonfat cappuccino	75
	135
Lunch	
Campbell's Chunky Microwavable Beef with Country Vegetables Soup	150
1 slice whole-wheat bread	110
Diet soda	0
	260
Afternoon Snack	
2 Lindt chocolate truffles	146
Coffee with 1% milk and Splenda	12
	158
Dinner	
Portobello Mushroom–Phyllo Packets (page 243)	221
Rapid Ratatouille (page 263)	59
1 (6-oz) glass red wine	145
1 cup strawberries	50
	475
	1,381

Your Calorie Countdown Choices: You lost 96 calories just by exchanging strawberries for Roasted Ginger Papaya at dinner, and 7 calories at breakfast by swapping out 1% milk for nonfat milk.

DAY 4: 1,400 to 1,500 calories

	CALORIES
Breakfast	
½ cup scrambled Egg Beaters	60
½ high-fiber English muffin	75
½ cup orange juice	56
Coffee or tea with 1% milk and Splenda	12
	203
Midmorning Snack	
½ cup Kashi Mighty Bites Honey Crunch Cereal	55
½ cup nonfat milk	45
	100
Lunch	
10-oz Corner Bakery Minestrone	140
Corner Bakery Tomato Fresca Salad	200
Iced tea	0
1 slice whole-wheat bread	110
	450
Afternoon Snack	
1 apple	80
1 Tall nonfat cappuccino	75
	155
Dinner	
Adobo-Roasted Pork Loin (page 183)	247
½ cup steamed broccoli	22
½ cup small baked sweet potato	79
Green salad with fat-free dressing	31
1 (6-oz) glass red wine	145
1 peach	37
	561
TOTALS	**1,469**

DAY 4: 1,250 to 1,400 calories

	CALORIES
Breakfast	
½ cup scrambled Egg Beaters	60
½ high-fiber English muffin	75
½ cup orange juice	56
Coffee or tea with 1% milk and Splenda	12
	203
Midmorning Snack	
½ cup Kashi Mighty Bites Honey Crunch Cereal	55
½ cup nonfat milk	45
	100
Lunch	
10-oz Corner Bakery Minestrone	140
Corner Bakery Tomato Fresca Salad	200
Iced tea	0
	340
Afternoon Snack	
1 apple	80
1 Tall nonfat cappuccino	75
	155
Dinner	
Adobo-Roasted Pork Loin (page 183)	247
½ cup steamed broccoli	22
Green salad with fat-free dressing	31
1 (6-oz) glass red wine	145
1 peach	37
	482
TOTALS	**1,280**

Your Calorie Countdown Choices: You lost 79 calories by giving up the sweet potato with your dinner and 110 calories by giving up the bread at lunch. You could keep the sweet potato and give up the wine instead.

DAY 5: 1,400 to 1,500 calories

	CALORIES
Breakfast	
1 cup Kashi Organic Promise Cranberry Sunshine cereal	120
1 cup 1% milk	53
½ cup orange juice	56
Coffee or tea with 1% milk and Splenda	12
	241
Midmorning Snack	
½ cup 1% cottage cheese	82
5 Melba toasts	60
	142
Lunch	
California roll sushi	361
Iced tea	0
	361
Afternoon Snack	
12-oz V8 juice	70
1 string cheese	80
	150
Dinner	
Garlic Shrimp Scampi (page 223)	359
Green salad with fat-free dressing	31
1 (6-oz) glass wine	145
Brownie (page 281)	92
	627
TOTALS	**1,521**

DAY 5: 1,250 to 1,400 calories

	CALORIES
Breakfast	
1 cup Kashi Organic Promise Cranberry Sunshine cereal	120
½ cup nonfat milk	46
½ cup orange juice	56
Coffee or tea with 1% milk and Splenda	12
	234
Midmorning Snack	
½ cup 1% cottage cheese	82
5 Melba toasts	60
	142
Lunch	
California roll sushi	361
Iced tea	0
	361
Afternoon Snack	
12-oz V8 juice	70
1 string cheese	80
	150
Dinner	
Braised Shrimp (page 219)	246
Green salad with fat-free dressing	31
1 (6-oz) glass wine	145
1 tangerine	37
	459
TOTALS	**1,346**

Your Calorie Countdown Choices: You saved 168 calories at dinner by choosing the Braised Shrimp instead of the Garlic Shrimp Scampi, and by choosing a tangerine over a brownie for dessert. If you need chocolate you still have room for a Dove Promises bar. You also knocked off a few calories at breakfast by having nonfat milk instead of 1% milk with your cereal.

DAY 6: 1,400 to 1,500 calories

	CALORIES
Breakfast	
Blueberry Ricotta Pancakes (page 145)	277
½ cup orange juice	56
Coffee or tea with 1% milk and Splenda	12
	345
Midmorning Snack	
6-oz Dannon Light 'n Fit yogurt	60
1 banana	105
	165
Lunch	
Strawberry–Toasted Pecan Chicken Salad (page 174)	230
	230
Afternoon Snack	
100-Calorie Snack Pack	100
1 Tall nonfat cappuccino	75
	175
Dinner	
Calorie Countdown Baked Beans (page 255)	255
Air Fries (page 250)	92
Green salad with fat-free ranch dressing	31
1 (12-oz) light beer	110
1 peach	37
	525
TOTALS	**1,440**

DAY 6: 1,250 to 1,400 calories

	CALORIES
Breakfast	
Blueberry Ricotta Pancakes (page 145)	277
½ cup orange juice	56
Coffee or tea with 1% milk and Splenda	12
	345
Midmorning Snack	
6-oz Dannon Light 'n Fit yogurt	60
1 banana	105
	165
Lunch	
Strawberry–Toasted Pecan Chicken Salad (page 174)	230
	230
Afternoon Snack	
100-Calorie Snack Pack	100
1 Tall nonfat cappuccino	75
	175
Dinner	
Calorie Countdown Baked Beans (page 255)	255
Air Fries (page 250)	92
Green salad with fat-free ranch dressing	31
1 peach	37
	415
TOTALS	**1,330**

Your Calorie Countdown Choices: You lost 110 calories by giving up the light beer at dinner.

DAY 7: 1,400 to 1,500 calories

	CALORIES
Breakfast	
2 poached eggs	160
1 small whole-wheat bagel	154
1 T low-fat cream cheese	35
½ cup orange juice	56
Coffee or tea with 1% milk and Splenda	12
	417
Midmorning Snack	
1 Tall Frappuccino	113
	113
Lunch	
Small roast beef sandwich	290
Diet Snapple (noncaloric)	0
	290
Afternoon Snack	
12-oz V8 juice	70
1 string cheese	80
	150
Dinner	
Chicken Parmesan (page 190)	331
½ cup steamed broccoli	22
Mixed Salad Greens with Balsamic Vinaigrette (page 169)	89
Chocolate-Chip Cookie (page 285)	68
	510
TOTALS	**1,480**

DAY 7: 1,250 to 1,400 calories

	CALORIES
Breakfast	
1 poached egg	80
½ small whole-wheat bagel	77
1 T low-fat cream cheese	35
½ cup orange juice	56
Coffee or tea with 1% milk and Splenda	12
	260
Midmorning Snack	
1 Tall Frappuccino	113
	113
Lunch	
Small roast beef sandwich	290
Diet Snapple (noncaloric)	0
	290
Afternoon Snack	
12-oz V8 juice	70
1 string cheese	80
	150
Dinner	
Chicken Parmesan (page 190)	331
½ cup steamed broccoli	22
Mixed Salad Greens with Balsamic Vinaigrette (page 169)	89
Chocolate-Chip Cookie (page 285)	68
	510
	1,323

Your Calorie Countdown Choices: You lost 157 calories at breakfast by losing one egg and half a bagel. If you crave a sweet in the afternoon you could have the cookie then instead of at dinner, or something else, like a 42-calorie Dove bar.

1,300 to 1,100 Calorie Countdown

DAY 1: **1,200 to 1,300 calories**	CALORIES
Breakfast	
½ cup All-Bran cereal	80
½ cup nonfat milk	45
½ cup orange juice	56
Coffee or tea with 1% milk and Splenda	12
	193
Midmorning Snack	
1 banana	105
6-oz Dannon Light 'n Fit yogurt	60
	165
Lunch	
Koo-Koo-Roo Ten Vegetable Soup (10-oz serving)	188
Koo-Koo-Roo Cucumber Salad	41
Iced tea	0
	229
Afternoon Snack	
1 Dove Promises bar	42
1 Tall nonfat cappuccino	75
	117
Dinner	
Spaghetti Squash with Roasted Garlic Pesto (page 241)	240
Cheese-Roasted Broccoli (page 257)	87
Green salad with fat-free dressing	31
1 (6-oz) glass red wine	145
1 cup strawberries	50
	553
TOTALS	**1,257**

DAY 1: **1,100 to 1,200 calories**	CALORIES
Breakfast	
½ cup All-Bran cereal	80
½ cup nonfat milk	45
½ cup orange juice	56
Coffee or tea with 1% milk and Splenda	12
	193
Midmorning Snack	
1 banana	105
6-oz Dannon Light 'n Fit yogurt	60
	165
Lunch	
Koo-Koo-Roo Ten Vegetable Soup (10-oz serving)	188
Koo-Koo-Roo Cucumber Salad	41
Iced tea	0
	229
Afternoon Snack	
1 Dove Promises bar	42
1 Tall nonfat cappuccino	75
	117
Dinner	
Spaghetti Squash with Roasted Garlic Pesto (page 241)	240
Cheese-Roasted Broccoli (page 257)	87
Green salad with fat-free dressing	31
1 cup strawberries	50
	408
TOTALS	**1,112**

Your Calorie Countdown Choices: You lost 145 calories just by losing the glass of red wine with dinner. If you really want the wine, lose the strawberries and the afternoon cappuccino.

DAY 2: **1,200 to 1,300 calories**	CALORIES	DAY 2: **1,100 to 1,200 calories**	CALORIES
Breakfast		**Breakfast**	
2-egg omelet	202	2 poached eggs	160
½ cup orange juice	56	½ cup orange juice	56
1 slice whole-wheat toast	110	1 slice whole-wheat toast	110
Coffee or tea with 1% milk and Splenda	12	Coffee or tea with 1% milk and Splenda	12
	380		**338**
Midmorning Snack		**Midmorning Snack**	
100-Calorie Snack Pack	100	100-Calorie Snack Pack	100
Diet soda	0	Diet soda	0
	100		**100**
Lunch		**Lunch**	
Shrimp Cocktail (page 155)	134	Shrimp Cocktail (page 155)	134
1 slice whole-wheat bread	110	1 slice whole-wheat bread	110
	244		**244**
Afternoon Snack		**Afternoon Snack**	
1 Babybel	70	1 Babybel	70
5 Melba toasts	60	5 Melba toasts	60
1 Tall nonfat cappuccino	75	1 Tall nonfat cappuccino	75
	205		**205**
Dinner		**Dinner**	
Tequila Chicken Fajita (page 213)	168	Tequila Chicken Fajita (page 213)	168
Green salad with fat-free dressing	31	Green salad with fat-free dressing	31
1 (12-oz) light beer	110		
1 peach	37	1 peach	37
	346		**236**
TOTALS	**1,275**		**1,123**

Your Calorie Countdown Choices: You dropped 110 calories by losing the beer at dinner. You lost another 42 calories by opting for poached eggs over an omelet at breakfast.

DAY 3: 1,200 to 1,300 calories

	CALORIES
Breakfast	
Kashi Heart to Heart™ Raisin Spice Oatmeal	150
½ cup nonfat milk	45
1 banana	105
Coffee or tea with 1% milk and Splenda	12
	312
Midmorning Snack	
1 Kashi GOLEAN Waffle	80
6-oz Dannon Light 'n Fit yogurt	60
	140
Lunch	
Club Salad (page 175)	271
Iced tea	0
	271
Afternoon Snack	
1 apple	80
1 Tall nonfat cappuccino	75
	155
Dinner	
Wild Mushroom Manicotti (page 248)	193
Green salad with Creamy Italian Dressing (page 180)	100
1 (6-oz) glass red wine	145
	438
TOTALS	**1,316**

DAY 3: 1,100 to 1,200 calories

	CALORIES
Breakfast	
Kashi Heart to Heart Raisin Spice Oatmeal	150
½ cup nonfat milk	45
1 banana	105
Coffee or tea with 1% milk and Splenda	12
	312
Midmorning Snack	
1 Kashi GOLEAN Waffle	80
6-oz Dannon Light 'n Fit yogurt	60
	140
Lunch	
Club Salad (page 175)	271
Iced tea	0
	271
Afternoon Snack	
1 apple	80
1 Dove Promises bar	42
	122
Dinner	
Wild Mushroom Manicotti (page 248)	193
Green salad with Creamy Italian dressing (page 180)	100
	293
	1,138

Your Calorie Countdown Choices: You lost 145 calories at dinner by dropping the wine. You had a Dove Promises bar in the afternoon instead of a cappuccino and dropped another 33 calories.

DAY 4: 1,200 to 1,300 calories

	CALORIES
Breakfast	
½ cup scrambled Egg Beaters	60
½ high-fiber English muffin	75
1 T I Can't Believe It's Not Butter!	60
½ cup orange juice	56
Coffee or tea with 1% milk and Splenda	12
	263
Midmorning Snack	
½ cup Kashi Mighty Bites Honey Crunch cereal	55
½ cup nonfat milk	45
	100
Lunch	
Saladworks Shrimp Caesar	353
Mineral water	0
	353
Afternoon Snack	
100-Calorie Snack Pack	100
Iced tea	0
	100
Dinner	
Spicy Seared Scallops (page 229)	187
Kashi 7 Whole Grain Pilaf	170
Green salad with fat-free dressing	31
Iced tea or mineral water	0
Fat Free Fudgsicle	71
	459
TOTALS	**1,275**

DAY 4: 1,100 to 1,200 calories

	CALORIES
Breakfast	
½ cup scrambled Egg Beaters	60
½ high-fiber English muffin	75
1 T I Can't Believe It's Not Butter!	60
½ cup orange juice	56
Coffee or tea with 1% milk and Splenda	12
	263
Midmorning Snack	
½ cup Kashi Mighty Bites Honey Crunch cereal	55
½ cup nonfat milk	45
	100
Lunch	
Saladworks Shrimp Caesar	353
Mineral water	0
	353
Afternoon Snack	
100-Calorie Snack Pack	100
Iced tea	0
	100
Dinner	
Spicy Seared Scallops (page 229)	187
½ cup steamed rice	103
Green salad with fat-free dressing	31
Iced tea or mineral water	0
	321
TOTALS	**1,137**

Your Calorie Countdown Choices: By having rice instead of the Kashi 7 Whole Grain Pilaf for dinner you lost 67 calories. You lost another 71 by giving up the Fudgsicle for dessert. If you've really gotta have chocolate, have a couple of Dove Promises bars or the Fat Free Fudgsicle instead of the snack pack in the afternoon.

DAY 5: 1,200 to 1,300 calories

	CALORIES
Breakfast	
1 cup plain nonfat yogurt	127
½ cup blueberries	41
Coffee or tea with 1% milk and Splenda	12
	180
Midmorning Snack	
1 Babybel	70
	70
Lunch	
Subway 6-inch Turkey Breast sandwich	280
Mineral water	0
	280
Afternoon Snack	
16-oz Jamba Juice Enlightened Berry Fulfilling smoothie	160
	160
Dinner	
Chili con Carne (page 195)	378
Green salad with fat-free dressing	31
1 (12-oz) light beer	110
1 cup strawberries	50
	569
TOTALS	**1,259**

DAY 5: 1,100 to 1,200 calories

	CALORIES
Breakfast	
1 cup plain nonfat yogurt	127
½ cup blueberries	41
Coffee or tea with 1% milk and Splenda	12
	180
Midmorning Snack	
1 Babybel	70
5 Melba toasts	60
	130
Lunch	
Subway 6-inch Turkey Breast sandwich	280
Mineral water	0
	280
Afternoon Snack	
16-oz Jamba Juice Enlightened Berry Fulfilling smoothie	160
	160
Dinner	
Crab and Avocado Quesadilla (page 221)	263
Green salad with fat-free dressing	31
1 cup strawberries	50
	344
TOTALS	**1,094**

Your Calorie Countdown Choices: You traded Chili con Carne for Crab and Avocado Quesadillas and lost 115 calories in the transaction. You also lost the light beer at dinner for another 110 calories. You added 60 calories' worth of Melba toast with your midmorning snack and still ended up consuming 165 fewer calories.

DAY 6: 1,200 to 1,300 calories

	CALORIES
Breakfast	
1 cup Kashi Organic Promise Strawberry Fields™ cereal	120
½ cup nonfat milk	45
½ cup blueberries	41
Coffee or tea with 1% milk and Splenda	12
	218
Midmorning Snack	
1 banana	105
	105
Lunch	
Portobello Mushroom–Phyllo Packet (page 243)	221
Mineral water	0
	221
Afternoon Snack	
1 Dove Promises bar	42
1 Tall nonfat cappuccino	75
	117
Dinner	
Tea-Smoked Chicken (page 212)	285
Creamy Coleslaw (page 176)	122
Broccoli with Garlic Chili Sauce (page 254)	48
1 (6-oz) glass white wine	145
	600
TOTALS	**1,261**

DAY 6: 1,100 to 1,200 calories

	CALORIES
Breakfast	
1 cup Kashi Organic Promise Strawberry Fields cereal	120
½ cup nonfat milk	45
½ cup blueberries	41
Coffee or tea with 1% milk and Splenda	12
	218
Midmorning Snack	
1 banana	105
	105
Lunch	
Portobello Mushroom–Phyllo Packet (page 243)	221
Mineral water	0
	221
Afternoon Snack	
1 Dove Promises bar	42
1 Tall nonfat cappuccino	75
	117
Dinner	
Tea-Smoked Chicken (page 212)	285
Creamy Coleslaw (page 176)	122
Broccoli with Garlic Chili Sauce (page 254)	48
	455
TOTALS	**1,116**

Your Calorie Countdown Choices: You lost 145 calories with the glass of white wine you gave up at dinner.

DAY 7: 1,200 to 1,300 calories

	CALORIES
Breakfast	
Cinnamon-Pear Stuffed French Toast (page 146)	242
½ cup orange juice	56
Coffee or tea with 1% milk and Splenda	12
	310
Midmorning Snack	
1 Tall Frappuccino	113
	113
Lunch	
Open-Faced Chili Dog (page 150)	314
Mineral water	0
	314
Afternoon Snack	
1 apple	80
	80
Dinner	
Kalamata Halibut (page 226)	238
½ cup steamed broccoli	22
½ cup white rice	103
Brownie (page 281)	92
	455
TOTALS	**1,272**

DAY 7: 1,100 to 1,200 calories

	CALORIES
Breakfast	
Cinnamon-Pear Stuffed French Toast (page 146)	242
½ cup orange juice	56
Coffee or tea with 1% milk and Splenda	12
	310
Midmorning Snack	
1 Tall Frappuccino	113
	113
Lunch	
Breakfast Taco (page 144)	231
Mineral water	0
	231
Afternoon Snack	
1 apple	80
	80
Dinner	
Kalamata Halibut (page 226)	238
½ cup steamed broccoli	22
½ cup white rice	103
	363
TOTALS	**1,097**

Your Calorie Countdown Choices: Instead of the Open-Faced Chili Dog you had a Breakfast Taco for lunch and saved 83 calories. You more than doubled this savings by losing the Brownie at dinner.

Six Weekly Menus
for the Non-Cook

1,900 to 1,650 CALORIE COUNTDOWN

DAY 1: 1,850 to 1,900 calories

	CALORIES
Breakfast	
1 cup Kashi Organic Promise Strawberry Fields cereal	120
½ cup 1% milk	53
1 banana	105
Coffee or tea with 1% milk and Splenda	12
	290
Midmorning Snack	
Campbell's Chunky microwavable bowl: Grilled Chicken with Vegetables & Pasta Soup	110
1 slice whole-wheat bread	110
	220
Lunch	
Subway 6-inch Cold Cut Combo sandwich	410
Iced tea	0
	410
Afternoon Snack	
2 Dove Promises bars	84
1 Tall nonfat cappuccino	75
	159
Dinner	
Lean Cuisine Lemon Garlic Shrimp	280
Green salad with vinaigrette	120
1 slice French bread	75
1 (6-oz) glass white wine	145
2 Chocolate-Chip Cookies (page 285)	136
	756
TOTALS	**1,835**

DAY 1: 1,650 to 1,800 calories

	CALORIES
Breakfast	
1 cup Kashi Organic Promise Strawberry Fields cereal	120
½ cup 1% milk	53
1 banana	105
Coffee or tea with 1% milk and Splenda	12
	290
Midmorning Snack	
Campbell's Chunky microwavable bowl: Grilled Chicken with Vegetables & Pasta Soup	110
1 slice whole-wheat bread	110
	220
Lunch	
Subway 6-inch Turkey Breast and Ham sandwich	280
Iced tea	0
	280
Afternoon Snack	
2 Dove Promises bars	84
1 Tall nonfat cappuccino	75
	159
Dinner	
Lean Cuisine Lemon Garlic Shrimp	280
Green salad with vinaigrette	120
1 slice French bread	75
1 (6-oz) glass white wine	145
2 Chocolate-Chip Cookies (page 285)	136
	756
	1,705

Your Calorie Countdown Choices: You lost 130 calories by trading in a Subway Cold Cut Combo sandwich for a Turkey Breast and Ham sandwich.

DAY 2: 1,850 to 1,900 calories

	CALORIES
Breakfast	
¾ cup raisin bran	150
6-oz Dannon Light 'n Fit Yogurt	60
1 banana	105
Coffee or tea with 1% milk & Splenda	12
	327
Midmorning Snack	
1 string cheese	80
12 almonds	85
1 apple	80
	245
Lunch	
Quiznos Turkey Ranch Swiss sandwich	691
Iced tea	0
	691
Afternoon Snack	
Campbell's Select™ microwavable bowl: Beef with Portobello Mushrooms and Rice Soup	90
	90
Dinner	
Lean Cuisine Creamy Basil Chicken Bowl	310
Green salad with fat-free dressing	31
1 (6-oz) glass white wine	145
Fat Free Fudgsicle	71
	557
TOTALS	**1,910**

DAY 2: 1,650 to 1,800 calories

	CALORIES
Breakfast	
¾ cup raisin bran	150
6-oz Dannon Light 'n Fit Yogurt	60
1 banana	105
Coffee or tea with 1% milk & Splenda	12
	327
Midmorning Snack	
1 string cheese	80
12 almonds	85
1 apple	80
	245
Lunch	
Quiznos Small Honey Bourbon Chicken sandwich	359
Iced tea	0
	359
Afternoon Snack	
Campbell's Select microwavable bowl: Beef with Portobello Mushrooms and Rice Soup	90
	90
Dinner	
Lean Cuisine Creamy Basil Chicken	310
Green salad with fat-free dressing	31
1 (6-oz) glass white wine	145
1 slice country bread	110
Fat Free Fudgsicle	71
	667
	1,688

Your Calorie Countdown Choices: You saved 332 calories when you chose a Quiznos Small Honey Bourbon Chicken sandwich instead of their Turkey Ranch & Swiss sandwich. This leaves you room to add a "chocolate-chip cookie" such as bread to your dinner.

DAY 3: 1,850 to 1,900 calories

	CALORIES
Breakfast	
1 English muffin	150
1 T I Can't Believe It's Not Butter!	60
1 soft-boiled egg	80
Coffee or tea with 1% milk and Splenda	12
	302
Midmorning Snack	
6-oz Dannon Light 'n Fit yogurt	60
	60
Lunch	
Boston Market Chicken Tortilla Soup with toppings	170
Boston Market Caesar Side Salad	300
Mineral water	0
	470
Afternoon Snack	
2 Babybels	140
5 Melba toasts	60
	200
Dinner	
Cedarlane™ Eggplant Parmesan (10-oz)	320
Green salad with vinaigrette	120
2 slices French bread	150
1 (6-oz) glass red wine	145
¾ cup frozen low-fat yogurt	150
	885
TOTALS	**1,917**

DAY 3: 1,650 to 1,800 calories

	CALORIES
Breakfast	
1 English muffin	150
1 T I Can't Believe It's Not Butter!	60
1 soft-boiled egg	80
Coffee or tea with 1% milk and Splenda	12
	302
Midmorning Snack	
6-oz Dannon Light 'n Fit yogurt	60
	60
Lunch	
Boston Market Chicken Tortilla Soup without toppings	80
Boston Market Caesar Side Salad	300
Mineral water	0
	380
Afternoon Snack	
2 Babybels	140
5 Melba toasts	60
	200
Dinner	
Cedarlane Eggplant Parmesan (10-oz)	320
Green salad with vinaigrette	120
1 slice French bread	75
1 (6-oz) glass red wine	145
¾ cup frozen low-fat yogurt	150
	810
TOTALS	**1,752**

Your Calorie Countdown Choices: You lost 90 calories at lunch by having the tortilla soup without the toppings. At dinner you lost another 75 calories by dropping 1 slice of the French bread.

DAY 4: **1,850 to 1,900 calories** | DAY 4: **1,650 to 1,800 calories**

	CALORIES		CALORIES
Breakfast		**Breakfast**	
1 cup oatmeal	150	1 cup oatmeal	150
1 cup 1% milk	105	1 cup 1% milk	105
½ grated apple	40	½ grated apple	40
½ cup orange juice	56	½ cup orange juice	56
Coffee or tea with 1% milk and Splenda	12	Coffee or tea with 1% milk and Splenda	12
	363		**363**
Midmorning Snack		**Midmorning Snack**	
Campbell's Select™ microwavable bowl: Minestrone Soup	100	Campbell's Select microwavable bowl: Minestrone Soup	100
	100		**100**
Lunch		**Lunch**	
Koo-Koo-Roo BBQ Chicken Sandwich	562	Koo-Koo-Roo BBQ Chicken Salad (no dressing)	365
Iced tea	0	Iced tea	0
	562		**365**
Afternoon Snack		**Afternoon Snack**	
1 banana	105	1 banana	105
1 Tall nonfat cappuccino	75	1 Tall nonfat cappuccino	75
	180		**180**
Dinner		**Dinner**	
Gardenburger Original	90	Gardenburger Original	90
Whole-wheat bun	140	Whole-wheat bun	140
Corn on the cob with butter	155	Corn on the cob with butter	155
Koo-Koo-Roo Tangy Tomato Salad	60	Koo-Koo-Roo Tangy Tomato Salad	60
1 (12-oz) regular beer	150	1 (12-oz) regular beer	150
	595		**595**
TOTALS	**1,800**		**1,603**

Your Calorie Countdown Choices: At lunch you had the Koo-Koo-Roo BBQ Chicken Salad instead of the sandwich and lost 197 calories.

DAY 5: 1,850 to 1,900 calories

	CALORIES
Breakfast	
1 small whole-wheat bagel	110
2 T low-fat cream cheese	70
½ cup orange juice	56
Coffee or tea with 1% milk and Splenda	12
	248
Midmorning Snack	
Nabisco Honey Maid Cinnamon Thin Crisps Snack Pack	100
	100
Lunch	
Wendy's Classic Single, no mayo	390
Diet Coke	0
	390
Afternoon Snack	
1 apple	80
1 Tall nonfat cappuccino	75
	155
Dinner	
Olive Garden Linguine alla Marinara	551
Olive Garden Minestrone	164
1 (6-oz) glass red wine	145
1 Tall cappuccino	150
	1,010
TOTALS	**1,903**

DAY 5: 1,650 to 1,800 calories

	CALORIES
Breakfast	
1 small whole-wheat bagel	110
2 T low-fat cream cheese	70
½ cup orange juice	56
Coffee or tea with 1% milk and Splenda	12
	248
Midmorning Snack	
Nabisco Honey Maid Cinnamon Thin Crisps Snack Pack	100
	100
Lunch	
Wendy's Classic Single, no mayo	390
Diet Coke	0
	390
Afternoon Snack	
1 apple	80
1 Tall nonfat cappuccino	75
	155
Dinner	
Olive Garden Linguine alla Marinara	551
Olive Garden Minestrone	164
1 (6-oz) glass red wine	145
	860
	1,753

Your Calorie Countdown Choices: Just by eliminating the after-dinner cappuccino you lost 150 calories.

DAY 6: 1,850 to 1,900 calories

	CALORIES
Breakfast	
2 Kashi GOLEAN Blueberry Waffles	170
1 T I Can't Believe It's Not Butter!	60
2 T light syrup	50
Coffee or tea with 1% milk and Splenda	12
½ cup orange juice	56
	348
Midmorning Snack	
Post-Workout Shake (page 275)	200
	200
Lunch	
California Pizza Kitchen Grilled Vegetarian Sandwich	651
Mineral water	0
	651
Afternoon Snack	
1 cup cantaloupe	53
6-oz Dannon Light 'n Fit yogurt	60
	113
Dinner	
Lean Cuisine Jumbo Rigatoni with Meatballs	390
Green salad with fat-free ranch dressing	31
Fat Free Fudgsicle	71
	492
TOTALS	**1,804**

DAY 6: 1,650 to 1,800 calories

	CALORIES
Breakfast	
2 Kashi GOLEAN Blueberry Waffles	170
1 T I Can't Believe It's Not Butter!	60
2 T light syrup	50
Coffee or tea with 1% milk and Splenda	12
½ cup orange juice	56
	348
Midmorning Snack	
16-oz Jamba Juice Matcha Green Tea Mist	190
	190
Lunch	
Baja Fresh Baja Ensalada with Charbroiled Steak and Salsa	465
Mineral water	0
	465
Afternoon Snack	
1 cup cantaloupe	53
6-oz Dannon Light 'n Fit yogurt	60
	113
Dinner	
Lean Cuisine Jumbo Rigatoni with Meatballs	390
Green salad with fat-free ranch dressing	31
Fat Free Fudgsicle	71
	492
	1,608

Your Calorie Countdown Choices: You went to Baja Fresh instead of California Pizza Kitchen for lunch and lost 186 calories eating Baja Charbroiled Steak and Salsa instead of a California Pizza Kitchen Vegetarian Sandwich. You lost another 10 calories when you chose the Jamba Juice over the Post-Workout Shake. But beware of Jamba Juice—they have only a few low-calorie selections.

DAY 7: 1,850 to 1,900 calories

	CALORIES
Breakfast	
1 Egg Beaters Southwestern omelet	60
2 slices whole-wheat toast	220
1 T I Can't Believe It's Not Butter!	60
1 Tall nonfat cappuccino	75
½ cup orange juice	56
	471
Midmorning Snack	
16-oz Jamba Juice Passion Berry Breeze	150
	150
Lunch	
Lean Cuisine Chicken Club Panini	320
Mineral water	0
	320
Afternoon Snack	
Tall Frappuccino	113
1 Dove Promises bar	42
	155
Dinner	
11-oz Cedarlane Three Layer Enchilada Pie	430
Green salad with fat-free ranch	31
1 (12-oz) light beer	105
1 cup low-fat soft frozen yogurt	200
	766
TOTALS	**1,862**

DAY 7: 1,650 to 1,800 calories

	CALORIES
Breakfast	
1 Egg Beaters Southwestern omelet	60
1 slice whole-wheat toast	110
1 T I Can't Believe It's Not Butter!	60
1 Tall nonfat cappuccino	75
½ cup orange juice	56
	361
Midmorning Snack	
16-oz Jamba Juice Passion Berry Breeze	150
	150
Lunch	
Lean Cuisine Chicken Club Panini	320
Mineral water	0
	320
Afternoon Snack	
Tall Frappuccino	113
1 Dove Promises bar	42
	155
Dinner	
11-oz Cedarlane Three Layer Enchilada Pie	430
Green salad with fat-free ranch	31
1 (12-oz) light beer	105
½ cup low-fat soft frozen yogurt	100
	666
TOTALS	**1,652**

Your Calorie Countdown Choices: You had ½ cup frozen yogurt for dessert at dinner instead of 1 cup, and lost 100 calories. You gave up another 110 calories with the second slice of toast at breakfast.

1,700 to 1,450 CALORIE COUNTDOWN

DAY 1: **1,600 to 1,700 calories**	CALORIES
Breakfast	
1 cup Kashi GOLEAN cereal	190
½ cup 1% milk	53
1 banana	105
Coffee or tea with 1% milk and Splenda	12
	360
Midmorning Snack	
100-Calorie Snack Pack	100
Noncaloric flavored water	0
	100
Lunch	
Baja Fresh Grilled Mahi Mahi Taco	300
Diet soda or mineral water	0
	300
Afternoon Snack	
2 Dove Promises bars	84
1 Tall nonfat cappuccino	75
	159
Dinner	
Koo-Koo-Roo Rotisserie Chicken, leg & thigh	300
Koo-Koo-Roo Mashed Potatoes	186
Koo-Koo-Roo Green Beans	62
Koo-Koo-Roo Tangy Tomato Salad	60
Rainbow Ice Fruit Popsicle	40
	648
TOTALS	**1,567**

DAY 1: **1,450 to 1,600 calories**	CALORIES
Breakfast	
1 cup Kashi GOLEAN cereal	190
½ cup 1% milk	53
1 banana	105
Coffee or tea with 1% milk and Splenda	12
	360
Midmorning Snack	
100-Calorie Snack Pack	100
Noncaloric flavored water	0
	100
Lunch	
Baja Fresh Grilled Mahi Mahi Taco	300
Diet soda or mineral water	0
	300
Afternoon Snack	
2 Dove Promises bars	84
1 Tall nonfat cappuccino	75
	159
Dinner	
Koo-Koo-Roo Rotisserie Chicken, leg & thigh	300
Koo-Koo-Roo Butternut Squash	66
Koo-Koo-Roo Green Beans	62
Koo-Koo-Roo Tangy Tomato Salad	60
Rainbow Ice Fruit Popsicle	40
	528
	1,447

Your Calorie Countdown Choices: You lost 120 calories by substituting Koo-Koo-Roo Butternut Squash for their mashed potatoes.

DAY 2: 1,600 to 1,700 calories

	CALORIES
Breakfast	
2 poached eggs	160
2 slices whole-wheat toast	220
½ cup fresh orange juice	56
Coffee or tea with 1% milk and Splenda	12
	448
Midmorning Snack	
1 banana	105
6-oz Dannon Light 'n Fit yogurt	60
	165
Lunch	
Subway 6-inch Veggie Delite sandwich	230
Iced tea	0
	230
Afternoon Snack	
1 Peanut Butter–Banana Cookie (page 293)	137
1 cup 1% milk	105
	242
Dinner	
Lean Cuisine Salisbury Steak with chive potatoes and honey-glazed carrots	270
Baby spinach with fat-free ranch dressing	31
1 cup Dreyer's/Edy's Fat Free Caramel Crunch Frozen Yogurt	200
	501
TOTALS	**1,586**

DAY 2: 1,450 to 1,600 calories

	CALORIES
Breakfast	
1 Egg Beaters Southwestern omelet	60
2 slices whole-wheat toast	220
½ cup fresh orange juice	56
Coffee or tea with 1% milk and Splenda	12
	348
Midmorning Snack	
1 banana	105
6-oz Dannon Light 'n Fit yogurt	60
	165
Lunch	
Subway 6-inch Veggie Delite sandwich	230
Iced tea	0
	230
Afternoon Snack	
1 Peanut Butter–Banana Cookie (page 293)	137
1 cup nonfat milk	91
	228
Dinner	
Lean Cuisine Salisbury Steak with chive potatoes and honey-glazed carrots	270
Baby spinach with fat-free ranch dressing	31
½ cup Dreyer's/Edy's Fat Free Caramel Crunch Frozen Yogurt	100
	401
TOTALS	**1,372**

Your Calorie Countdown Choices: For breakfast you saved yourself 100 calories by substituting the Egg Beaters Southwestern omelet for the 2 poached eggs. You lost another 100 calories at dinner by having ½ cup of frozen yogurt instead of 1 cup. You could have gotten away with ¾ cup of yogurt and still remained under 1,500 calories.

DAY 3: 1,600 to 1,700 calories

	CALORIES
Breakfast	
2 Kashi GOLEAN Waffles	170
1 T I Can't Believe It's Not Butter!	60
2 T light syrup	50
½ cup orange juice	56
Coffee or tea with 1% milk and Splenda	12
	348
Midmorning Snack	
1 Babybel	70
½ high-fiber English muffin	75
	145
Lunch	
Koo-Koo-Roo BBQ Chicken Salad	365
with vinaigrette	120
	485
Afternoon Snack	
100-Calorie Snack Pack	100
1 Tall nonfat cappuccino	75
	175
Dinner	
Lean Cuisine Baked Fish with Cheddar Cheese & Shells	310
½ cup broccoli	22
1 (6-oz) glass white wine	145
Fat Free Fudgsicle	71
	548
TOTALS	**1,701**

DAY 3: 1,450 to 1,600 calories

	CALORIES
Breakfast	
2 Kashi GOLEAN Waffles	170
1 T I Can't Believe It's Not Butter!	60
2 T light syrup	50
½ cup orange juice	56
Coffee or tea with 1% milk and Splenda	12
	348
Midmorning Snack	
1 Babybel	70
½ high-fiber English muffin	75
	145
Lunch	
Koo-Koo-Roo BBQ Chicken Salad	365
with fat-free ranch dressing	31
	396
Afternoon Snack	
100-Calorie Snack Pack	100
1 Tall nonfat cappuccino	75
	175
Dinner	
Lean Cuisine Baked Fish with Cheddar Cheese & Shells	310
½ cup broccoli	22
Fat Free Fudgsicle	71
	403
	1,467

Your Calorie Countdown Choices: You lost 89 calories by switching to fat-free dressing on your lunchtime salad. You dropped another 145 calories by dropping the wine at dinner.

DAY 4: 1,600 to 1,700 calories

	CALORIES
Breakfast	
1 boiled egg	80
1 high-fiber English muffin	150
2 T light cream cheese	70
½ cup orange juice	56
Coffee or tea with 1% milk and Splenda	12
	368
Midmorning Snack	
¾ cup nonfat cottage cheese	120
12 almonds	85
	205
Lunch	
Arby's Regular Roast Beef Sandwich	320
Iced tea	0
	320
Afternoon Snack	
1 apple	80
1 string cheese	80
	160
Dinner	
Steak Escape® Ragin' Cajun Chicken sandwich	418
Side salad with ranch dressing	113
Diet Coke	0
Fruit Popsicle®	40
	571
TOTALS	**1,624**

DAY 4: 1,450 to 1,600 calories

	CALORIES
Breakfast	
1 boiled egg	80
½ high-fiber English muffin	75
2 T light cream cheese	70
½ cup orange juice	56
Coffee or tea with 1% milk and Splenda	12
	293
Midmorning Snack	
½ cup nonfat cottage cheese	80
12 almonds	85
	165
Lunch	
Campbell's Chunky™ microwavable bowls: Beef with Country Vegetable	150
French bread	150
Iced tea	0
	300
Afternoon Snack	
1 apple	80
1 string cheese	80
	160
Dinner	
Steak Escape Ragin' Cajun Chicken sandwich	418
Side salad with fat-free ranch dressing	57
Diet Coke	0
Fruit Popsicle	40
	515
	1,433

Your Calorie Countdown Choices: At breakfast you lost 75 calories by giving up half an English muffin. You lost 40 calories by giving up ¼ cup cottage cheese as a snack. At lunch you had a bowl of Campbell's microwavable soup instead of going out to Arby's for a sandwich, and got to add bread but still saved 20 calories. You saved 56 calories at dinner by requesting fat-free ranch dressing.

DAY 5: 1,600 to 1,700 calories

	CALORIES
Breakfast	
1 packet Kashi GOLEAN Hot Cereal	150
½ cup blueberries	41
1 cup 1% milk	105
Coffee or tea with 1% milk and Splenda	12
	308
Midmorning Snack	
1 cup grapes	100
6-oz Dannon Light 'n Fit yogurt	60
	160
Lunch	
Baja Fresh Baja Ensalada with Charbroiled Steak and Salsa	465
Iced tea	0
	465
Afternoon Snack	
100-Calorie Snack Pack	100
1 Tall nonfat cappuccino	75
	175
Dinner	
Ethnic Gourmet Bowl Pad Thai with Tofu	460
1 (12-oz) light beer	110
	570
TOTALS	**1,678**

DAY 5: 1,450 to 1,600 calories

	CALORIES
Breakfast	
1 packet Kashi GOLEAN Hot Cereal	150
½ cup blueberries	41
1 cup 1% milk	105
Coffee or tea with 1% milk and Splenda	12
	308
Midmorning Snack	
1 cup grapes	100
6-oz Dannon Light 'n Fit yogurt	60
	160
Lunch	
Applebee's Grilled Shrimp Skewer Salad	210
Iced tea	0
	210
Afternoon Snack	
100-Calorie Snack Pack	100
1 Tall nonfat cappuccino	75
	175
Dinner	
Ethnic Gourmet Bowl Pad Thai with Tofu	460
1 (12-oz) light beer	110
	570
	1,423

Your Calorie Countdown Choices: You saved yourself 255 calories at lunch by going to Applebee's for their Shrimp Skewer Salad instead of to Baja Fresh for their Baja Salad with Charbroiled Steak.

DAY 6: 1,600 to 1,700 calories

	CALORIES
Breakfast	
1 small whole-wheat bagel	110
2 T low-fat cream cheese	70
½ cup orange juice	56
Coffee or tea with 1% milk and Splenda	12
	248
Midmorning Snack	
1 banana	105
½ cup nonfat cottage cheese	80
	185
Lunch	
Campbell's Chunky microwavable bowl: Firehouse Hot and Spicy Beef & Bean Chili	220
1 slice whole-wheat bread	110
1 cup nonfat milk	91
	421
Afternoon Snack	
2 Lindt chocolate truffles	146
1 Tall nonfat cappuccino	75
	221
Dinner	
Applebee's Grilled Tilapia with Mango Salsa	320
1 (6-oz) glass white wine	145
Green salad with vinaigrette	120
	585
TOTALS	**1,660**

DAY 6: 1,450 to 1,600 calories

	CALORIES
Breakfast	
1 small whole-wheat bagel	110
2 T low-fat cream cheese	70
½ cup orange juice	56
Coffee or tea with 1% milk and Splenda	12
	248
Midmorning Snack	
1 banana	105
½ cup nonfat cottage cheese	80
	185
Lunch	
Campbell's Microwavable Soup bowl: Chicken Noodle Soup	70
1 slice whole-wheat bread	110
1 cup nonfat milk	91
	271
Afternoon Snack	
2 Lindt chocolate truffles	146
1 Tall nonfat cappuccino	75
	221
Dinner	
Applebee's Grilled Tilapia with Mango Salsa	320
1 (6-oz) glass white wine	145
Green salad with vinaigrette	120
	585
	1,510

Your Calorie Countdown Choices: You lost 150 calories at lunch by choosing the Chicken Noodle Soup instead of the Firehouse Hot and Spicy Beef & Bean Chili.

DAY 7: 1,600 to 1,700 calories

	CALORIES
Breakfast	
McDonald's Egg McMuffin®	300
½ cup orange juice	56
Coffee or tea with 1% milk and Splenda	12
	368
Midmorning Snack	
100-Calorie Snack Pack	100
Small blended coffee drink	113
	213
Lunch	
Campbell's Chunky microwavable bowl: Grilled Chicken & Sausage Gumbo	120
1 slice whole-wheat bread	110
	230
Afternoon Snack	
Pringles 100-Calorie Pack	100
Diet soda	
	100
Dinner	
Lean Cuisine Lemon Garlic Shrimp	280
Green salad with vinaigrette	120
1 slice French bread	75
1 (6-oz) glass white wine	145
1 Chocolate-Chip Cookie (page 285)	68
	688
TOTALS	**1,599**

DAY 7: 1,450 to 1,600 calories

	CALORIES
Breakfast	
McDonald's Egg McMuffin	300
½ cup orange juice	56
Coffee or tea with 1% milk and Splenda	12
	368
Midmorning Snack	
100-Calorie Snack Pack	100
Small blended coffee drink	113
	213
Lunch	
Campbell's Chunky microwavable bowl: Grilled Chicken & Sausage Gumbo	120
	120
Afternoon Snack	
Pringles 100-Calorie Pack	100
Diet soda	
	100
Dinner	
Lean Cuisine Lemon Garlic Shrimp	280
Green salad with vinaigrette	120
1 slice French bread	75
1 (6-oz) glass white wine	145
1 Chocolate-Chip Cookie (page 285)	68
	688
	1,489

Your Calorie Countdown Choices: You lost the bread at lunch and saved 110 calories.

1,500 to 1,300 CALORIE COUNTDOWN

DAY 1: **1,400 to 1,500 calories**	CALORIES	DAY 1: **1,300 to 1,400 calories**	CALORIES
Breakfast		**Breakfast**	
1 boiled egg	80	1 boiled egg	80
1 small whole-wheat bagel	154	1 small whole-wheat bagel	154
1 T low-fat cream cheese	35	1 T low-fat cream cheese	35
½ cup orange juice	56	½ cup orange juice	56
Coffee or tea with 1% milk and Splenda	12	Coffee or tea with 1% milk and Splenda	12
	337		**337**
Midmorning Snack		**Midmorning Snack**	
1 banana	105	1 banana	105
6-oz Dannon Light 'n Fit yogurt	60	6-oz Dannon Light 'n Fit yogurt	60
	165		**165**
Lunch		**Lunch**	
Campbell's Chunky microwavable bowl: Beef with Country Vegetable	150	Campbell's Chunky microwavable bowl: Beef with Country Vegetable	150
1 string cheese	80	1 string cheese	80
	230		**230**
Afternoon Snack		**Afternoon Snack**	
2 Dove Promises bars	84	2 Dove Promises bars	84
1 Tall nonfat cappuccino	75	1 Tall nonfat cappuccino	75
	159		**159**
Dinner		**Dinner**	
Lean Cuisine Roasted Turkey Breast	280	Lean Cuisine Roasted Turkey Breast	280
Green salad with vinaigrette	120	Green salad with vinaigrette	120
1 (6-oz) glass white wine	145		
1 cup cantaloupe	56	1 cup cantaloupe	56
	601		**456**
TOTALS	**1,492**		**1,347**

Your Calorie Countdown Choices: You lost the wine and with it 145 calories at dinner. You could lose another 42 by having only 1 Dove Promises bar in the afternoon.

DAY 2: 1,400 to 1,500 calories

	CALORIES
Breakfast	
1 packet Kashi Hot Cereal	150
½ cup blueberries	41
½ cup 1% milk	53
Coffee or tea	12
	256
Midmorning Snack	
1 string cheese	80
12 almonds	85
	165
Lunch	
Panda Express Chicken with String Beans	160
½ cup steamed rice	103
Green Tea	0
	263
Afternoon Snack	
Ritz 100-Calorie Snack Mix	100
1 Tall nonfat cappuccino	75
	175
Dinner	
Lean Cuisine Beef Pot Roast	190
Green salad with vinaigrette	120
1 (6-oz) glass red wine	145
1 slice French bread	75
Roasted Pineapple (page 301)	82
	612
TOTALS	**1,471**

DAY 2: 1,300 to 1,400 calories

	CALORIES
Breakfast	
1 packet Kashi Hot Cereal	150
½ cup blueberries	41
½ cup 1% milk	53
Coffee or tea	12
	256
Midmorning Snack	
1 string cheese	80
12 almonds	85
	165
Lunch	
Panda Express Chicken with String Beans	160
½ cup steamed rice	103
Green Tea	0
	263
Afternoon Snack	
Ritz 100-Calorie Snack Mix	100
1 Tall nonfat cappuccino	75
	175
Dinner	
Lean Cuisine Beef Pot Roast	190
Green salad with fat-free dressing	31
1 (6-oz) glass red wine	145
Roasted Pineapple (page 301)	82
	448
	1,307

Your Calorie Countdown Choices: You lost 75 calories by omitting the bread with your dinner. You lost another 89 by trading fat-free dressing for vinaigrette.

DAY 3: 1,400 to 1,500 calories

	CALORIES
Breakfast	
1 cup Kashi GOLEAN cereal	190
½ cup nonfat milk	45
1 banana	105
Coffee or tea with 1% milk and Splenda	12
	352
Midmorning Snack	
6-oz Dannon Light 'n Fit yogurt	60
1 Tall nonfat cappuccino	75
	135
Lunch	
Subway 6-inch Cheesesteak Sandwich	360
Mineral water	0
	360
Afternoon Snack	
2 Lindt chocolate truffles	146
Coffee or tea	12
	158
Dinner	
½ Linda McCartney Spicy Thai Veggie Pizza	320
Green salad with fat-free dressing	31
1 (6-oz) glass red wine	145
	496
TOTALS	**1,501**

DAY 3: 1,300 to 1,400 calories

	CALORIES
Breakfast	
1 cup Kashi GOLEAN cereal	190
½ cup nonfat milk	45
1 banana	105
Coffee or tea with 1% milk and Splenda	12
	352
Midmorning Snack	
6-oz Dannon Light 'n Fit yogurt	60
1 Tall nonfat cappuccino	75
	135
Lunch	
Subway Grilled Chicken & Baby Spinach Salad	140
Mineral water	0
	140
Afternoon Snack	
2 Lindt chocolate truffles	146
Coffee or tea	12
	158
Dinner	
½ Linda McCartney Spicy Thai Veggie Pizza	320
Green salad with fat-free dressing	31
1 (6-oz) glass red wine	145
	496
TOTALS	**1,281**

Your Calorie Countdown Choices: You dropped more than 200 calories just by switching from a Subway 6-inch Cheesesteak Sandwich to their Grilled Chicken & Baby Spinach Salad.

DAY 4: 1,400 to 1,500 calories

	CALORIES
Breakfast	
½ cup scrambled Egg Beaters	60
½ high-fiber English muffin	75
½ cup orange juice	56
Coffee or tea with 1% milk and Splenda	12
	203
Midmorning Snack	
½ cup Kashi Mighty Bites Honey Crunch cereal	55
½ cup nonfat milk	45
	100
Lunch	
10-oz Corner Bakery Minestrone	140
Corner Bakery Tomato Fresca Salad	200
Iced tea	0
	340
Afternoon Snack	
1 apple	80
1 Tall nonfat cappuccino	75
	155
Dinner	
Amy's Black Bean Chili & Cornbread	340
Green salad with vinaigrette	120
1 (12-oz) regular beer	150
1 peach	37
	647
TOTALS	**1,445**

DAY 4: 1,300 to 1,400 calories

	CALORIES
Breakfast	
½ cup scrambled Egg Beaters	60
½ high-fiber English muffin	75
½ cup orange juice	56
Coffee or tea with 1% milk and Splenda	12
	203
Midmorning Snack	
½ cup Kashi Mighty Bites Honey Crunch cereal	55
½ cup nonfat milk	45
	100
Lunch	
10-oz Corner Bakery Minestrone	140
Corner Bakery Tomato Fresca Salad	200
Iced tea	0
	340
Afternoon Snack	
1 apple	80
1 Tall nonfat cappuccino	75
	155
Dinner	
Amy's Black Bean Chili & Cornbread	340
Green salad with fat-free ranch dressing	31
1 (12-oz) light beer	110
1 peach	37
	513
TOTALS	**1,316**

Your Calorie Countdown Choices: You gave up 89 calories by switching from a regular vinaigrette to a fat-free dressing with your salad at dinner. You dropped another 40 by switching to light beer.

DAY 5: 1,400 to 1,500 calories

	CALORIES
Breakfast	
2 Kashi Heart to Heart Honey Oat Waffles	160
2 T light syrup	50
1 T I Can't Believe It's Not Butter!	60
½ cup orange juice	56
Coffee or tea with 1% milk and Splenda	12
	338
Midmorning Snack	
½ cup 1% cottage cheese	82
5 Melba toasts	60
	142
Lunch	
California roll sushi	361
1 peach	37
Iced tea	0
	398
Afternoon Snack	
12-oz V8 juice	70
1 string cheese	80
	150
Dinner	
Applebee's Grilled Tilapia with Mango Salsa	320
1 (6-oz) glass white wine	145
	465
TOTALS	**1,493**

DAY 5: 1,300 to 1,400 calories

	CALORIES
Breakfast	
2 Kashi Heart to Heart Honey Oat Waffles	160
2 T light syrup	50
1 T I Can't Believe It's Not Butter!	60
½ cup orange juice	56
Coffee or tea with 1% milk and Splenda	12
	338
Midmorning Snack	
½ cup 1% cottage cheese	82
5 Melba toasts	60
	142
Lunch	
California roll sushi	361
1 peach	37
Iced tea	0
	398
Afternoon Snack	
12-oz V8 juice	70
1 string cheese	80
	150
Dinner	
Applebee's Grilled Tilapia with Mango Salsa	320
Mineral water	0
	320
TOTALS	**1,348**

Your Calorie Countdown Choices: You lost 145 calories by trading in wine for mineral water at dinner.

DAY 6: 1,400 to 1,500 calories

	CALORIES
Breakfast	
1 cup Kashi Organic Promise cereal	190
½ cup 1% milk	53
½ cup blueberries	41
Coffee or tea with 1% milk and Splenda	12
	296
Midmorning Snack	
6-oz Dannon Light 'n Fit yogurt	60
1 banana	105
	165
Lunch	
Applebee's Grilled Shrimp Skewer Salad	210
Iced tea	0
	210
Afternoon Snack	
100-Calorie Snack Pack	100
1 Tall nonfat cappuccino	75
	175
Dinner	
3 slices Pizza Hut Lower Fat Fit 'n Delicious Pizza	420
Green Salad with fat-free ranch	31
1 (12-oz) light beer	110
	561
TOTALS	**1,407**

DAY 6: 1,300 to 1,400 calories

	CALORIES
Breakfast	
1 cup Kashi Organic Promise cereal	190
½ cup 1% milk	53
½ cup blueberries	41
Coffee or tea with 1% milk and Splenda	12
	296
Midmorning Snack	
6-oz Dannon Light 'n Fit yogurt	60
1 banana	105
	165
Lunch	
Applebee's Grilled Shrimp Skewer Salad	210
Iced tea	0
	210
Afternoon Snack	
100-Calorie Snack Pack	100
1 Tall nonfat cappuccino	75
	175
Dinner	
Panda Express Beef with Broccoli	150
½ cup steamed rice	103
1 (12-oz) light beer	110
	363
TOTALS	**1,209**

Your Calorie Countdown Choices: You lost 198 calories by choosing Chinese take-out over pizza. This doesn't always work, but you went for one of the Panda Express light options. Always check these options online.

DAY 7: 1,400 to 1,500 calories

	CALORIES
Breakfast	
2 poached eggs	160
½ small whole-wheat bagel	77
1 T low-fat cream cheese	35
½ cup orange juice	56
Coffee or tea with 1% milk and Splenda	12
	340
Midmorning Snack	
1 Tall Frappuccino	113
	113
Lunch	
Lean Cuisine Chicken Club Panini	320
Mineral water	0
	320
Afternoon Snack	
12-oz V8® juice	70
1 string cheese	80
	150
Dinner	
Lean Cuisine Steak Tips Dijon	320
Green salad with fat-free dressing	31
1 (6-oz) glass red wine	145
1 cup strawberries	50
	546
TOTALS	**1,469**

DAY 7: 1,300 to 1,400 calories

	CALORIES
Breakfast	
2 poached eggs	160
½ small whole-wheat bagel	77
1 T low-fat cream cheese	35
½ cup orange juice	56
Coffee or tea with 1% milk and Splenda	12
	340
Midmorning Snack	
1 Tall Frappuccino	113
	113
Lunch	
Campbell's Chunky Microwavable Chicken and Dumplings Soup	190
Mineral water	0
	190
Afternoon Snack	
12-oz V8 juice	70
1 string cheese	80
	150
Dinner	
Lean Cuisine Steak Tips Dijon	320
Green salad with fat-free dressing	31
1 (6-oz) glass red wine	145
1 cup strawberries	50
	546
TOTALS	**1,339**

Your Calorie Countdown Choices: You lost 130 calories by choosing a ready-to-eat Campbell's soup for lunch instead of the Lean Cuisine Chicken Club Panini.

THE
CALORIE
COUNTDOWN
RECIPES

Breakfasts and Sandwiches

Appetizers, Salads, Salsas, Sauces, and Dips

Main Dishes

Side Dishes

Snacks

Desserts

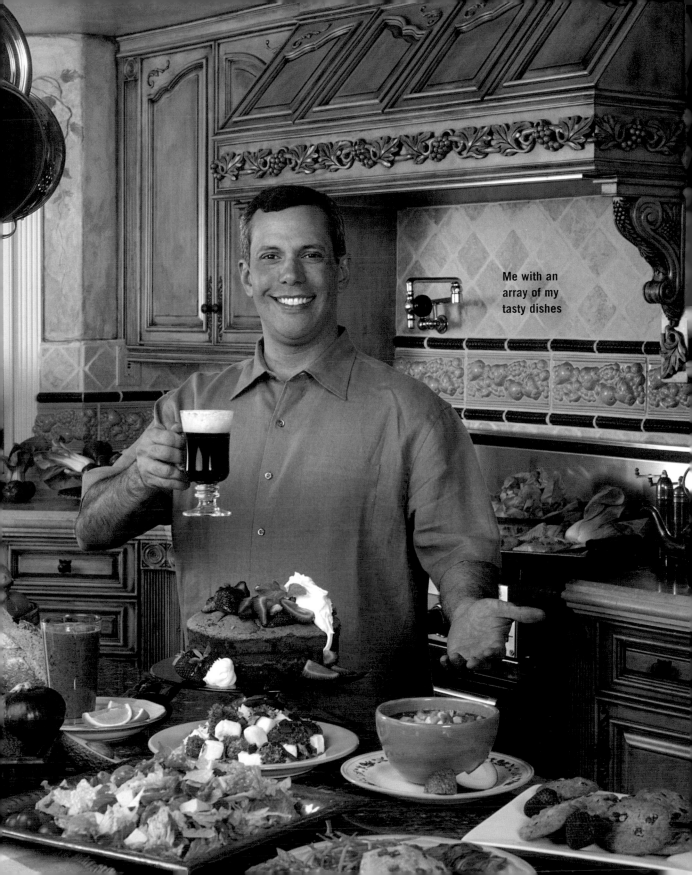

Me with an
array of my
tasty dishes

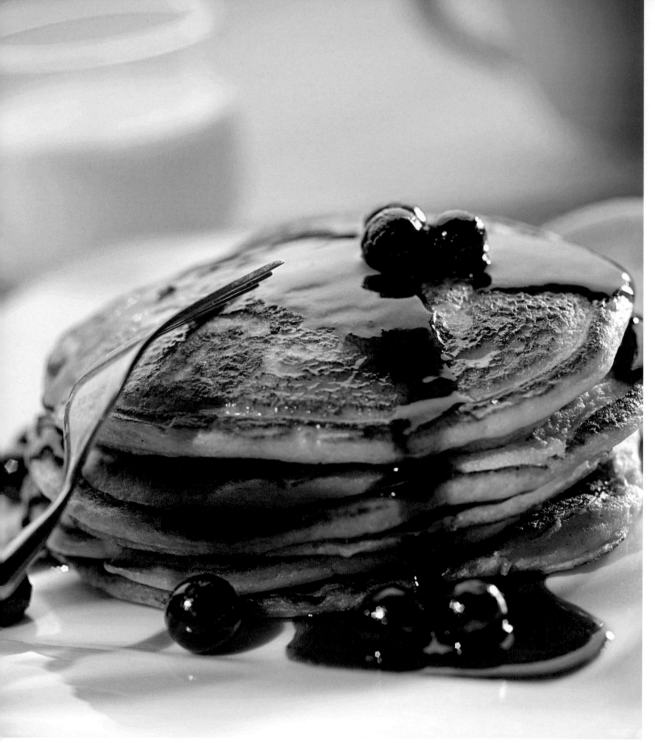

Blueberry Ricotta Pancakes

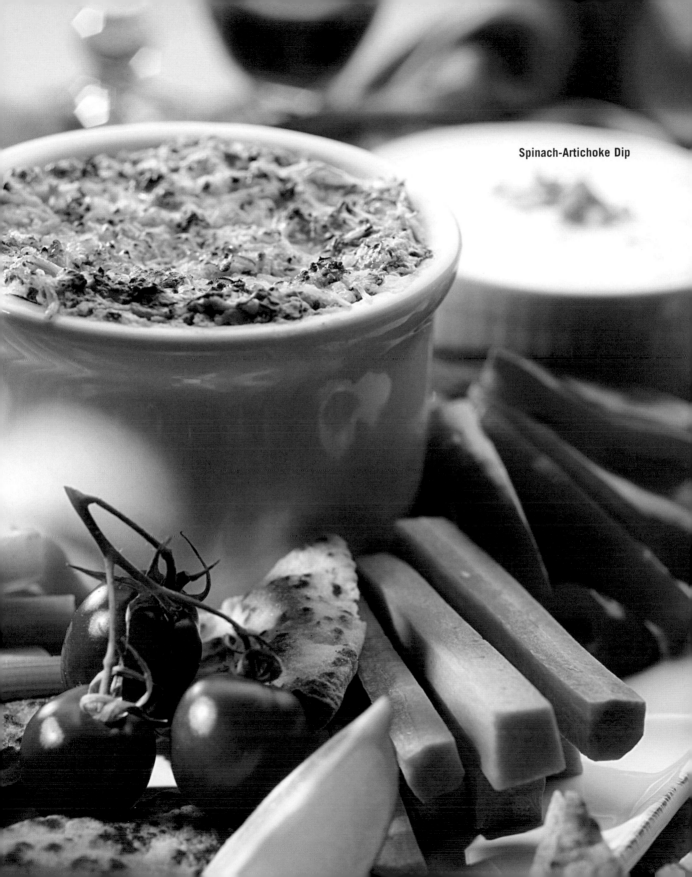

Spinach-Artichoke Dip

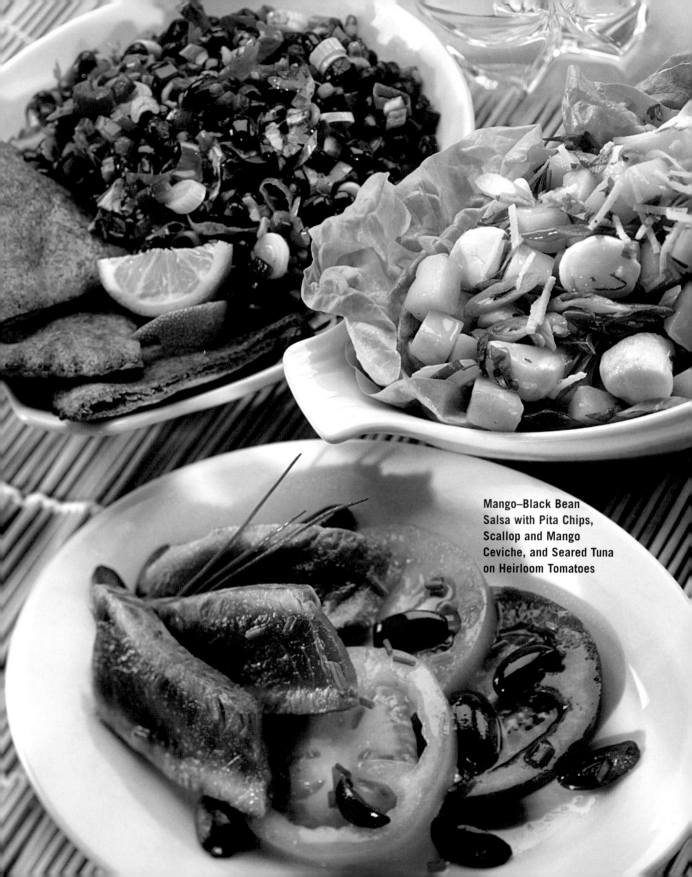

Mango–Black Bean
Salsa with Pita Chips,
Scallop and Mango
Ceviche, and Seared Tuna
on Heirloom Tomatoes

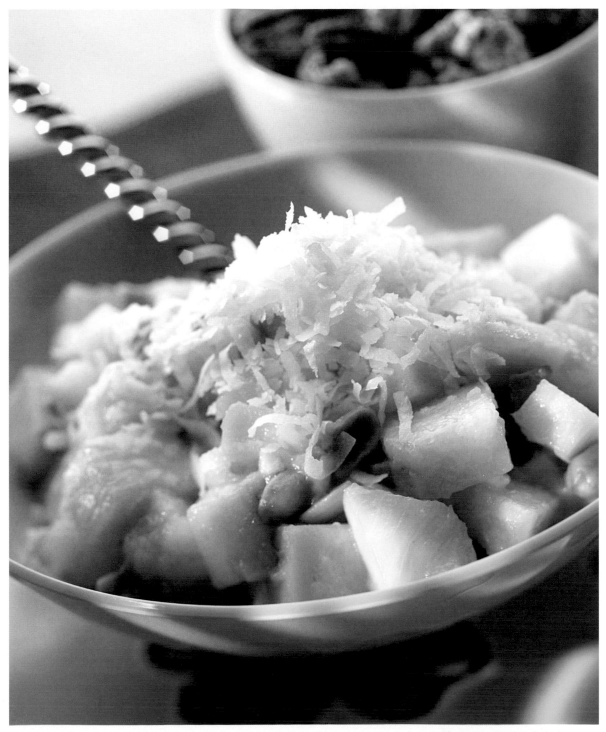

Pineapple-Peanut Salad

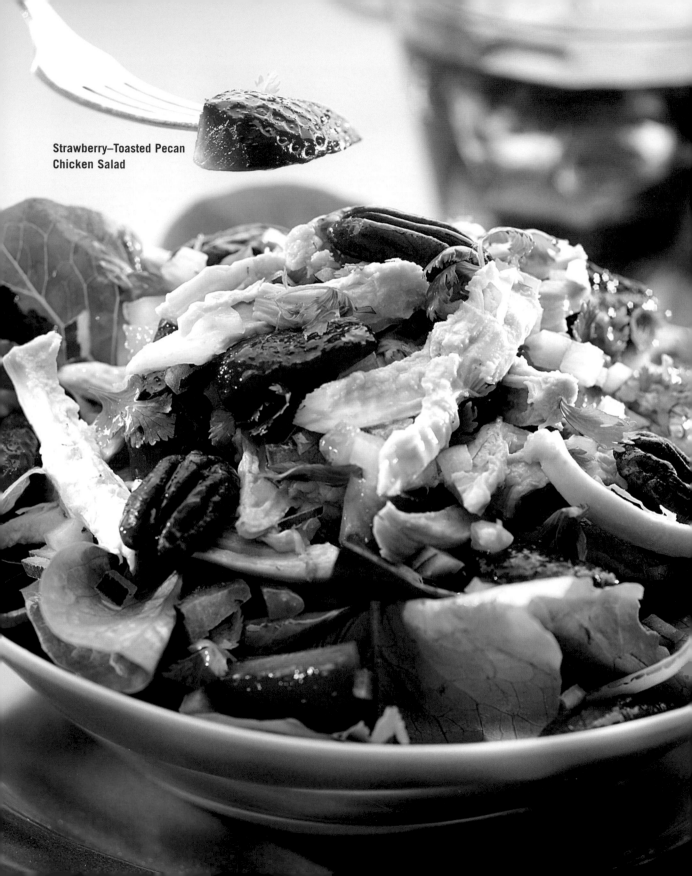

Strawberry–Toasted Pecan
Chicken Salad

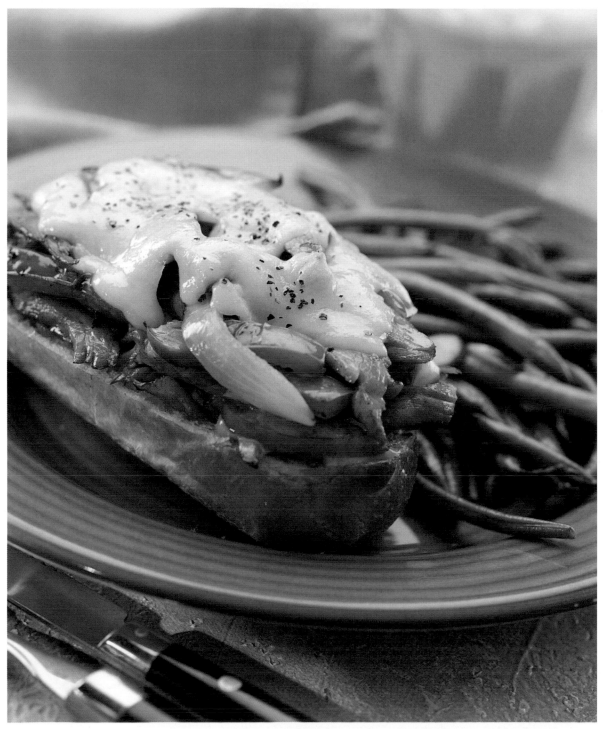

Cali Cheesesteak with Toasted Almond Green Beans

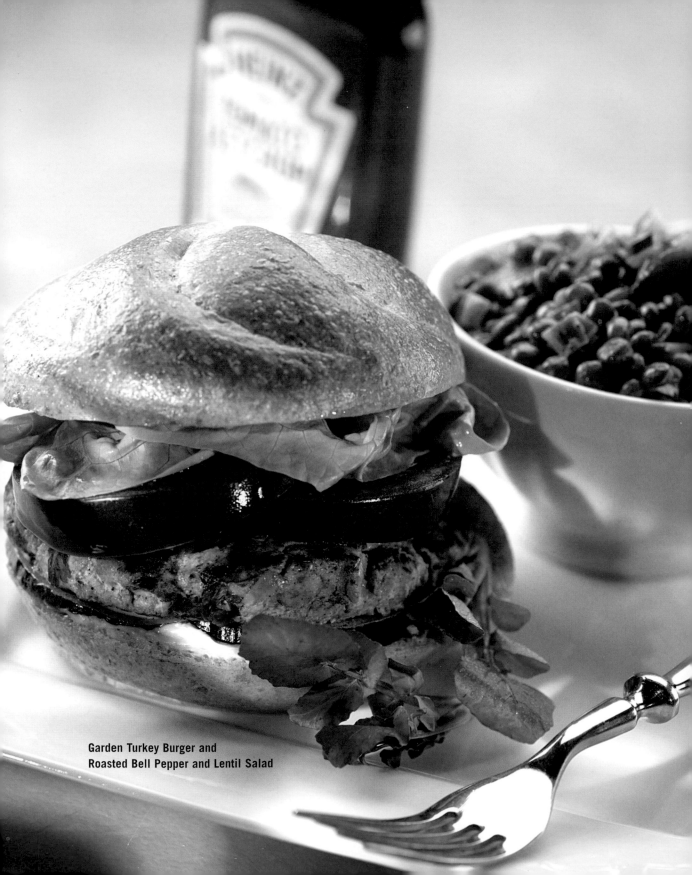

Garden Turkey Burger and
Roasted Bell Pepper and Lentil Salad

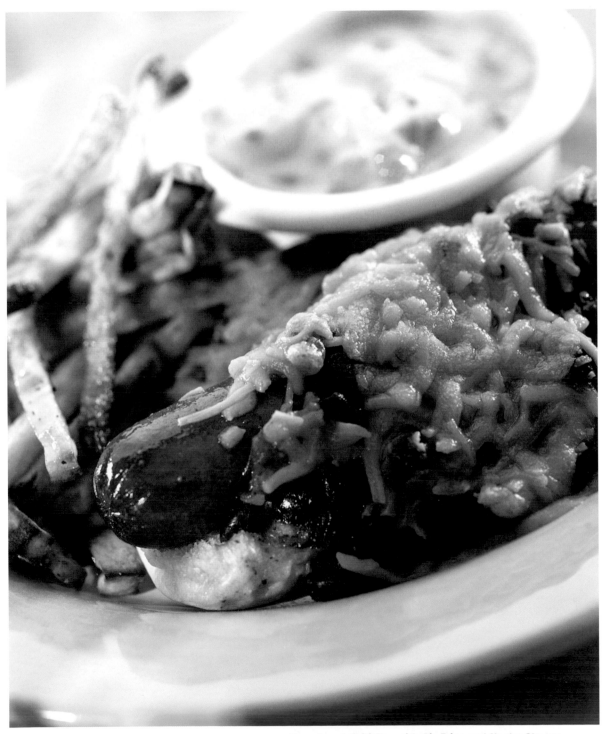

Open-Faced Chili Dog with Air Fries and Nacho Cheese

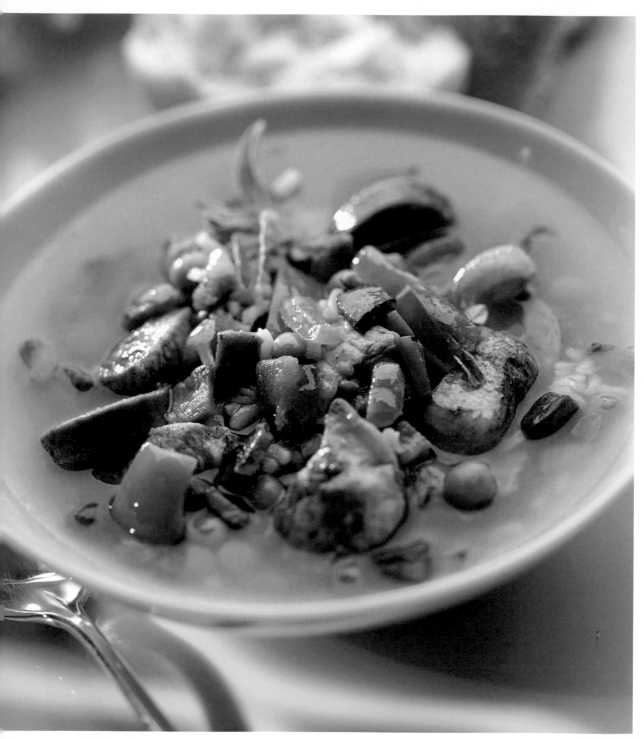

Chicken Asopa

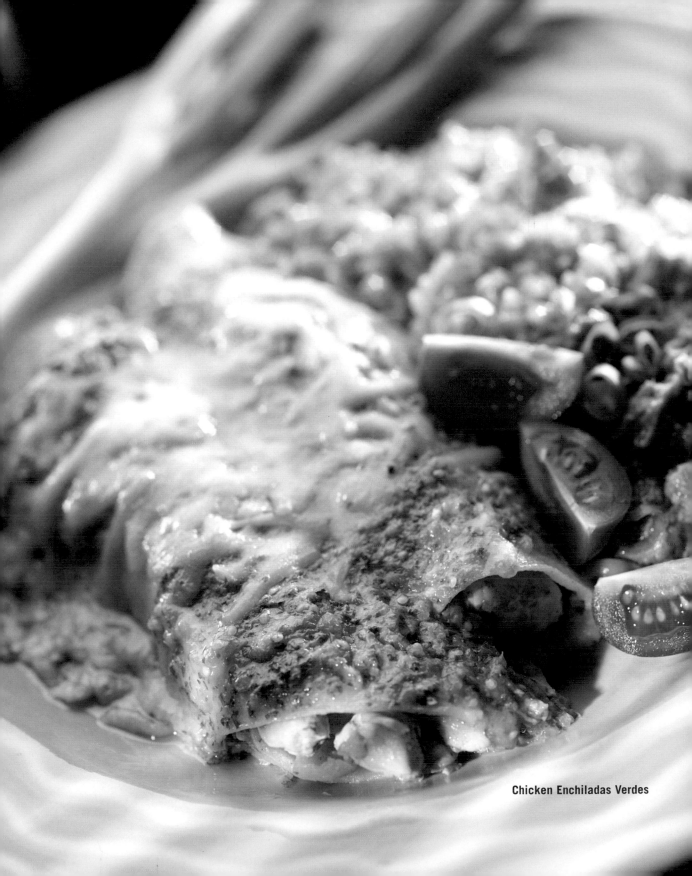

Chicken Enchiladas Verdes

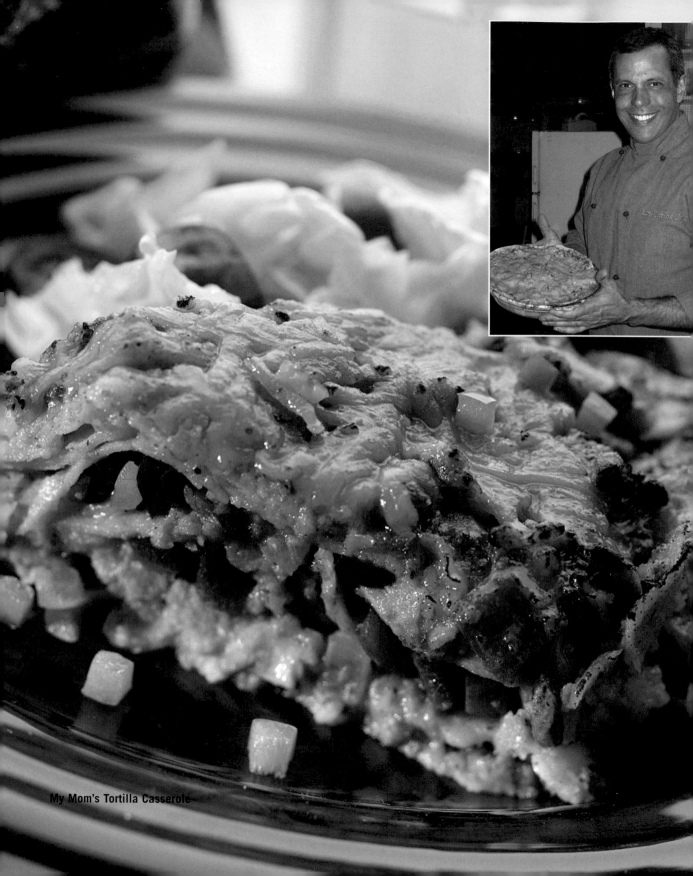

My Mom's Tortilla Casserole

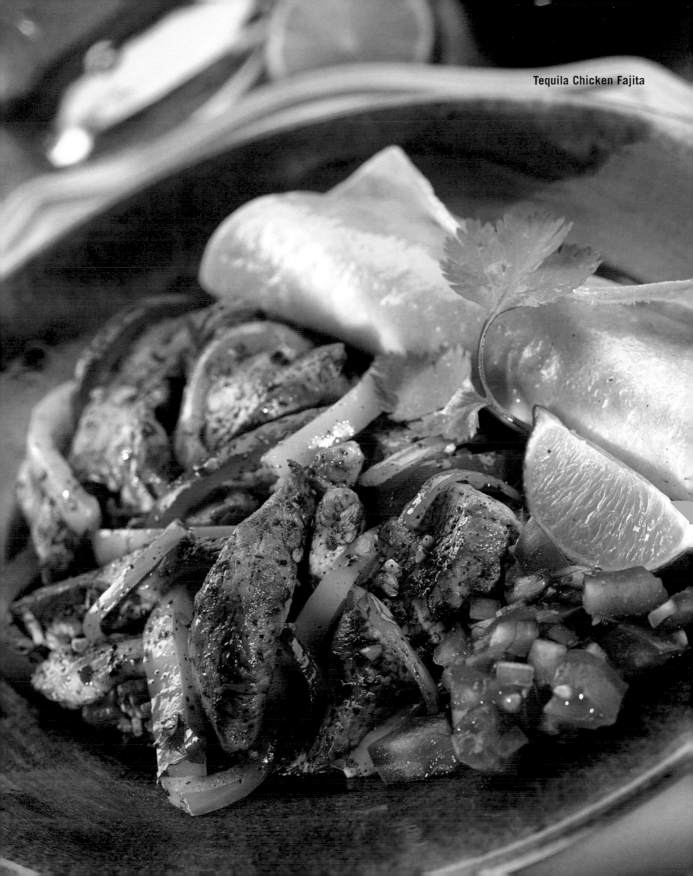

Tequila Chicken Fajita

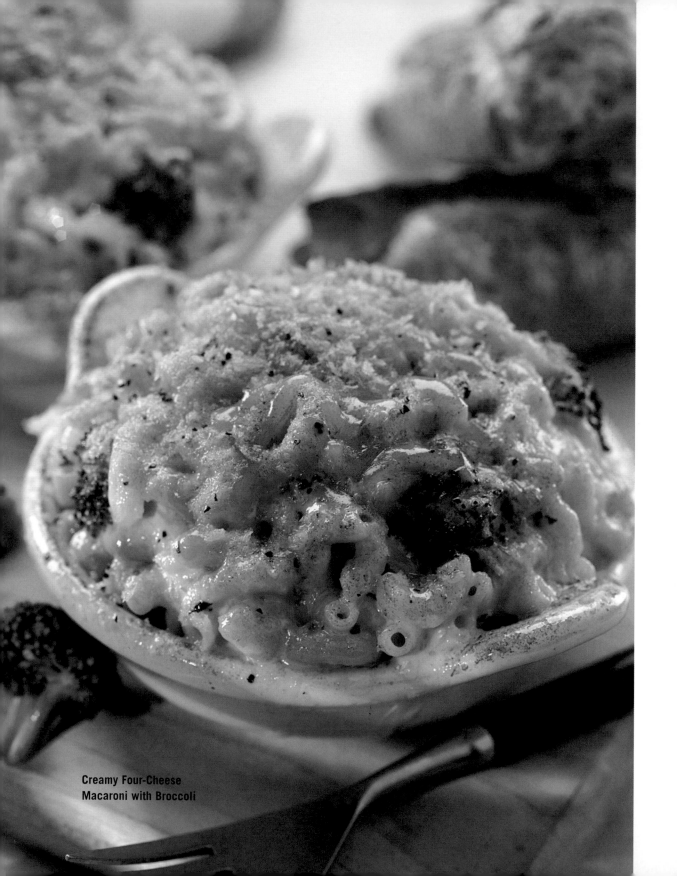

Creamy Four-Cheese
Macaroni with Broccoli

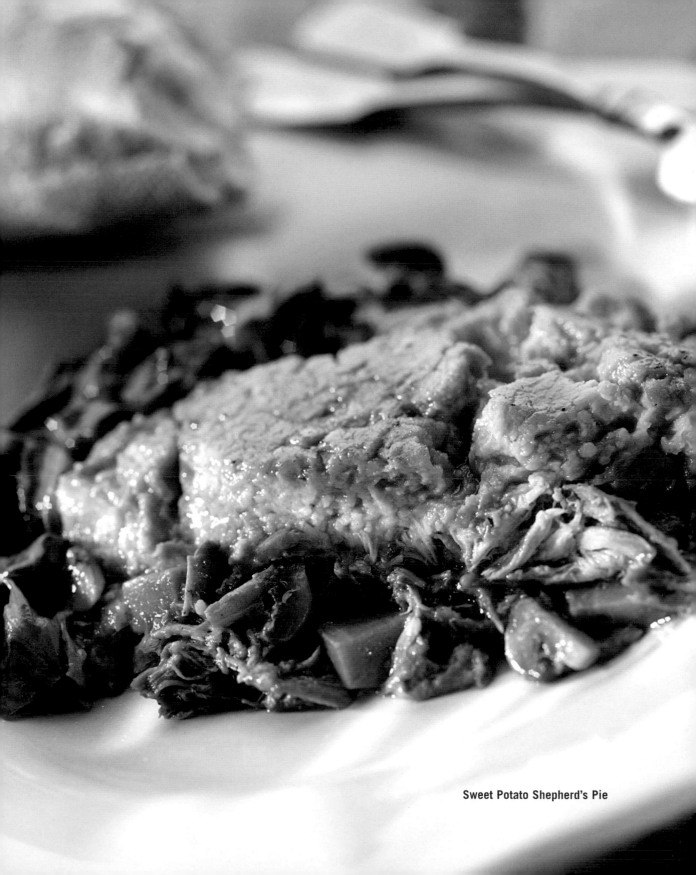

Sweet Potato Shepherd's Pie

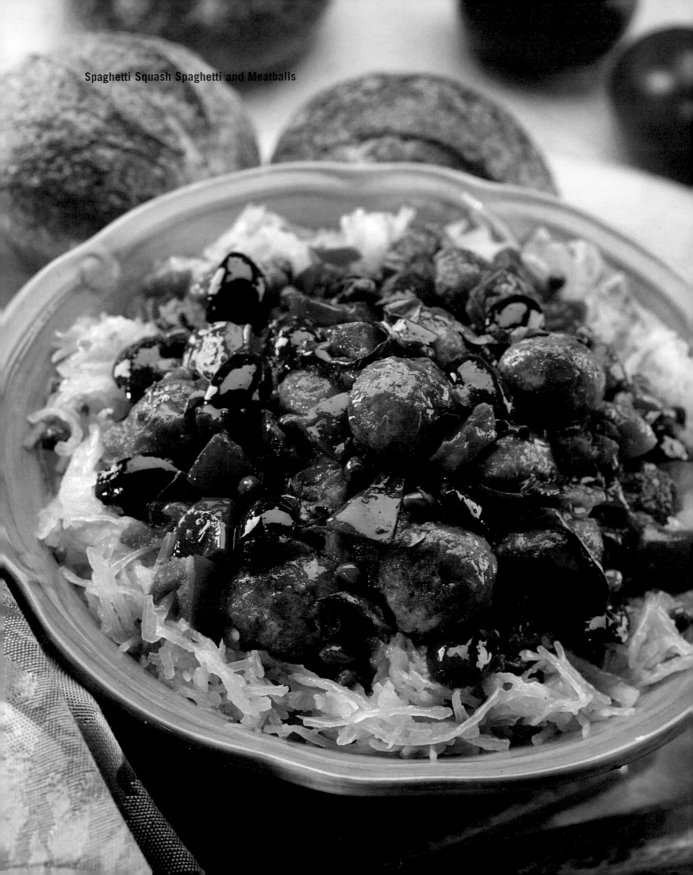

Spaghetti Squash Spaghetti and Meatballs

Introduction
to the Recipes

People are always asking me, "What's going to be in the book? What style of food? California? Hearty? Light? Fancy??" I nod my head in response and say, "It's a little of everything." What I'm trying to show people is that all kinds of cuisines have a place in the Calorie Countdown. My palate is eclectic, and I don't like to get stuck in any particular cuisine. I've had the same kinds of conversations you guys have had on Friday nights: "What are we going to eat? Thai or Chinese? Italian? Mexican?" So that's how I set up the recipes. When you're in the mood for something with south-of-the-border flavors

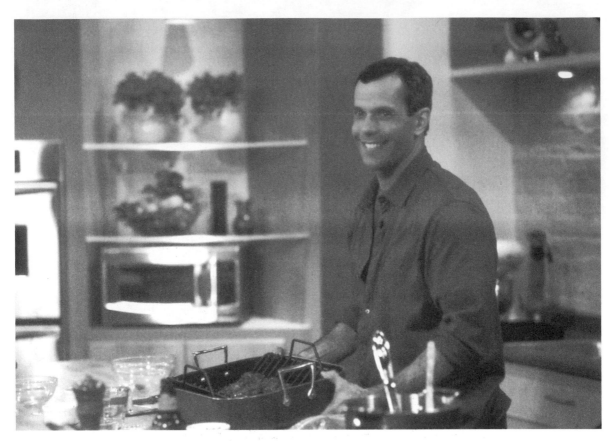

Yes, you can still eat your favorite dishes if you use my recipes.

you'll find lots of dishes that you may have thought you were going to have to say good-bye to, like Chiles Rellenos (page 193), Tequila Chicken Fajitas (page 213), and Chile-Cheese Rice Burritos (page 192). Feel like something Asian? Try Spicy Orange Chicken Lo Mein (page 200), Broccoli-Halibut Stir-Fry (page 220), or Pork Fried Rice (page 203). Like you, I love anything Italian, and have found ways to make low-calorie versions of favorites like Eggplant Parmesan (page 237), Spaghetti Squash Spaghetti and Meatballs (page 244), and even Fettuccine Alfredo (page 240). And if you just want something comforting like macaroni and cheese (page 233) or chicken and rice (page 187), you'll have plenty of choices here. What all of these dishes have in common is an abundance of flavors, because it's my firm belief that you make up on lost calories by putting a lot of flavor in the food.

You'll be surprised, maybe even dumbfounded, to find some of the dishes I've included here. You might expect that Garden Turkey Burgers (page 196)

QUICK TIP

Use smaller plates whenever you're at a buffet, and for eating at home too, for portion control.

would be included in the Calorie Countdown, but Tiramisu? You'll find it on page 302. The Sunset Fish Skewers on page 230 is a dish that you would expect to show up in a book like this, but what about Cali Cheesesteak sandwich? The one on page 147 certainly doesn't taste like something you would normally find in a book on healthy eating. It doesn't taste like diet food because it *isn't* diet food.

Do remember to use portion control, though, because this is good stuff. I don't know how many times I've worked with people who have said to me: "If the recipe has half the calories, then we can eat twice as much, right?" This is how *not* to follow the Calorie Countdown. If the recipe says "serves 8," then make it serve eight. If there are only four of you eating, eat the rest the next day. Everything in this book makes a good leftover, and many of the recipes are perfect for batch cooking.

TECHNIQUES

Look at these recipes as a course on how to cook healthier. Then you can use the techniques for lightening up food on other family favorites (but of course you're still going to buy my next cookbook!). You'll learn a lot of them here. Your hand blender will become your best friend. You'll thicken sauces with root vegetables instead of a roux, enrich dishes with roasted garlic instead of butter (the garlic will also keep the vampires away), and experience the joy of using spray oil along with your nonstick pan, which is not only a great way to save tons of calories, but also a heck of a lot easier to clean up.

I use a number of techniques that you might not have thought of before. There's a Tea-Smoked Chicken Breast on page 212 that you could swear is a fatty meal because it comes out so juicy. Once you get this technique down, you can use it on tomatoes, trout, any light protein. Just remember to unplug your smoke alarm and use a cheap pan! And you may have never thought about roasting fruit, but it makes for a terrific low-cal dessert (and, guys, it'll give you something else to throw on the barbecue).

You'll also see that your microwave is not just for making popcorn or warming up coffee and soup. The microwave is one of the best tools in the kitchen for healthy cooking—a high-tech steamer that will make it possible for you to cook up a bowl of spicy, flavorful vegetables in minutes.

I think you'll be surprised that not all the cheeses in the recipes are nonfat cheeses. I mix low-fat cheeses and some nonfat cheeses with full-fat cheeses because, let's face it, a cuisine without cheese, what's the point? Full-fat cheeses will

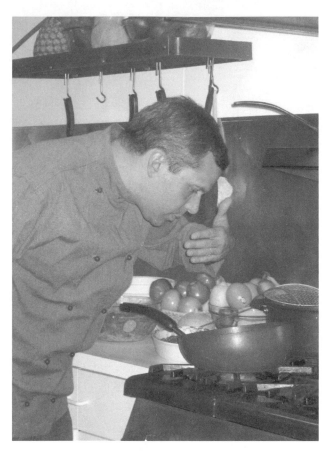

All kinds of recipes have a place in the Calorie Countdown.

contribute to the flavor and richness of a dish like the Feta-Artichoke Lasagne on page 239, or the Garlic Pesto–Stuffed Chicken Breast on page 197, but a little goes a long way. I love the variety of products available to us, like Splenda, nonfat cheeses, and low-fat salad dressings. But sometimes I like to throw some of the real stuff in, to keep the flavor and texture of the original.

I've tried to make the dishes easy and accessible. You don't have to have a culinary degree to make them, and you don't have to have tons of time. It's all about taste and convenience, and of course, calorie count. Healthy cooking doesn't make sense if it takes forever to make and then you don't want to eat it.

You may also be surprised by the number of desserts in this collection. Well, you can't expect a recovering pastry chef not to have lots of desserts. I had a sweet tooth when I was a pastry chef, and I have a sweet tooth now. I'm not about to deprive it, and neither should you. So get in there and try that Tiramisu (page 302)—it rocks!

Breakfasts and Sandwiches

Breakfast Taco

Blueberry Ricotta Pancakes

Cinnamon-Pear Stuffed French Toast

Cali Cheesesteak

Black Forest Ham and White Bean Panini

Herb Turkey Wraps

Open-Faced Chili Dogs

Pita Steak Sandwich with Dill Sauce

Quick String Cheese Quesadillas

BREAKFAST TACO

I reduced the calories in this traditional-tasting breakfast taco by using **Egg Beaters** instead of eggs and a corn tortilla instead of a huge flour tortilla. You could further reduce the calories if you use soy chorizo, one of my favorite soy products.

SERVES 4

Cooking spray

4 ounces regular or soy chorizo

½ red onion, chopped fine

3 cloves garlic, chopped

1 (4-ounce) can chopped green chiles, drained

½ cup chopped cilantro leaves

1 cup egg substitute, such as Egg Beaters

Salt to taste

4 (6-inch) corn tortillas

½ cup shredded low-fat Cheddar cheese

1. Heat a medium, heavy nonstick skillet and lightly spray with the cooking spray. Add the chorizo and break up into small pieces with a wooden spoon. Cook thoroughly. Drain grease if any has accumulated.

2. Add the red onions and cook, stirring, for 3 to 5 minutes, until tender. Add the garlic, green chiles, and cilantro to the pan, and sauté for another 3 minutes. Add the egg substitute and salt to taste. Stir with a wooden spoon until the egg substitute is scrambled and thoroughly cooked. Taste and adjust seasonings.

3. Warm the tortillas in a toaster oven, microwave, or on top of a stove burner. Place on plates. Divide the taco mixture equally among the 4 tortillas and top each with one-quarter of the cheese. Serve hot.

Nutritional Analysis per serving ▪ Calories 231 ▪ Fat (g) 12 ▪ Saturated Fat (g) 5 ▪ Carbohydrate (g) 12 ▪ Protein (g) 18 ▪ Cholesterol (mg) 28 ▪ Fiber (g) 2

BLUEBERRY RICOTTA PANCAKES

This dish so rocks. Make sure to use a nonstick pan. You might not think it's going to work, but it does. You save so many calories using so little flour and egg whites that you can use real maple syrup to top them.

SERVES 4

1 cup fresh or frozen blueberries

¼ cup real maple syrup

¾ cup all-purpose flour

½ teaspoon baking soda

¾ teaspoon baking powder

¼ teaspoon salt

1¼ cups low-fat ricotta cheese

¾ cup buttermilk

1 tablespoon honey

¾ teaspoon finely grated orange zest

2 large egg whites

Butter-flavored cooking spray

1. Combine the blueberries and maple syrup in a small saucepan. Cook over medium heat until the berries begin to pop. Keep warm for serving.

2. In a medium bowl, sift together the flour, baking soda, baking powder, and salt. In another large bowl, mix together the ricotta, buttermilk, honey, and orange zest. Fold the flour mixture into the ricotta mixture until just combined. In a clean mixing bowl or in the bowl of a standing electric mixer fitted with the whisk attachment, beat the egg whites to soft peaks. Gently fold into the batter.

3. Heat a nonstick griddle or a large nonstick pan over medium-low heat and lightly spray once with cooking spray. Spoon ⅓ cup of batter per pancake onto the hot griddle. When the pancakes are covered with bubbles and the edges are golden brown, about 1½ minutes, flip. Cook for another 30 to 45 seconds, or until golden brown. If cooking the pancakes in batches, lightly spray your griddle with additional cooking spray as needed.

4. Place two pancakes on each plate and serve with the blueberry syrup.

Nutritional Analysis per serving ▪ Calories 277 ▪ Fat (g) 4 ▪ Saturated Fat (g) 2 ▪ Carbohydrate (g) 47 ▪ Protein (g) 12 ▪ Cholesterol (mg) 21 ▪ Fiber (g) 2

QUICK TIP

Muffins are just cake, even the ones that are fat-free. Have a look at the calorie count on the fat-free muffins and you'll find they are not much better than the full-fat versions. They still average around 500 calories per muffin. That goes for bagels too.

CINNAMON-PEAR STUFFED FRENCH TOAST

This is a Sunday brunch kind of dish. It takes a couple of steps, and what you end up with is French toast with a surprise inside. There's lots of sweetness and fiber in the pears, and more fiber in the whole-grain toast. You could substitute Egg Beaters for the egg.

SERVES 4

2 teaspoons canola oil

1 teaspoon butter

1½ cups peeled, diced (¼-inch dice) firm pears

1 teaspoon ground cinnamon

2 tablespoons light cream cheese

4 (1½-inch-thick) slices whole-grain bread

2 large egg whites

1 large egg

¼ teaspoon vanilla extract

Pinch of salt

Butter-flavored cooking spray

1. Heat the canola oil and butter over medium-high heat in a 10-inch nonstick skillet. Once the foam from the butter has subsided, add the pears and ½ teaspoon cinnamon. Sear the pears for about 4 minutes, until slightly softened. Remove from the heat and add the cream cheese; stir until the cream cheese is melted and scrape into a bowl.

2. Lay a bread slice on a cutting board and make a 2-inch incision into the side to form a pocket inside the bread. Be careful not to pierce the other side of the bread. Repeat for each slice of bread. Spoon 2 tablespoons of the pear mixture into each pocket and set aside.

3. Combine the egg whites, egg, vanilla extract, salt, and remaining ½ teaspoon cinnamon; whisk together. Transfer the egg mixture to a shallow bowl or a small baking dish.

4. Heat a nonstick griddle over medium heat for 1 minute. Lightly spray the griddle with cooking spray. Take one stuffed bread slice and lightly dip both sides into the egg mixture, and then lightly dip each edge. Place the bread on the griddle and cook for 1½ minutes. Flip and cook for another 1½ minutes on the other side. While each piece of French toast is cooking on its first side, repeat the dipping process with the next one. Once the toast is golden brown, remove from the heat. (You can keep the toast warm in a low-temperature oven while you are making the rest.) Serve with maple syrup, if desired.

Nutritional Analysis per serving ▪ Calories 242 ▪ Fat (g) 8 ▪ Saturated Fat (g) 2 ▪ Carbohydrate (g) 35 ▪ Protein (g) 10 ▪ Cholesterol (mg) 59 ▪ Fiber (g) 6

CALI CHEESESTEAK

This popular deli sandwich fulfills all sorts of cravings at a fraction of the calorie and fat cost of the original. I substitute smoked turkey for beef, and throw out more than half the bread. But you'd never know this is a Calorie Countdown dish! The dish calls for light processed American cheese (such as Velveeta Light®), which you may wonder about; but it gives the dish the texture you want at a very low calorie cost.

SERVES 4

2 tablespoons canola oil

1 large yellow onion, thinly sliced

1 large green bell pepper, thinly sliced

2 cloves garlic, minced

¾ pound thinly sliced smoked turkey, preferably pepper turkey

Seasoned salt to taste

2 teaspoons Worcestershire sauce

2 ounces light processed American brick cheese such as Velveeta Light, cut into small cubes

4 (6-inch) Italian sandwich rolls

4 slices light provolone cheese

1. Preheat the broiler.

2. Heat the canola oil over medium heat in a medium heavy nonstick frying pan. Add the onions and bell peppers and sauté until well caramelized, about 10 minutes. Add the garlic and stir until just mixed.

3. Push the onion mixture to the side of the pan. On the other side of the pan, place the smoked turkey. Shred the turkey with 2 nylon spatulas and toss in the pan until warm. Stir the turkey together with the onion mixture. Add the seasoned salt and Worcestershire sauce. Add the American cheese and stir until the cheese is melted. Remove from the heat.

4. Cut the sandwich rolls in half and dig out the insides of the rolls without puncturing the crust. Discard the excess bread and the top crusts. Divide the turkey mixture evenly among the bottom half of the rolls and top with the provolone cheese slices.

5. Place under broiler just until the cheese is melted. Serve warm.

   VARIATION Substitute whole-wheat pita bread for the sandwich rolls. Fill the pockets with the filling and warm in a toaster oven until the cheese melts.

Nutritional Analysis per serving ▪ Calories 344 ▪ Fat (g) 14 ▪ Saturated Fat (g) 4 ▪ Carbohydrate (g) 28 ▪ Protein (g) 27 ▪ Cholesterol (mg) 46 ▪ Fiber (g) 3

BLACK FOREST HAM AND WHITE BEAN PANINI

These are substantial sandwiches that taste like they have much more cheese in them than they do. The Black Forest ham is so flavorful, all you need is a small amount of Parmesan. Try to find thick pitas for this. Thin ones can fall apart.

SERVES 4

1 (15-ounce) can white beans, drained and rinsed

1 tablespoon extra virgin olive oil

2 tablespoons freshly grated Parmesan

½ teaspoon dried oregano

½ teaspoon kosher salt (or to taste)

Freshly ground black pepper

4 (6-inch) whole-wheat pita breads, halved lengthwise and separated

8 ounces thinly sliced Black Forest ham

1 or 2 plum tomatoes, as needed, thinly sliced

Olive oil cooking spray

1. In a food processor, puree the beans with the olive oil. Stir in the Parmesan, oregano, salt and pepper to taste.

2. Spread the bean mixture over the bottom half of each pita, then layer the ham and tomato slices. Top with the remaining pita halves.

3. Heat a large nonstick griddle or panini grill. Lightly spray the sandwiches if using a panini grill, or a griddle with olive oil spray. Grill in the panini maker for 3 minutes. If using a griddle, place each of the sandwiches, with the bean side down, onto the hot griddle. Place a sheet of aluminum foil over the sandwiches and weight with a heavy pan. Grill for about 1½ minutes on the first side. Flip the sandwiches and grill for about another minute. Remove from griddle, cut into halves or quarters, and serve hot.

Nutritional Analysis per serving ▪ Calories 356 ▪ Fat (g) 9 ▪ Saturated Fat (g) 2 ▪ Carbohydrate (g) 51 ▪ Protein (g) 25 ▪ Cholesterol (mg) 32 ▪ Fiber (g) 10

HERB TURKEY WRAPS

Wraps sometimes look like a better alternative to a sandwich, but you have to be careful about what's in them. If you use a nonfat tortilla, this will be lower in calories. If you want to take it to work, roll it up and wrap tightly in plastic wrap.

SERVES 4

2 tablespoons light cream cheese

2 teaspoons minced fresh dill

4 herb tortilla wraps or plain low-fat tortilla wraps
(if you can't find herb variety)

8 leaves butter lettuce

12 ounces deli sliced turkey breast

1 tomato, thinly sliced (8 slices)

½ avocado, sliced

1 cup bean sprouts

Combine the cream cheese and dill in a small bowl. Spread ½ tablespoon of cream cheese mixture on each wrap and top with 2 lettuce leaves. Stack one-quarter of the turkey on the lettuce and then place 2 tomato slices on each stack of turkey. Divide the avocado slices evenly among the wraps on top of the tomato slices. Divide the bean sprouts evenly among the wraps on top of the avocado. Fold the bottom of wrap toward the top, and roll until the filling is encased in the wrap. Serve immediately, or wrap tightly in plastic and refrigerate.

Nutritional Analysis per serving ▪ Calories 262 ▪ Fat (g) 7 ▪ Saturated Fat (g) 1 ▪ Carbohydrate (g) 30 ▪ Protein (g) 21 ▪ Cholesterol (mg) 34 ▪ Fiber (g) 4

OPEN-FACED CHILI DOGS

These chili dogs call for half the bread and low-fat Cheddar for easy calorie reduction. The chili is a quick bean chili, so you can throw these together at half-time and serve them on Superbowl Sunday.

SERVES 4

2 teaspoons canola oil

1 small onion, finely diced

1 red bell pepper, diced

2 cloves garlic, crushed

1 tablespoon chili powder

1 (15-ounce) can black beans, wth liquid

2 tomatoes, diced

4 low-fat turkey hot dogs

2 hot dog buns, separated to make 4 halves

½ cup shredded low-fat Cheddar cheese

1. Preheat the broiler.

2. Heat the canola oil in a large nonstick skillet over medium heat. Add the onions and bell peppers. Sauté until soft, about 5 minutes, then add the garlic and chili powder. Cook until well blended, about 30 seconds. Add the black beans. Cook until warmed through, about 3 minutes. Add the tomatoes. Bring to a simmer and reduce heat. Cook until the chili thickens, 10 to 15 minutes.

3. While the chili is simmering, in a medium saucepan, cover the hot dogs in water. Over medium heat, bring to a boil. Reduce heat to a simmer. Cook for 4 minutes or until heated through.

4. Remove 1 hot dog from the saucepan and place on 1 bun half on a baking sheet. Top with one-quarter of the chili and one-quarter of the cheese. Repeat for remaining 3 hot dogs. Place hot dogs in the broiler for about 1 minute, until the cheese begins to melt. Serve hot.

Nutritional Analysis per serving ▪ Calories 314 ▪ Fat (g) 12 ▪ Saturated Fat (g) 3 ▪ Carbohydrate (g) 35 ▪ Protein (g) 18 ▪ Cholesterol (mg) 44 ▪ Fiber (g) 9

PITA STEAK SANDWICH WITH DILL SAUCE

For this dish I was looking for a quick, easy sandwich with lots of fiber and herbal flavors. The light steak sandwich I came up with will keep you going all afternoon. Make sure you buy pita that is thick enough to hold the ingredients without falling apart.

SERVES 4

1 tablespoon minced garlic (3 cloves)

1 tablespoon chopped fresh oregano

⅓ cup plus 1 tablespoon fresh lemon juice

Salt and freshly ground pepper

1 pound lean cube steak, cut into 4-ounce portions

Cooking spray

½ cup plain low-fat yogurt

1 tablespoon chopped fresh dill

1 tablespoon chopped fresh mint

1 Roma tomato, diced

1 small cucumber, peeled if desired, diced

1 green onion, sliced

4 (6-inch thick) whole-wheat pita breads

1. Mix together the garlic, oregano, and ⅓ cup of the lemon juice. Salt and pepper the steaks and place in a resealable plastic bag. Add the garlic, oregano, and lemon juice mixture, seal and refrigerate for 20 minutes to 6 hours.

2. Heat a large nonstick skillet over high heat and spray lightly with cooking spray. Remove the steaks from the bag and pat dry. Sear on each side for 2 minutes. Remove from the heat and cut in half.

3. Mix together the yogurt, dill, mint, tomato, cucumber, green onion, and the remaining 1 tablespoon lemon juice. Season to taste with salt and pepper. Cut the pita breads in half, then open them up and place a piece of steak in each pocket. Spoon in the dressing, and serve.

Nutritional Analysis per serving ▪ Calories 341 ▪ Fat (g) 6 ▪ Saturated Fat (g) 2 ▪ Carbohydrate (g) 40 ▪ Protein (g) 34 ▪ Cholesterol (mg) 66 ▪ Fiber (g) 5

QUICK STRING CHEESE QUESADILLAS

This is a snack or a side dish that you can throw together when you think you have no food on hand. You rummage around in the refrigerator and find the string cheese, then you remember that you have corn tortillas in the freezer, so you thaw a couple. Here's what you do next:

SERVES 1 (2 QUESADILLAS)

2 corn tortillas   2 string cheeses

Heat a nonstick frying pan or a griddle over medium-high heat. Meanwhile, shred the string cheeses. Place the tortillas on the pan and heat until they begin to blister. Turn them over and place a shredded string cheese down the middle of each. When the cheese begins to melt, fold the tortilla in half, and flip over. Heat through until the cheese has melted, and serve, with salsa.

Nutritional Analysis per serving (1 serving per recipe) ▪ Calories 269 ▪ Fat (g) 13 ▪ Saturated Fat (g) 8 ▪ Carbohydrate (g) 22 ▪ Protein (g) 17 ▪ Cholesterol (mg) 40 ▪ Fiber (g) 3

Appetizers, Salads, Salsas, Sauces, and Dips

Spinach-Artichoke Dip

Shrimp Cocktail

Gazpacho

Seared Tuna on Heirloom Tomatoes

Scallop and Mango Ceviche

Baked Stuffed Clams

Pigs in a Blanket

Southeast Asian–Inspired Char-Roasted Eggplant Dip and Pita Chips

Crab Dip

Nacho Cheese

Green Chile Black Beans

Caramelized Onion Dip

Mango-Coconut Salsa

Mango–Black Bean Salsa

Apple-Pear Slaw

Mixed Salad Greens with Balsamic Vinaigrette

Arugula and Tomato Salad

Potato Salad

Roasted Bell Pepper and Lentil Salad

Cranberry-Walnut-Quinoa Salad

Strawberry–Toasted Pecan Chicken Salad

Club Salad

Creamy Coleslaw

Cucumber-Dill Salad

Tuna Salad

Roasted Garlic Pesto

Creamy Italian Dressing

SPINACH-ARTICHOKE DIP

When I take this to a potluck dinner, nobody can believe that it's low-fat. The traditional artichoke dip has lots of full-fat cheese, which is yummy but packs on the pounds. I swap it here for reduced-fat cheese, and bulk out the artichokes with spinach. I also save a lot of fat and calories by substituting water-packed artichokes for the oil-packed ones.

SERVES 6

Olive oil cooking spray

4 cloves garlic, crushed

1 (14-ounce) can water-packed artichoke hearts, drained

1 (10-ounce) box frozen chopped spinach, thawed and moisture squeezed out

1 cup light sour cream

¾ cup freshly grated Parmesan cheese

½ cup grated part-skim mozzarella

8 ounces reduced-fat cream cheese

½ teaspoon ground black pepper

½ to 1 teaspoon Tabasco sauce or hot sauce, to taste

Salt

1. Preheat the oven to 350°F. Spray a 1½-quart baking dish with olive oil cooking spray.

2. Turn on a food processor fitted with the steel blade and drop in the garlic. Process until the garlic is chopped and adhering to the sides of the bowl. Stop the machine and scrape down the sides. Add the drained artichokes and spinach and pulse a few times, until coarsely chopped. Add the sour cream, ½ cup of the Parmesan, the mozzarella, cream cheese, pepper, and Tabasco, and salt to taste, then process until blended but still slightly lumpy. Taste and adjust the seasoning.

3. Scrape the mixture into the baking dish. Top with the ¼ cup remaining grated Parmesan. Place in the oven and bake for 30 minutes, until bubbling. Serve warm, as a dip with carrot sticks, celery sticks, jicama sticks, baked tortilla chips, or warm Pita Chips (see page 161).

Nutritional Analysis per serving ▪ Calories 236 ▪ Fat (g) 14 ▪ Saturated Fat (g) 9 ▪ Carbohydrate (g) 11 ▪ Protein (g) 15 ▪ Cholesterol (mg) 46 ▪ Fiber (g) 2

QUICK TIP

Tank up before you fill up! Drink a couple of large glasses of water before every meal and you will feel fuller faster.

SHRIMP COCKTAIL

This makes a very healthy tapa. It's like a shrimp gazpacho, minus a lot of the olive oil.

SERVES 6

6 plum tomatoes, diced

8 green onions, sliced

1 green bell pepper, diced

1 cup peeled, diced cucumber

2 hard-boiled eggs, whites only, chopped

2 tablespoons olive oil

1 clove garlic, minced

2 tablespoons red wine vinegar

2 tablespoons chopped cilantro

Salt

¾ pound cooked shrimp, cleaned and chopped

1 head butter lettuce, leaves separated, washed, and dried

1. In a medium bowl, combine the tomatoes, green onions, bell pepper, cucumber, and egg whites. In a small bowl, whisk together the olive oil, garlic, vinegar, and cilantro, and salt to taste. Stir into the tomato mixture. Taste and adjust seasoning.

2. Add the shrimp to the tomato mixture and toss together. Distribute the lettuce leaves among plates, or line a platter with them. Spoon the shrimp mixture into the lettuce leaves and serve.

Nutritional Analysis per serving ▪ Calories 134 ▪ Fat (g) 5 ▪ Saturated Fat (g) 1 ▪ Carbohydrate (g) 7 ▪ Protein (g) 14 ▪ Cholesterol (mg) 111 ▪ Fiber (g) 3

GAZPACHO

This is like the previous recipe, without the shrimp, and with the addition of V8. It's very refreshing on a hot day and a great way to drink a salad.

SERVES 6

6 plum tomatoes, diced

½ small onion, coarsely chopped and rinsed

1 green bell pepper, diced

1 cup peeled, diced cucumber

1 clove garlic, minced

2 tablespoons olive oil

2 tablespoons red wine vinegar

2 tablespoons chopped fresh basil or cilantro (or to taste)

3 cups V8 juice

1 teaspoon paprika

Salt

OPTIONAL GARNISHES

1 small cucumber, peeled, seeded, and minced

½ green bell pepper, seeded and minced

2 hard-boiled egg whites, chopped

6 green onions, minced

1. Combine all of the ingredients except the garnishes in a bowl. Transfer in batches to a blender and blend until smooth. Transfer to a bowl and stir together. Taste and adjust seasonings after all of the ingredients have been blended. Chill for a few hours if possible.

2. Serve, adding the garnishes of your choice to each bowl.

Nutritional Analysis per serving ▪ Calories 87 ▪ Fat (g) 5 ▪ Saturated Fat (g) 1 ▪ Carbohydrate (g) 10 ▪ Protein (g) 2 ▪ Cholesterol (mg) 0 ▪ Fiber (g) 2

SEARED TUNA ON HEIRLOOM TOMATOES

Whenever I make this elegant appetizer for a party, the guests go nuts!

SERVES 6

2 fresh ripe heirloom tomatoes, sliced

6 ounces tuna steak

2 cloves garlic, minced

2 tablespoons olive oil

1 tablespoon red wine vinegar

¼ to ½ teaspoon red pepper flakes, to taste

8 large imported black olives, chopped

Salt and freshly ground pepper to taste

1 tablespoon chopped chives

1. Arrange the tomato slices on an attractive serving plate, or on individual plates.

2. Heat a heavy nonstick pan over high heat until very hot. Quickly sear the tuna for 1 minute on each side. Set aside.

3. Mix together the garlic, olive oil, vinegar, pepper flakes, and olives in a bowl. Season to taste with salt and pepper. Slice the tuna into thin strips and toss the strips in the olive oil mixture. Spoon onto the tomato slices, sprinkle with chives, and serve.

Nutritional Analysis per serving ▪ Calories 94 ▪ Fat (g) 6 ▪ Saturated Fat (g) 1 ▪ Carbohydrate (g) 3 ▪ Protein (g) 7 ▪ Cholesterol (mg) 13 ▪ Fiber (g) 1

SCALLOP AND MANGO CEVICHE

Ceviche is a dieter's dream dish. Lots of lean protein, next to no fat, and lots of zingy flavor.

SERVES 4

½ pound bay scallops

Juice of 3 limes (about ½ cup)

½ cup thinly sliced green onions

½ cup chopped cilantro

1½ teaspoons grated fresh ginger

Salt

1 large ripe mango, peeled and diced

1 head butter lettuce, leaves separated, washed, and dried

1. In a large bowl, toss the scallops with the lime juice, green onions, cilantro, and ginger. Cover and refrigerate for 1 hour to 5 hours, stirring the mixture from time to time.

2. Remove from the refrigerator and season to taste with salt. Add the mango and stir together until well combined.

3. Divide the butter lettuce leaves among 4 plates. Top the leaves with the ceviche, and serve.

Nutritional Analysis per serving ▪ Calories 97 ▪ Fat (g) 1 ▪ Saturated Fat (g) 0 ▪ Carbohydrate (g) 14 ▪ Protein (g) 10 ▪ Cholesterol (mg) 19 ▪ Fiber (g) 2

BAKED STUFFED CLAMS

Here we're saving calories by substituting Canadian bacon for fatty bacon, and by doing without the tons of butter that the traditional dish would have.

SERVES 4 AS AN APPETIZER

12 cherrystone clams, scrubbed and purged of sand

2 ounces Canadian bacon, cut in small dice

Olive oil cooking spray

¼ cup finely diced onion

¼ cup finely diced parsnip

1 to 2 garlic cloves (to taste), minced

½ cup chopped flat-leaf parsley

⅛ to ¼ teaspoon cayenne pepper

½ cup freshly grated Parmesan

1. Bring 1 cup of water to a boil in a saucepan or stock pot fitted with a steamer. Place the clams in the steamer and set above the boiling water. Cover tightly and steam until the clams open, about 5 minutes. Remove from the pot and when cool enough to handle, remove the clams from the shells, rinse them briefly with cold water, and set aside. Separate the shells and set aside. Strain the clam water through a cheesecloth-lined strainer, measure out ¼ cup, and set aside.

2. Heat a nonstick frying pan over medium heat and add the Canadian bacon. Cook, stirring, until the bacon is browned, about 5 minutes. Transfer the bacon to a bowl. Wipe the pan dry and spray for about 1 second with olive oil spray. Heat over medium heat and add the onion and parsnips. Cook, stirring, until tender, 3 to 5 minutes. Add the garlic and cook for another 30 seconds to a minute, until fragrant. Stir in the reserved clam water, the parsley, and the cayenne, and remove from the heat. Allow to cool slightly and transfer to the bowl with the bacon. Stir in the Parmesan.

3. Preheat the broiler. Place 12 clam shells on a baking sheet, and place a clam in each one. Top with the onion and parsley mixture. Place under the broiler until browned, 2 to 3 minutes.

Nutritional Analysis per serving ▪ Calories 105 ▪ Fat (g) 4 ▪ Saturated Fat (g) 2 ▪ Carbohydrate (g) 5 ▪ Protein (g) 12 ▪ Cholesterol (mg) 31 ▪ Fiber (g) 1

QUICK TIP

Keep an arsenal of cooking sprays in the kitchen. There are now many flavored ones, like olive oil spray and butter-flavored spray. Using cooking sprays is a great way of controlling portions of fat calories.

PIGS IN A BLANKET

When you wrap hot dogs in phyllo instead of using buns you save a lot of calories. Plus your family will have fun making these.

SERVES 4

12 sheets phyllo dough

Butter-flavored cooking spray

Salt and freshly ground black pepper

4 low-fat turkey hot dogs

1. Preheat the oven to 400°F. Place a wire rack over a baking sheet.

2. Lay a sheet of phyllo dough in front of you with the short side facing you. Spray for 6 seconds with cooking spray and sprinkle with salt and pepper. Lay a second sheet of dough over the first and repeat. Repeat one more time with the third sheet of phyllo.

3. Place a hot dog on one end of the dough and roll up tightly. Slice off the overhanging phyllo at the ends and discard. Cut each roll into three equal pieces and arrange on the wire rack–covered baking sheet. Spray lightly with the butter-flavored spray. Place in the oven and bake 10 minutes. Turn and bake another 5 to 10 minutes, until uniformly browned. Serve with the Mustard Dipping Sauce below.

Nutritional Analysis per serving ▪ Calories 193 ▪ Fat (g) 7 ▪ Saturated Fat (g) 2 ▪ Carbohydrate (g) 25 ▪ Protein (g) 7 ▪ Cholesterol (mg) 41 ▪ Fiber (g) 1

Mustard Dipping Sauce

½ cup hot grainy mustard

¼ cup buttermilk

Mix together the mustard and buttermilk, and chill in the refrigerator for 30 minutes or longer.

SOUTHEAST ASIAN–INSPIRED CHAR-ROASTED EGGPLANT DIP AND PITA CHIPS

I once made this for a vegetarian client who forgot to tell me that he didn't like eggplant. But with all the Southeast Asian flavor in the dish, even he liked it. Pita chips are the perfect low-fat answer when you crave chips. They are virtually fat-free, but they have that satisfying crispiness.

SERVES 8

FOR THE PITA CHIPS

8 whole-wheat pita breads, cut into eight wedges

FOR THE DIP

1½ pounds eggplant (1 large or 2 medium)

1 to 2 teaspoons garlic chili sauce (I like Lee Kum Kee), to taste

2 tablespoons lemon juice

½ teaspoon salt

½ cup golden raisins (optional)

2 tablespoons finely chopped fresh basil leaves

2 tablespoons finely chopped fresh mint leaves

¼ cup sliced green onions

2 tablespoons chopped roasted peanuts

1. Make the Pita Chips: Preheat the oven to 400°F. Place the pita triangles on a sheet pan, place in the oven, and bake for about 10 minutes, until crispy. Check carefully so they don't burn. Remove from the oven and allow to cool.

2. Either preheat the broiler and cover a baking sheet with foil, or place the eggplant over a burner with the flame on high. Cook the eggplant under the broiler or over the burner, turning until all of the sides are charred black. Remove from the heat and allow to cool until you can handle it. Scrape or lift off and discard the skin. Cut away the stem, roughly chop the eggplant, and place it in a microwave-safe bowl. Cover with plastic, pierce the plastic in a few places, and microwave on high for 2 to 3 minutes, until thoroughly soft. Remove from the microwave and carefully remove the plastic. Allow to cool slightly.

3. Transfer the eggplant to a food processor fitted with the steel blade and add the garlic chili sauce, lemon juice, and ½ teaspoon salt. Process until smooth. Scrape into a bowl and stir in the raisins (if using), basil, and mint. Taste and adjust seasonings.

4. Scrape into an attractive serving dish and top with the green onions and peanuts. Serve with the Pita Chips.

Nutritional Analysis per serving ▪ Calories 219 ▪ Fat (g) 3 ▪ Saturated Fat (g) 0 ▪ Carbohydrate (g) 45 ▪ Protein (g) 7 ▪ Cholesterol (mg) 0 ▪ Fiber (g) 7

CRAB DIP

I made this once for a bunch of guys who came over to watch *Monday Night Football.* I saved lots of calories by using nonfat cream cheese and low-fat sour cream, but bulked up on flavor with the spices and Worcestershire sauce. I'm not sure the guys cared about this calorie savings, but I certainly did. It must not have tasted like diet food to them, because the whole dish was gone in about 15 minutes.

MAKES 3 CUPS, SERVING 10

½ cup low-fat sour cream

2 tablespoons reduced-calorie mayonnaise

1 tablespoon nonfat milk

1 tablespoon prepared horseradish

½ teaspoon dry mustard

½ teaspoon Worcestershire sauce

¼ teaspoon Tabasco sauce

½ pound nonfat cream cheese

½ pound lump crabmeat

Salt

⅛ teaspoon paprika

1. Place the sour cream, mayonnaise, milk, horseradish, dry mustard, Worcestershire sauce, Tabasco sauce, and cream cheese in the bowl of a food processor fitted with the steel blade. Blend until smooth.

2. Stir in the crabmeat. Add salt to taste. Cover and chill until ready to serve. Transfer to an attractive bowl, sprinkle with the paprika, and serve with Pita Chips (page 161) or low-calorie crackers.

Nutritional Analysis per serving ▪ Calories 77 ▪ Fat (g) 2 ▪ Saturated Fat (g) 1 ▪ Carbohydrate (g) 3 ▪ Protein (g) 9 ▪ Cholesterol (mg) 26 ▪ Fiber (g) 0

NACHO CHEESE

Velveeta is what nacho cheese is, and Velveeta Light is what makes these nachos a possibility for you. We're stretching it with salsa, so if you use air-baked chips you can have your nachos and eat them too!

MAKES 1 CUP, SERVING 6

8 ounces Velveeta Light, diced   **½ cup salsa**

Combine the Velveeta and the salsa in a microwave-safe bowl and microwave on 50% power for 1 to 3 minutes. Stir and microwave again for a minute or two if not completely melted. Serve with baked tortilla chips or Air Fries (page 250).

Nutritional Analysis per serving ■ Calories 90 ■ Fat (g) 4 ■ Saturated Fat (g) 3 ■ Carbohydrate (g) 6 ■ Protein (g) 7 ■ Cholesterol (mg) 16 ■ Fiber (g) 0

GREEN CHILE BLACK BEANS

Canned legumes are an essential pantry food for the Calorie Countdown diet. This dish is simple enough for a guy who doesn't cook to make. The beans contribute lots of fiber and protein, and the chiles add flavor and zip.

SERVES 6 AS AN APPETIZER

2 tablespoons olive oil

1 red bell pepper, chopped

2 cloves garlic, minced

1 (4 ounce) can chopped mild green chiles

1 (15-ounce) can black beans, with their liquid

Salt

3 tablespoons nonfat sour cream

2 tablespoons chopped cilantro

1. Heat the olive oil over medium heat in a medium nonstick skillet. Add the bell pepper and sauté for a couple of minutes, until it begins to soften. Add the garlic and sauté for another minute, until fragrant.

2. Add the can of chiles with their juice and the beans. Stir together and bring to a simmer. Simmer 5 minutes, stirring occasionally. Add salt, taste, and adjust seasoning. Remove from the heat and transfer to an attractive bowl. Garnish with the sour cream and cilantro, and serve warm, with air-baked chips.

Nutritional Analysis per serving ▪ Calories 98 ▪ Fat (g) 3 ▪ Saturated Fat (g) 0 ▪ Carbohydrate (g) 13 ▪ Protein (g) 5 ▪ Cholesterol (mg) 1 ▪ Fiber (g) 5

CARAMELIZED ONION DIP

This is incredibly tasty, especially if you use a sweet onion like Vidalia. Serve it with air-baked chips, and your guests won't even ask you if it's low-fat.

MAKES 1 1/2 CUPS, SERVING 12

1 tablespoon canola oil

1/2 large sweet onion, chopped fine

1 tablespoon balsamic vinegar

1 cup low-fat sour cream

1/2 to 1 teaspoon garlic powder

1/2 to 1 teaspoon seasoned salt or regular salt

1. Heat a heavy nonstick sauté pan over medium heat and add the canola oil and the onions. Stir until the onions are coated with oil. Allow to cook, stirring only occasionally, until the onions are golden brown, about 5 to 6 minutes. Add the balsamic vinegar and continue to cook, stirring and scraping the bottom of the pan with a wooden spoon, until the liquid has evaporated. Remove from the heat.

2. Stir in the sour cream, garlic powder, and salt to taste. Stir together. Transfer to a bowl. Cover and place in the refrigerator for 30 minutes or longer, to allow the flavors to mellow and the dip to thicken. Serve with air-baked chips (tortilla or pita) and/or crudités.

Nutritional Analysis per serving ▪ Calories 41 ▪ Fat (g) 3 ▪ Saturated Fat (g) 1 ▪ Carbohydrate (g) 2 ▪ Protein (g) 1 ▪ Cholesterol (mg) 7 ▪ Fiber (g) 0

MANGO-COCONUT SALSA

Try this sweet and spicy salsa with fish or chicken breasts, or serve it with air-baked tortilla chips.

MAKES 4 SERVINGS

¼ cup thinly sliced green onions

¼ cup chopped cilantro

1 teaspoon minced jalapeño

1 large mango, peeled, seeded, and finely diced

¼ cup finely diced red bell pepper

½ to 1 tablespoon fresh lemon or lime juice

¼ cup shredded coconut

Salt to taste

Mix together all of the ingredients in a large bowl. Cover and refrigerate for at least one hour.

Nutritional Analysis per serving ▪ Calories 57 ▪ Fat (g) 2 ▪ Saturated Fat (g) 2 ▪ Carbohydrate (g) 11 ▪ Protein (g) 1 ▪ Cholesterol (mg) 0 ▪ Fiber (g) 2

MANGO–BLACK BEAN SALSA

This salsa is so substantial you could eat it as a high-protein side dish.

SERVES 8 (MAKES ABOUT 3 CUPS)

¼ cup thinly sliced green onions

¼ cup chopped cilantro

1 teaspoon minced jalapeño

1 large mango, peeled and diced

¼ cup minced fresh red bell pepper

½ teaspoon fresh lemon or lime juice

1 (15-ounce) can black beans, drained and rinsed

Salt to taste

Mix together all of the ingredients in a large bowl. Cover and refrigerate for at least one hour. Enjoy with baked corn tortilla or pita chips, or as a garnish for fish or chicken.

Nutritional Analysis per serving for 8 servings ▪ Calories 65 ▪ Fat (g) 0 ▪ Saturated Fat (g) 0 ▪ Carbohydrate (g) 12 ▪ Protein (g) 3 ▪ Cholesterol (mg) 0 ▪ Fiber (g) 4

APPLE-PEAR SLAW

This is an excellent Thanksgiving salad. It's sweet and crunchy, with lots of fiber.

SERVES 4

¼ cup apple cider vinegar

1 tablespoon light brown sugar

¼ teaspoon salt, or to taste

Freshly ground pepper

1 cup grated or julienned peeled apple

1 cup grated or julienned peeled pear or Asian pear

¼ cup dried cranberries

3 Belgian endives, broken into leaves

1. In a bowl, mix together the vinegar, brown sugar, salt, and pepper to taste. Toss with the apples, pears, and cranberries.

2. Line 4 plates with endive leaves. Top with the apple mixture, and serve.

Nutritional Analysis per serving ▪ Calories 72 ▪ Fat (g) 0 ▪ Saturated Fat (g) 0 ▪ Carbohydrate (g) 18 ▪ Protein (g) 0 ▪ Cholesterol (mg) 0 ▪ Fiber (g) 2

MIXED SALAD GREENS WITH BALSAMIC VINAIGRETTE

I call those bags of prewashed salad greens *yuppie chow,* and I don't mean this disparagingly. Those bags are a godsend to dieters everywhere.

SERVES 4

1 large clove garlic, finely chopped	2 tablespoons olive oil
Salt	Freshly ground black pepper
¼ cup balsamic vinegar	2 (5-ounce) bags salad greens

In a glass bowl or salad bowl, mash together the garlic and salt to taste. Add the vinegar and oil and whisk together. Add pepper to taste. Just before serving, toss with the salad greens.

Nutritional Analysis per serving ▪ Calories 89 ▪ Fat (g) 7 ▪ Saturated Fat (g) 1 ▪ Carbohydrate (g) 6 ▪ Protein (g) 1 ▪ Cholesterol (mg) 0 ▪ Fiber (g) 2

QUICK TIP

Beware of salad dressing! You can build this great salad with all kinds of healthy ingredients and then dump on 700 calories' worth of dressing in just a couple level tablespoons. If you must have full-fat dressing, then dip your fork into the dressing first and then spear some salad. You'll save a tremendous number of calories.

ARUGULA AND TOMATO SALAD

I think my favorite "yuppie green" is arugula, and this is a perfect way to use it. Make it in summer when tomatoes are at their best.

SERVES 4

1 (7-ounce) bag prewashed baby arugula

2 ripe tomatoes, cut in wedges, or 1 cup cherry tomatoes, cut in half

1 ounce Parmesan cheese, shaved into thin slivers with a vegetable peeler

2 tablespoons balsamic vinegar

Salt and freshly ground black pepper

2 tablespoons olive oil

Combine the arugula, tomatoes, and Parmesan in a salad bowl. Toss with the balsamic vinegar, salt and pepper (to taste), and the olive oil, and serve.

Nutritional Analysis per serving ▪ Calories 123 ▪ Fat (g) 9 ▪ Saturated Fat (g) 2 ▪ Carbohydrate (g) 7 ▪ Protein (g) 5 ▪ Cholesterol (mg) 6 ▪ Fiber (g) 2

POTATO SALAD

To make a lower-carb potato salad I substituted lots of vegetables for some of the potatoes. This contributed crunch, which means fiber. And fiber makes you feel full for a long time. The light mayo makes a good base for the dressing, but you need a little Dijon mustard to give it some kick.

SERVES 4

¾ pound red new potatoes, scrubbed

1 teaspoon salt

¼ cup nonfat mayonnaise

1½ teaspoons Dijon mustard

1 tablespoon sweet pickle relish

1 tablespoon chopped fresh parsley

⅛ teaspoon ground white pepper

½ cup sliced green onions

½ cup frozen peas, thawed

¼ cup finely diced carrot

¼ cup finely diced green bell pepper

¼ cup finely diced celery

1. Place the potatoes in a saucepan and cover with water. Add 1 teaspoon salt and bring to a boil. Turn down the heat and boil gently until tender when pierced with a knife, about 20 minutes. Drain, cool, then quarter the potatoes.

2. Mix together the mayonnaise, Dijon mustard, and pickle relish. Toss with the potatoes. Add the parsley, pepper, and vegetables, and toss together well. Taste, adjust seasonings, and serve.

Nutritional Analysis per serving ▪ Calories 110 ▪ Fat (g) 1 ▪ Saturated Fat (g) 0 ▪ Carbohydrate (g) 23 ▪ Protein (g) 3 ▪ Cholesterol (mg) 2 ▪ Fiber (g) 4

ROASTED BELL PEPPER AND LENTIL SALAD

Lentils have lots of flavor, and they're loaded with fiber as well. They also have a lot of iron, and the vitamin C in the peppers helps your body access this iron. This is a salad that I could eat for lunch or dinner every day.

SERVES 6

2 cups lentils, washed and picked over for hidden pebbles

2 teaspoons salt

3 bell peppers, preferably 1 red, 1 yellow, and 1 green

½ cup light sour cream

3 tablespoons grainy mustard

1 tablespoon balsamic vinegar

½ medium red onion, diced

Freshly ground black pepper

1. Bring 5 cups water to a boil in a large saucepan and add the lentils. Bring back to a boil, cover, reduce the heat and simmer 30 minutes. Add 2 teaspoons salt and continue to simmer another 15 minutes, or until the lentils are tender. Remove from the heat and drain.

2. Meanwhile, roast the peppers, either over an open flame or under the broiler, turning every few minutes, until they have blackened all over. Remove from the heat and place in a bowl. Cover tightly with plastic wrap or set a plate snugly over the top and allow to cool. Peel and discard the skins. Stem and seed the peppers, and cut into 1 × ½-inch slices. Set aside (if using bottled peppers, drain and dice).

3. Transfer the lentils to a large bowl. Stir in the sour cream, mustard, and vinegar. Add the roasted peppers and the diced onions. Season to taste with salt and pepper. Serve warm, at room temperature, or chilled.

NOTE You may substitute bottled roasted peppers for the fresh peppers.

Nutritional Analysis per serving ▪ Calories 294 ▪ Fat (g) 2 ▪ Saturated Fat (g) 1 ▪ Carbohydrate (g) 50 ▪ Protein (g) 22 ▪ Cholesterol (mg) 7 ▪ Fiber (g) 10

CRANBERRY-WALNUT-QUINOA SALAD

Quinoa (pronounced KEEN-wa) is a super-food, and I'm always looking for ways to use it. The tiny little grains are packed with nutrients, and they really fill you up. But the best part of all is that you can dress it up or down, so it's never the same. I needed a dish to bring to a barbecue, and came up with this one, which has a nice contrast of sweetness and texture, with the cranberries and crunchy walnuts. The salad became the main dish for some of the guests. Another great thing about this is that it's great for batch cooking. You can make it on Sunday and take it to work for lunch on Monday and Tuesday. The flavors just get better.

SERVES 6 AS A STARTER OR SIDE DISH, OR 4 AS A MAIN COURSE

1 cup quinoa

½ teaspoon salt or to taste

¾ cup dried cranberries

1 cup frozen green beans or peas, thawed, green beans cut in half if long

¼ cup chopped walnuts

¼ cup sliced green onions (optional)

¼ cup balsamic vinegar

1½ tablespoons olive oil

1 to 2 cloves garlic (to taste), minced

Freshly ground black pepper

1. Rinse the quinoa in several changes of water. Combine with 2 cups water and ½ teaspoon salt in a medium saucepan and bring to a boil over high heat. Reduce heat to a simmer, cover, and continue cooking until all water is absorbed, about 20 minutes. Remove from the heat, uncover, and allow to cool for 15 minutes.

2. In a medium bowl, combine the cooked quinoa, dried cranberries, green beans, walnuts, and green onions (if using) until well mixed. In a small bowl, whisk the balsamic vinegar, olive oil, and garlic until well blended. Pour over the quinoa mixture. Toss until well blended. Season with salt and pepper to taste. Chill in the refrigerator for at least 30 minutes before serving.

Nutritional Analysis per serving (4 main dishes) ▪ Calories 351 ▪ Fat (g) 12 ▪ Saturated Fat (g) 1 ▪ Carbohydrate (g) 55 ▪ Protein (g) 7 ▪ Cholesterol (mg) 0 ▪ Fiber (g) 5

Nutritional Analysis per serving (6 side dishes) ▪ Calories 234 ▪ Fat (g) 8 ▪ Saturated Fat (g) 1 ▪ Carbohydrate (g) 36 ▪ Protein (g) 5 ▪ Cholesterol (mg) 0 ▪ Fiber (g) 3

STRAWBERRY—TOASTED PECAN CHICKEN SALAD

One of my clients was complaining one day about how tired she was becoming of chicken breasts. I looked around her kitchen, saw what she had, and threw together this lovely, nutritious salad. She stopped complaining. Once you realize how much you can do with chicken breasts, they won't be boring anymore.

SERVES 4

2 cups skinned and boned roasted chicken breast, from a store-bought rotisserie chicken

¼ cup pecans, toasted

2 cups hulled and quartered strawberries

¼ cup finely diced red onion

¼ cup finely diced celery

¼ cup finely chopped cilantro leaves

2 tablespoons balsamic vinegar

2 teaspoons olive oil

4 cups salad greens

In a medium bowl, combine the chicken, pecans, strawberries, onion, celery, cilantro, vinegar, and oil. Cover and marinate in the refrigerator for 1 hour. Serve over salad greens.

Nutritional Analysis per serving ▪ Calories 230 ▪ Fat (g) 10 ▪ Saturated Fat (g) 1 ▪ Carbohydrate (g) 12 ▪ Protein (g) 24 ▪ Cholesterol (mg) 59 ▪ Fiber (g) 4

CLUB SALAD

This has everything you love about a club sandwich without the calories from the bread and the mayonnaise.

SERVES 4

⅓ cup buttermilk

2 tablespoons light mayonnaise

½ teaspoon Italian seasoning

¼ teaspoon dry mustard

¼ teaspoon garlic powder or 1 small clove garlic, minced or pressed

¼ teaspoon kosher salt (or to taste)

Freshly ground black pepper

½ head romaine lettuce, coarsely chopped

1 pound deli oven-roasted turkey breast cut into ¾-inch cubes

6 slices turkey bacon, cooked and crumbled

3 ribs celery, thinly sliced, or 1 red bell pepper, diced

¼ red onion, diced

3 slices multigrain bread, toasted

2 plum tomatoes, each cut into 6 wedges

1. Whisk together the buttermilk, light mayonnaise, Italian seasoning, dry mustard, garlic, powder, salt, and pepper to taste in a small bowl. Set aside.

2. Combine the lettuce, turkey, bacon, celery, and onions in a large bowl. Toss with the dressing, and season to taste. Cut each toast slice into 4 even triangles. Divide the salad among 4 plates, garnish with the tomato wedges and toast triangles, and serve.

Nutritional Analysis per serving ▪ Calories 271 ▪ Fat (g) 8 ▪ Saturated Fat (g) 2 ▪ Carbohydrate (g) 22 ▪ Protein (g) 28 ▪ Cholesterol (mg) 62 ▪ Fiber (g) 3

CREAMY COLESLAW

Coleslaw can be deceptive. People think they're ordering something healthy, but it can be filled with mayonnaise and cream. I like to add crunch whenever I can, and here I added it in the form of jicama. I cut the calories by using light mayonnaise, and added lots of flavor with cilantro and chili sauce. Use prepackaged shredded carrots for convenience.

SERVES 6

¼ cup apple cider vinegar

½ cup light mayonnaise

2 tablespoons poppy seeds

½ teaspoon celery salt

½ cup chopped fresh cilantro leaves

1 teaspoon chili sauce

2 cups shredded red cabbage (about ¼ head or use prepackaged)

2 cups prepackaged shredded carrots

½ cup thinly sliced green onions

1 medium red bell pepper, thinly sliced

1 cup finely julienned jicama (1 jicama, about the size of a softball)

1 teaspoon kosher salt

½ teaspoon crushed black pepper

In a small bowl, combine the vinegar, mayonnaise, poppy seeds, celery salt, cilantro, and chili sauce, stirring until well blended. In a medium bowl, toss together the cabbage, carrots, green onions, bell pepper, and jicama. Pour dressing over cabbage mixture and toss until vegetables are coated with dressing. Season with salt and pepper. Cover and refrigerate for at least 1 hour so that flavors meld. Serve chilled.

Nutritional Analysis per serving ▪ Calories 122 ▪ Fat (g) 8 ▪ Saturated Fat (g) 2 ▪ Carbohydrate (g) 11 ▪ Protein (g) 2 ▪ Cholesterol (mg) 7 ▪ Fiber (g) 4

CUCUMBER-DILL SALAD

This versatile salad makes a great appetizer with baked pita chips, and also a great side dish. I also use it in pita sandwiches.

SERVES 4

½ cup low-fat plain yogurt

1 tablespoon chopped fresh dill

1 garlic clove, minced

3 tablespoons fresh lemon juice (more to taste)

1 cucumber, peeled if desired, and diced

2 plum tomatoes, diced

2 green onions, sliced

1 tablespoon chopped fresh mint leaves

Salt and freshly ground black pepper

In a small bowl, mix the yogurt with the dill, garlic, and lemon juice. Cover and refrigerate for at least 30 minutes to let flavors blend. In another small bowl, mix cucumber with the tomatoes, green onions, and mint. Season with salt and pepper. Toss with the yogurt mixture and serve.

Nutritional Analysis per serving ▪ Calories 41 ▪ Fat (g) 1 ▪ Saturated Fat (g) 0 ▪ Carbohydrate (g) 7 ▪ Protein (g) 2 ▪ Cholesterol (mg) 2 ▪ Fiber (g) 1

TUNA SALAD

It's easy to make a low-fat tuna salad, just by substituting low-fat mayonnaise and yogurt for the regular mayonnaise, and pepping up the flavor with a little mustard and lemon juice. Give it lots of crunch with peppers and celery and you're good to go.

SERVES 2

1 (6-ounce) can water-packed tuna

1 tablespoon low-fat mayonnaise

1 tablespoon plain nonfat yogurt

1 teaspoon Dijon mustard

1 tablespoon fresh lemon juice

1 small red or green bell pepper, chopped

1 stalk celery, chopped

Drain the tuna and mash together with the mayonnaise, yogurt, mustard, and lemon juice. Stir in the chopped vegetables. Use for salads or sandwiches.

Nutritional Analysis per serving ▪ Calories 143 ▪ Fat (g) 3 ▪ Saturated Fat (g) 1 ▪ Carbohydrate (g) 6 ▪ Protein (g) 21 ▪ Cholesterol (mg) 36 ▪ Fiber (g) 1

ROASTED GARLIC PESTO

I use this as a stuffing for chicken breasts (page 197), as a topping for spaghetti squash (page 241), and whenever I need a creamy, pesto-like sauce without the fat calories of an authentic pesto.

MAKES ABOUT 1/2 CUP, SERVING 4

4 heads garlic

Olive oil cooking spray

2 cups fresh basil leaves, chopped

1 teaspoon pine nuts

2 teaspoons grated Parmesan

Salt

1. Preheat the oven to 375°F. Slice the tops off the 4 heads of garlic. Lightly spray the heads with olive oil cooking spray. Wrap in lightly oiled aluminum foil and roast 1 hour. Allow to cool before handling.

2. Separate the garlic cloves and squeeze the pulp out into the bowl of a food processor fitted with the stainless steel blade. Add the chopped basil and pine nuts. Puree until smooth. Stir in the Parmesan. Add salt to taste, and scrape into a jar.

Nutritional Analysis Per 2 tablespoons ▪ Calories 64 ▪ Fat (g) 1 ▪ Saturated Fat (g) 1 ▪ Carbohydrate (g) 11 ▪ Protein (g) 4 ▪ Cholesterol (mg) 44 ▪ Fiber (g) 2

CREAMY ITALIAN DRESSING

Since I'm a sucker for creamy salad dressings I'm always working on low-calorie versions. This one is worth having roasted garlic in your refrigerator for. The roasted garlic and buttermilk combo gives this the taste and mouth feel of the fattening dressings I love. Serve it with sturdy salads like spinach or endive, use it for coleslaws, or serve it as a dip.

MAKES ABOUT 1 ¹⁄₈ CUPS, SERVING 6

2 heads garlic, tops sliced off

Olive oil cooking spray

2 tablespoons chopped fresh herbs (any combination of parsley, basil, oregano, and thyme leaves)

½ cup light sour cream

⅓ cup buttermilk

2 tablespoons olive oil

¼ to ½ teaspoon salt

¼ teaspoon freshly ground black pepper

Juice of ½ lemon (more to taste)

1. Preheat the oven to 375°F.

2. Place the garlic heads on aluminum foil and lightly spray each head with 2 sprays of olive oil cooking spray. Wrap the aluminum foil around the garlic to form a tight package. Roast for 1 hour. Remove from the oven and place the whole heads of garlic in a food mill. Press the garlic through the food mill (see first note below). Transfer the garlic pulp to a bowl. Add the fresh herbs and sour cream and stir until completely blended. Whisk in the buttermilk and olive oil, adding just enough to give the dressing a consistency that is easy to pour. Add salt to taste, pepper, and lemon juice. Taste and adjust seasonings. Chill for at least 30 minutes to allow flavors to meld.

> **NOTE** Adding the whole garlic heads eliminates the step of removing the pulp from the cloves because the food mill squeezes the pulp out. If you don't have a food mill, squeeze the pulp from the skins and mash with a fork or in a food processor fitted with the steel blade.

Nutritional Analysis per serving ▪ Calories 89 ▪ Fat (g) 6 ▪ Saturated Fat (g) 2 ▪ Carbohydrate (g) 6 ▪ Protein (g) 2 ▪ Cholesterol (mg) 7 ▪ Fiber (g) 0

> **NOTE** 1 cup of salad greens contains about 11 calories, so a salad with this dressing would give you 100 calories.

Main Dishes

MEAT AND POULTRY

Adobo-Roasted Pork Loin

Air-Fried Pork Chops

Barbecued Pork Loin

Quick Black Bean–Lime Chili

Chicken Asopa

Chicken Enchiladas Verdes

Chicken Parmesan

Chilaquiles

Chile-Cheese Rice Burritos

Chiles Rellenos

Chili con Carne

Garden Turkey Burgers

Garlic Pesto–Stuffed Chicken Breast

Garlic-Roasted Tenderloin with
Horseradish Cream

Herb-Roasted Turkey Breast

Spicy Orange Chicken Lo Mein

Oven-Fried Chicken Breasts

Pork Fried Rice

Roast Beef with Root Veggie Gravy

Quick Shoyu Chicken

Slow-Braised Carnitas

Spicy Korean Rice with Flank Steak

Sweet Potato Shepherd's Pie

Light Beef Taco Wraps

Tea-Smoked Chicken

Tequila Chicken Fajitas

My Mom's Tortilla Casserole

Turkey or Chicken for One

Turkey Meatloaf

Turkey Tacos Fiesta

FISH

Braised Shrimp

Broccoli-Halibut Stir-Fry

Crab and Avocado Quesadillas

Fennel-Roasted Sea Bass

Garlic Shrimp Scampi

Ginger-Lime Snapper

Ginger Packet Salmon, Toaster Style

Kalamata Halibut

New England Clam Chowder

Spicy Garlic Shrimp with Bell Peppers

Spicy Seared Scallops

Sunset Fish Skewers

PASTA, PIZZA, AND VEGETARIAN

Calzones

Creamy Four-Cheese Macaroni with Broccoli

Curried Eggplant

Denver Quiche

Eggplant Parmesan

Feta-Artichoke Lasagne

Fettucine Alfredo

Spaghetti Squash with Roasted Garlic Pesto

Portobello Pizza

Portobello Mushroom–Phyllo Packets

Spaghetti Squash Spaghetti and Meatballs

Tuna Noodle Casserole

Whole-Wheat Pizza with Assorted Toppings

Wild Mushroom Manicotti

ADOBO-ROASTED PORK LOIN

This is one of my many dishes that I think of as a "guy's recipe," easy to make and full of big flavors. That said, it's a pretty delicate roast. It can be made on a grill (that's the guy thing) or roasted at 375°F. Enjoy it with a beer (light, of course), or a glass of red wine.

SERVES 6

1 (2-pound) boneless pork loin, trimmed of all visible fat

Salt

6 cloves garlic, minced

3 tablespoons chopped fresh oregano, or 1 tablespoon dried

10 green onions, thinly sliced

1 chipotle chile in adobo sauce, seeded and chopped

2 limes, cut in wedges

½ cup chopped cilantro

1. Salt the pork loin generously. Rub the pork loin all over with the minced garlic. Place in a shallow baking dish and toss with the oregano, half of the green onions, and the chopped chipotle. Cover with plastic and place in the refrigerator for 1 hour or longer.

2. Prepare a hot fire in a barbecue (or preheat a gas barbecue). Insert a programmable digital thermometer into the middle of the loin, and set the thermometer for 160°F. Place on the barbecue, just to the side of the direct heat, cover, and cook, turning periodically, until the thermometer registers 160°F, about 25 to 30 minutes. Alternatively, place on a rack in a roasting pan and roast in a preheated 375°F oven until your thermometer registers 160°F, about 40 minutes.

3. Remove the roast from the heat and allow to rest for 10 to 15 minutes. Slice and serve garnished with lime wedges, cilantro, and the remaining sliced green onions.

Nutritional Analysis per serving ▪ Calories 247 ▪ Fat (g) 10 ▪ Saturated Fat (g) 4 ▪ Carbohydrate (g) 5 ▪ Protein (g) 30 ▪ Cholesterol (mg) 85 ▪ Fiber (g) 2

AIR-FRIED PORK CHOPS

This low-fat version of an American classic also has the advantage of being faster to make and easier to clean up than the fried version. Air-frying means broiling the pork chops, after setting them on a rack above a baking sheet. The fat drips onto the baking sheet instead of being reabsorbed back into the meat. Give the chops a light spray of vegetable oil before broiling, for a crisper texture.

SERVES 4

1 cup plain or Italian-flavor bread crumbs

¾ teaspoon salt (to taste)

½ teaspoon freshly ground black pepper

¼ teaspoon cayenne pepper

4 pork loin chops, about ¾ inch thick

½ cup Dijon mustard

1. Preheat the broiler. Place a wire rack over a sheet pan. Combine the bread crumbs, ½ teaspoon salt, the pepper, and cayenne and place in a shallow dish.

2. Salt the pork chops and brush on both sides with a thick coating of mustard. Dredge in the bread crumb mixture and place on the wire rack. Place under the broiler about 3 to 4 inches from the flame. Broil for 5 to 8 minutes on each side, until the coating is dark golden brown.

Nutritional Analysis per serving ▪ Calories 321 ▪ Fat (g) 12 ▪ Saturated Fat (g) 4 ▪ Carbohydrate (g) 13 ▪ Protein (g) 39 ▪ Cholesterol (mg) 97 ▪ Fiber (g) 2

BARBECUED PORK LOIN

I love barbecue; boy, do I love it. As a cooking technique, barbecue isn't a bad choice for a dieter. Where it goes wrong is the cuts of meat that are usually used: the big fatty, juicy cuts that taste so great. They taste great because of the fat, and that's what will clog up your system. I've barbecued everything from salmon to prime rib, and have learned a few tricks about making barbecue taste, and feel, like it's got all of that fat when it doesn't. For this recipe I'm using center cut pork loin, which is very lean because today meat producers are raising leaner pigs. But lean meat can mean dry meat, unless you're very careful about how you cook it. I use a dry rub to add flavor, and stuff the loin with dried fruit, which will contribute moisture from the inside as the loin cooks.

SERVES 8

½ cup chopped dried apricots

½ cup raisins

½ cup Port wine

1 (2-pound) center cut boneless pork loin, or 2 (1-pound) pork loins

1 tablespoon five-spice powder

2 tablespoons ground ginger

2 tablespoons light brown sugar

1 teaspoon kosher salt

Freshly ground black pepper

1. In a bowl, combine the dried apricots, raisins, and Port wine and let sit for 20 to 30 minutes, or longer, until the fruit is soft and has absorbed most of the Port.

2. Using a clean knife-sharpening steel, make a hole running down the length of the pork loin by pushing the steel through the middle of the loin. Fill the hole with the fruit mixture, pushing it through using the knife steel (now put your steel in the dishwasher).

3. Mix together the five-spice powder, ginger, and brown sugar and spread all over the pork loin. Wrap in plastic and refrigerate for 2 hours or longer.

4. Rub the loin all over with salt and sprinkle with pepper. Prepare a medium-hot fire in a grill, preferably with some wood chips for flavor. Place the loin on the grill, a little off to the side so it isn't over the hottest coals, and cook, turning often, until the meat has an internal temperature of 160°F, about 45 minutes (I like to insert a probe thermometer that will go off when the meat reaches 160°F before I begin). Remove from the grill and let the meat rest for 10 minutes before carving.

5. Slice about ½ inch thick, arrange on a platter, and serve.

Nutritional Analysis per serving ▪ Calories 256 ▪ Fat (g) 8 ▪ Saturated Fat (g) 3 ▪ Carbohydrate (g) 20 ▪ Protein (g) 24 ▪ Cholesterol (mg) 64 ▪ Fiber (g) 1

QUICK BLACK BEAN–LIME CHILI

This is a great high-fiber chili that you can make in quantity and divide into batches. It may seem strange to include couscous in a chili, but it adds bulk to the dish without lots of calories.

SERVES 4

⅔ cup instant couscous

¼ teaspoon salt

2 tablespoons olive oil

1 Vidalia onion, chopped

1 red bell pepper, chopped

1 green bell pepper, chopped

3 cloves garlic, minced

1 tablespoon chili powder

1 (14-ounce) can stewed tomatoes, chopped, with liquid

1 (15-ounce) can black beans, with liquid

2 cups shredded cooked chicken, store-bought, skin discarded

2 to 4 tablespoons fresh lime juice (to taste)

¼ cup fresh cilantro leaves

1. Place the couscous in a bowl and combine with ¼ teaspoon salt. Heat 1 cup water in a small saucepan and pour over the couscous. Stir to prevent lumps. Cover and set aside for 15 minutes. Once the liquid is absorbed, fluff with a fork.

2. In a heavy-bottomed pot, heat the oil over medium heat. Add the onion and cook until beginning to soften, about 3 minutes. Add the peppers and cook, stirring often, until tender, 5 to 8 minutes. Add the garlic and cook for 1 minute, stirring. Add the chili powder and cook for another minute. Stir in the tomatoes and black beans and their liquid, and salt to taste; bring all to a simmer and simmer for 10 minutes, or until thick and fragrant. Add the chicken and heat through. Stir in the lime juice and cilantro and remove from heat. Taste and adjust seasonings. Serve over the fluffed couscous.

Nutritional Analysis per serving ▪ Calories 459 ▪ Fat (g) 13 ▪ Saturated Fat (g) 2 ▪ Carbohydrate (g) 51Protein (g) 32 ▪ Cholesterol (mg) 62 ▪ Fiber (g) 11

CHICKEN ASOPA

I'm 100 percent Caribbean, and I needed to develop a recipe that would be like arroz con pollo, minus lots of the calories. So I left out our traditional ham hocks and used chicken without the skin and Canadian bacon and a little bit of sausage for flavor. This is a dish that you can divide into batches and keep in the refrigerator for about 5 days. It will be better every day, too, as the flavors intensify.

SERVES 10

3 pounds boneless skinless chicken breast, cut into ½-inch cubes

2 teaspoons dried oregano

½ teaspoon freshly ground black pepper

1 tablespoon paprika

½ teaspoon salt

3 tablespoons olive oil

3 ounces Canadian bacon, chopped

1 clove garlic, chopped

1 medium onion, chopped

1 medium green bell pepper, chopped

1 medium tomato, chopped

½ medium-spicy cooked turkey sausage, cut into ½-inch-thick slices (about 2 ounces)

¼ cup pimiento-stuffed olives, chopped

1 tablespoon capers

1 cup long-grain white rice

3 cups water or chicken stock

½ cup frozen peas

1. Toss the chicken with the oregano, pepper, paprika, ½ teaspoon salt, and 2 tablespoons of the olive oil until evenly coated. Heat a large nonstick skillet over medium-high heat and add the chicken. Cook, stirring, until lightly browned, about 5 minutes. Remove from the heat and set aside.

2. Heat the remaining tablespoon of oil in a large nonstick pot or lidded frying pan. Add the Canadian bacon and garlic and sauté until fragrant, about 1 minute. Add the onion and bell pepper and sauté until the onion and pepper are tender, 5 to 8 minutes.

3. Add the browned chicken, tomato, and sausage. Cover, reduce the heat to medium-low, and simmer for 10 minutes, stirring occasionally. Add the olives, capers, rice, salt to taste, and water or chicken stock. Bring to a simmer, cover, and simmer over low heat for 20 minutes, or until the rice is tender and the chicken is cooked through. Add the frozen peas and simmer for 5 more minutes. Taste for seasoning and serve.

Nutritional Analysis per serving ▪ Calories 288 ▪ Fat (g) 7 ▪ Saturated Fat (g) 1 ▪ Carbohydrate (g) 18 ▪ Protein (g) 36 ▪ Cholesterol (mg) 87 ▪ Fiber (g) 1

CHICKEN ENCHILADAS VERDES

Everybody loves Tex-Mex or California-Mex chicken enchiladas. What's not to like? Lots of gooey cheese and sour cream, tortillas softened in oil, yum. You can get the same degree of pleasure from these. They've got the cheese and sour cream, it's just that they're all low-fat versions. And instead of softening the tortillas in oil, I dunk them very quickly into hot water. Serve these with beans and rice for a fabulous Tex-Mex meal.

SERVES 4

½ pound tomatillos, husked and quartered, or 1 (13-ounce) can, drained

¼ cup chopped cilantro

1 (4-ounce) can chopped mild green chiles

¼ cup egg substitute

Salt

2 teaspoons olive oil

1 medium onion, chopped

3 cloves garlic, minced

1 pound boneless, skinless chicken breasts, diced

½ teaspoon ground cumin

¼ teaspoon ground coriander

¾ cup beer

Olive oil cooking spray

8 corn tortillas

¾ cup shredded reduced-fat Cheddar cheese

½ cup shredded reduced-fat Monterey Jack cheese

2 tablespoons low-fat sour cream

1. If using fresh tomatillos, preheat the broiler. Cover a baking sheet with foil. Place the quartered green tomatoes on the rack and roast for 5 minutes, or until softened. Remove from the broiler and transfer to a blender (if using drained canned tomatillos, place directly in the blender). Add the cilantro, half the green chiles, and the egg substitute. Pulse until you have a salsa with a chunky consistency. Season to taste with salt. Set aside.

2. Heat the olive oil over medium heat in a large nonstick skillet. Add the onions and sauté until tender, 3 to 5 minutes, and stir in the garlic. Sauté for 30 seconds to a minute, until fragrant, and add the chicken breast, remaining green chiles, cumin, ground coriander, and salt to taste. Turn the heat to medium-high and sauté the chicken for 5 to 10 minutes, until cooked through. Transfer to a bowl. Add the beer to the pan and bring to a boil, stirring constantly with a wooden spoon to scrape up any tasty food particles clinging to the bottom of the pan. Boil until there is only about ¼ cup of liquid in the pan. Stir the chicken back into the pan and set aside.

3. Preheat the oven to 350°F. Lightly grease a casserole or 2-quart baking dish with olive oil spray. Fill a medium-size sauté pan halfway with water and bring to a simmer. Using tongs, dip a tortilla into the water, count to 2 and remove. You must dip the tortilla quickly—the aim is to soften it so that it's easy to roll, but not to moisten it so much that it falls apart. Place about ⅓ cup of filling on each tortilla and roll up. Place in the casserole. When all of the tortillas have been filled, pour the sauce over them and place in the oven. Bake 20 minutes. Remove from the oven, top with the cheeses, and return to the oven for 10 to 15 minutes, until the cheese has melted and the enchiladas are bubbling. Serve warm, garnishing each enchilada with a small dollop of low-fat sour cream.

Nutritional Analysis per serving ▪ Calories 385 ▪ Fat (g) 12 ▪ Saturated Fat (g) 5 ▪ Carbohydrate (g) 24 ▪ Protein (g) 41 ▪ Cholesterol (mg) 87 ▪ Fiber (g) 4

CHICKEN PARMESAN

The traditional version of this dish would have you frying chicken breasts—sometimes with the skin on—in lots of olive oil or butter. In this version I'm giving your arteries a break by air-frying the chicken in the oven. The chicken breasts are incredibly moist when prepared this way.

SERVES 4

1 cup panko (Japanese bread crumbs, found in most supermarkets)

½ cup freshly grated Parmesan

2 teaspoons fresh thyme leaves or 1 teaspoon dried thyme

½ cup egg substitute

½ cup all-purpose flour

4 boneless, skinless chicken breast halves

Salt and freshly ground black pepper

1 cup marinara sauce for serving, or 1 lemon, quartered

1. Preheat the oven to 350°F. Place a wire rack over a baking sheet.

2. Mix together the panko, cheese, and thyme in a shallow bowl. Place the egg substitute in another shallow bowl and the flour in another.

3. Place the chicken breasts in a heavy plastic freezer bag, and one at a time, pound with a rolling pin, a mallet, or the palm of your hand until thin. Season each pounded chicken breast with salt and pepper, then dredge each one first in the flour, then in the egg substitute, and then in the panko mix. Place the breasts on the wire rack.

4. Bake in the oven for 15 to 20 minutes, until cooked through and crispy. Remove from the oven and serve with marinara sauce or a squeeze of lemon.

Nutritional Analysis per serving (without the marinara) ▪ Calories 295 ▪ Fat (g) 4 ▪ Saturated Fat (g) 2 ▪ Carbohydrate (g) 23 ▪ Protein (g) 37 ▪ Cholesterol (mg) 77 ▪ Fiber (g) 1

Nutritional Analysis per serving (with the marinara) ▪ Calories 331 ▪ Fat (g) 6 ▪ Saturated Fat (g) 2 ▪ Carbohydrate (g) 29 ▪ Protein (g) 38 ▪ Cholesterol (mg) 77 ▪ Fiber (g) 2

CHILAQUILES

This is my version of a south-of-the-border favorite. It's kind of like a Mexican version of lasagne and makes a great one-dish meal. I use lean ground turkey as a substitute for beef, and low-fat cheeses. For convenience I use canned tomatoes, and the dish is quickly put together.

SERVES 8

2 tablespoons canola oil

1 pound lean ground turkey

Salt

1 red onion, chopped

4 garlic cloves, minced

1½ teaspoons chili powder

½ teaspoon ground cumin

2 (15-ounce) cans tomatoes with green chiles, with juice

½ to 1 (4-ounce) can chopped mild green chiles

Cooking spray

12 corn tortillas

½ pound light cream cheese, softened

2 cups shredded low-fat Cheddar cheese

1 bunch green onions, sliced

1. Heat a large nonstick pan over medium-high heat, add 1 tablespoon of the canola oil and add the ground turkey. Brown the meat, breaking it up as it cooks, until there is no trace of pink, about 7 minutes. Drain off liquid from the pan and transfer the meat to a bowl. Season to taste with salt.

2. Add the remaining 1 tablespoon of canola oil to the pan and turn the heat to medium. Add the onion and cook, stirring often, until tender, 3 to 5 minutes. Add the garlic, chili powder, and cumin and stir together for about 30 seconds or until fragrant. Return the meat to the pan and stir together with the onions and spices until well coated. Add the tomatoes and juice and additional chiles (to taste) and simmer for 15 minutes, or until thick.

3. Preheat the oven to 350°F. Spray a 2-quart casserole with cooking spray and line with half the tortillas. Top with half the meat sauce. Add half the cream cheese, using a spoon to dollop it over the sauce, then sprinkle on half the Cheddar and half the green onions. Repeat the layers. Spray the top layer of cheese with 1 second's worth of pan spray.

4. Bake 30 minutes, until bubbling. Serve hot or warm.

Nutritional Analysis per serving ▪ Calories 290 ▪ Fat (g) 11 ▪ Saturated Fat (g) 5 ▪ Carbohydrate (g) 21 ▪ Protein (g) 25 ▪ Cholesterol (mg) 58 ▪ Fiber (g) 4

QUICK TIPS

Buy lean ground turkey breast. Regular ground turkey can include the skin and can have as much fat as ground beef.

CHILE-CHEESE RICE BURRITOS

I made these for a meat lover who needed proof that you could make a satisfying vegetarian burrito. He loved them, of course.

SERVES 6

Vegetable or olive oil cooking spray

1½ cups shredded zucchini (1 medium)

Salt

1½ cups thinly sliced green onions

2 cups cooked rice (1 cup uncooked)

¾ cup shredded fat-free Monterey Jack cheese with jalapeño peppers

2 to 4 tablespoons canned chopped green chiles, drained

¾ cup fat-free sour cream

¼ teaspoon freshly ground black pepper (to taste)

6 large burrito-style flour tortillas, preferably low-fat

1½ cups shredded lettuce

1½ cups diced fresh tomatoes

6 tablespoons salsa

1. Spray a large nonstick skillet with cooking spray and heat over medium-high heat until hot. Add the zucchini and onions and sauté 3 to 5 minutes, until tender. Add salt to taste. Turn the heat down to medium.

2. Add the rice, Monterey Jack, and chopped green chiles to taste, and stir together for 1 minute. Remove from the heat and stir in the sour cream. Add pepper, taste, and adjust seasonings.

3. Warm the tortillas in a dry skillet until flexible. Top each with one-sixth of the rice mixture, ¼ cup shredded lettuce, and ¼ cup diced tomato. Fold the sides over the filling and roll up the burrito.

4. Serve warm, with salsa.

Nutritional Analysis per serving ▪ Calories 310 ▪ Fat (g) 1 ▪ Saturated Fat (g) 0 ▪ Carbohydrate (g) 60 ▪ Protein (g) 14 ▪ Cholesterol (mg) 6 ▪ Fiber (g) 6

QUICK TIP

Since low-fat and nonfat cheeses are not easy to grate, always buy the pre-grated kind.

CHILES RELLENOS

This is "guy cooking." You get to burn things over an open flame. Chiles rellenos are traditionally deep-fried or pan-fried in a lot of oil, and stuffed with a lot of high-fat cheese and ground beef. We use ground turkey breast and low-fat cheese instead, and season it with lots of spice and chiles.

SERVES 4

4 fresh poblano chiles

1 tablespoon canola oil

½ small red onion, diced

½ pound ground turkey breast

1½ teaspoons ground cumin

1½ teaspoons dried oregano

½ teaspoon garlic powder

Salt and freshly ground black pepper

1 (14-ounce) can fire-roasted tomatoes, drained and chopped

1 (4-ounce) can chopped green chiles, drained

1 cup frozen corn kernels, thawed

1 cup grated low-fat Cheddar cheese

2 large egg whites

1 large egg

Cooking spray

1 cup tomato salsa

1. Place a wire rack over a burner. Turn on the burner and place one or two chiles on the rack. Roast, turning regularly with tongs, until the chiles are blackened all over. Repeat with the remaining chiles. Remove from the heat and allow to cool while you prepare the filling.

2. Heat a heavy nonstick skillet over medium heat and add the canola oil. Add the onion and sauté until tender, about 5 minutes. Add the ground turkey and cook, breaking up with a wooden spoon, until there are no traces of pink left in the meat. Add the spices, salt and pepper, tomatoes, chiles, and corn, and continue to cook until almost dry, about 15 to 20 minutes. Taste and adjust seasonings. Remove from the heat and stir in the grated cheese.

3. Using paper towels, scrape away the charred skin from the poblanos. Rinse under cold water if necessary, and pat dry. With the point of a paring knife, make an incision on one side of the poblano, and remove seeds and membranes, trying to keep the peppers intact. Wear rubber gloves to avoid irritating your skin.

4. Fill the peppers with the ground turkey mixture. In a wide, shallow bowl or pan, whisk together the egg whites and the whole egg. Clean and dry your sauté pan, heat over medium-high heat, and spray with pan spray. Carefully dip the stuffed peppers into the egg mixture and roll from side to side to coat evenly. Place in the hot sauté pan and sear on each side for approximately 2 minutes, until nicely browned. Serve warm, with tomato salsa.

Nutritional Analysis per serving ▪ Calories 300 ▪ Fat (g) 8 ▪ Saturated Fat (g) 2 ▪ Carbohydrate (g) 31 ▪ Protein (g) 28 ▪ Cholesterol (mg) 97 ▪ Fiber (g) 6

CHILI CON CARNE

Just by substituting lean ground turkey for ground beef here you'll be getting a huge savings on fat and calories. But make sure it's lean ground turkey, otherwise you might as well use beef. Since absence of fat can equal absence of flavor, I make sure to punch up the flavor with lots of spice and a little bit of cocoa and espresso. This sounds weird but it really adds depth of flavor. Finally, I air-bake the tortilla chips that are always served with a bowl of chili.

SERVES 4

1 tablespoon canola oil

1 pound lean ground turkey

½ red onion, diced

1 green bell pepper, diced

2 teaspoons cumin

4 cloves garlic, minced

1½ teaspoons chili powder

¼ teaspoon cinnamon (optional)

1 teaspoon cocoa powder

2 shots espresso or ½ cup coffee

1 (28-ounce) can chopped tomatoes

1 (14-ounce) can beef stock

½ to 1 teaspoon salt

8 (6-inch) corn tortillas

1 cup grated reduced-fat Cheddar cheese

1. Heat the canola oil over medium-high heat in a heavy nonstick saucepan or wide, straight-sided sauté pan. Add the ground turkey and sauté, stirring and breaking up the turkey with a wooden spoon. Sauté until all the pink has disappeared from the turkey, 5 to 8 minutes. Drain off any liquid from the pan and add the onions, bell pepper, 1 teaspoon of the cumin, the garlic, chili powder, cinnamon (if using), and the cocoa powder. Sauté together until the meat and onions are well coated and the onions become slightly translucent, about 6 minutes.

2. Add the espresso or coffee, tomatoes, and stock. Stir until well mixed. Add salt to taste, bring the mixture to a boil, then lower heat to medium-low. Simmer uncovered for 30 to 40 minutes, until thick. Taste and adjust seasonings.

3. While the chili is simmering, make the tortilla chips. Preheat the oven to 350°F. Slice the tortillas into wedges and arrange on a cookie sheet. Sprinkle the wedges with the remaining cumin. Bake until the tortilla wedges have crisped, about 10 minutes.

4. Serve the chili hot, topping each bowl with grated Cheddar and passing the tortilla chips in a bowl.

Nutritional Analysis per serving ▪ Calories 378 ▪ Fat (g) 11 ▪ Saturated Fat (g) 4 ▪ Carbohydrate (g) 28 ▪ Protein (g) 41 ▪ Cholesterol (mg) 92 ▪ Fiber (g) 6

GARDEN TURKEY BURGERS

I guarantee you that this will become a family favorite. The secret to making tasty burgers with ground turkey, which is so much lower in fat than ground beef but has so much less flavor, is to put the flavor into the turkey. I do this with teriyaki sauce and jerk seasonings. (You might want to go easy on the jerk seasonings if you're making it for the kids.) I add peppers, onions, and watercress, so the vegetables are already in the burger, and your kids won't even know the difference.

SERVES 6

1 pound lean ground turkey breast

1 cup finely chopped red onion, rinsed

½ cup finely chopped red bell pepper

1 large egg white

¼ cup chopped watercress leaves

3 tablespoons teriyaki sauce

1 to 2 teaspoons jerk seasoning (to taste)

Salt and freshly ground black pepper

Canola oil cooking spray

6 whole-wheat buns

¼ cup reduced-calorie mayonnaise

1 large tomato, sliced

Ketchup (optional)

1. In a large bowl, combine the ground turkey, chopped red onion, bell pepper, egg white, watercress leaves, teriyaki sauce, jerk seasoning, and salt and pepper to taste. Stir until well blended. Form the turkey mixture into 6 equal patties.

2. Heat a nonstick griddle or large nonstick skillet over medium-high heat and spray twice lightly with canola oil cooking spray. Place each patty on the griddle, in batches if necessary, and cook for 3 to 5 minutes on each side. The burgers should not be pink in the middle. (You can also do this on an outdoor grill.)

3. Remove the burgers from the heat. Spread the bottom half of each bun with low-fat mayonnaise and place a burger on top. Top the burger with a slice of tomato and the remaining bun. All right, pass the ketchup if you have to.

Nutritional Analysis per serving ▪ Calories 267 ▪ Fat (g) 6 ▪ Saturated Fat (g) 1 ▪ Carbohydrate (g) 30 ▪ Protein (g) 23 ▪ Cholesterol (mg) 55 ▪ Fiber (g) 4

GARLIC PESTO–STUFFED CHICKEN BREAST

"Chicken, chicken, chicken. I want to stay on the program, but I want to make something fancy." That was the statement that inspired this dish. The gentleman who was getting awfully tired of plain old chicken breasts loved pesto on anything. Truth be told, I love pesto too, but it's a very high-energy sauce with a lot of fat calories. So instead of responding that you can never have pesto and that you'll be eating plain chicken breasts forever, I took my lighter garlic pesto sauce and stuffed it inside a skinless breast of chicken. It came out like the chic dishes I've made in some of the fancier restaurants I've worked in. If you're hesitant to try stuffing the chicken breast, then just serve the sauce as a topping.

SERVES 4

4 boneless, skinless chicken breasts
1 batch Roasted Garlic Pesto (page 179)
¼ cup crumbled goat cheese

Salt and freshly ground black pepper
Vegetable cooking spray

1. Heat a cast iron griddle or skillet over high heat. Preheat the oven to 350°F.

2. Meanwhile, using a sharp paring knife or boning knife, make a crosswise slit at the end of each chicken breast, cutting through the middle to form a pocket and being careful not to cut through the outside of the chicken breast. Fill each of the pockets with 2 heaped tablespoons of the Roasted Garlic Pesto and 1 tablespoon goat cheese. Press the cut ends together, and season the chicken breasts with salt and pepper.

3. Spray the hot griddle lightly with cooking spray and add the chicken breasts. If your pan is not large enough to hold all of the chicken breasts without crowding, sauté the chicken in batches. Let the meat cook undisturbed for a few minutes. Sear to a golden brown, about 4 minutes, and turn the breasts over and cook on the other side until golden brown, about 4 minutes. Place the pan in the oven and allow the chicken to sizzle slowly for 5 to 7 minutes, or until the breasts are cooked through. They should feel firm but not hard when you press on them. Remove from the pan and serve, either whole or sliced crosswise into three pieces each.

Nutritional Analysis per serving ▪ Calories 230 ▪ Fat (g) 5 ▪ Saturated Fat (g) 2 ▪ Carbohydrate (g) 13 ▪ Protein (g) 33 ▪ Cholesterol (mg) 77 ▪ Fiber (g) 2

GARLIC-ROASTED TENDERLOIN WITH HORSERADISH CREAM

I developed this flavorful recipe as a replacement dish for standing rib roast, the type I used to prepare for Friday night buffet lines when I worked at country clubs. Tenderloin is much lower in saturated fats than standing rib, but when you eat this you'll feel like you've had a real meal, a feeling that too many diets deprive you of.

SERVES 8

6 cloves garlic, crushed

2 tablespoons freshly cracked black pepper

1 tablespoon sea salt

2 tablespoons prepared horseradish

5 tablespoons finely chopped fresh thyme

2 (3-pound) beef tenderloins, trimmed of all visible fat

Horseradish Cream (below)

1. Preheat the oven to 400°F.

2. In a small food processor or (preferably) in a mortar and pestle, puree the garlic, pepper, salt, horseradish, and thyme until smooth. Place the tenderloins on a clean work surface and rub all over with the horseradish paste. Place on a rack in a roasting pan.

3. Roast until a meat thermometer inserted into the center of the meat registers 120°F for rare, 125°F to 130°F for medium rare, or 135°F to 140°F for medium, 45 to 60 minutes. Remove from the oven and allow to rest for 10 to 15 minutes before slicing. Serve warm, with the Horseradish Cream below.

Horseradish Cream

MAKES ¾ CUP, SERVING 8

2 tablespoons prepared horseradish (to taste)

¼ cup nonfat plain yogurt

¼ cup buttermilk

Salt to taste

In a small bowl, mix together the horseradish, yogurt, and buttermilk. Add salt to taste. Cover and place in refrigerator for at least 30 minutes.

Nutritional Analysis per serving ▪ Calories 447 ▪ Fat (g) 16 ▪ Saturated Fat (g) 6 ▪ Carbohydrate (g) 4 ▪ Protein (g) 68 ▪ Cholesterol (mg) 157 ▪ Fiber (g) 1

HERB-ROASTED TURKEY BREAST

I developed this dish for a healthy holiday buffet. It's a great dish to do for a Super Bowl Sunday party.

SERVES 16

2 teaspoons salt

2 tablespoons dried thyme

2 tablespoons dried sage

2 tablespoons poultry seasoning

4 cloves garlic, minced

2 tablespoons canola oil

1 large boneless, skinless turkey breast, about 5 pounds

1 onion, chopped

4 carrots, chopped

4 stalks celery, chopped

1 (14-ounce) can chicken broth

1. Preheat the oven to 375°F. Mix together the salt, thyme, sage, poultry seasoning, and garlic with the canola oil. Rub all over the turkey breast.

2. Place the chopped onion, carrots, and celery on the bottom of a roasting pan and top with the breast. Pour the chicken broth over the vegetables. Insert a meat thermometer and place in the oven.

3. Roast until the internal temperature of the breast reaches 160°F, about 1½ hours. Remove from the oven and allow to rest for 20 minutes before carving.

Nutritional Analysis per serving ▪ Calories 178 ▪ Fat (g) 3 ▪ Saturated Fat (g) 1 ▪ Carbohydrate (g) 1 ▪ Protein (g) 34 ▪ Cholesterol (mg) 96 ▪ Fiber (g) 0

SPICY ORANGE CHICKEN LO MEIN

When I was going to culinary school in San Francisco, I worked in a mall and had lunch almost every day at a Chinese chain restaurant that served a wonderful spicy chicken lo mein. I loved the crunchy deep-fried chicken, and the sweet flavors in the lo mein. My body didn't like the calories and fat, however. So I've reworked the recipe, and still get that walk down memory lane when I eat it. But this time I marinate the chicken in concentrated orange juice for the sweet orange flavor, and instead of deep-frying the chicken I coat it with cornstarch and stir-fry it, drastically reducing the fat. You could reduce the carbs even further here by using low-carb tofu noodles instead of lo mein noodles. Try them—they're really good!

SERVES 2 AS A MAIN DISH

FOR THE CHICKEN AND MARINADE

1 cup orange juice from frozen concentrate

1 tablespoon garlic chili sauce (to taste)

½ pound boneless, skinless chicken breasts, cut in thin strips

1 tablespoon cornstarch

FOR THE LO MEIN

2 ounces lo mein noodles, either dry or frozen

¼ cup chicken stock

2 tablespoons frozen orange juice concentrate, thawed

1½ tablespoons oyster sauce

1 tablespoon soy sauce

1½ teaspoons cornstarch

1½ teaspoons grated fresh ginger

1 teaspoon garlic chili sauce

8 ounces mixed stir-fry vegetables, either fresh or frozen

1 tablespoon peanut oil

Salt and freshly ground black pepper

½ bunch green onions, sliced on the diagonal

1. Mix together the orange juice and garlic chili sauce in a medium bowl and toss with the chicken. Place in the refrigerator for 1 hour, stirring every once in a while.

2. Cook the noodles according to the instructions on the package. Drain and hold in a bowl of cold water.

3. For the sauce, mix together the chicken stock, orange juice concentrate, oyster sauce, soy sauce, cornstarch, ginger, and garlic chili sauce. Set aside.

4. Place the vegetables in a microwave-safe bowl, cover, and microwave on high until the vegetables are just crisp, about 2 to 3 minutes. This is actually steaming, my favorite way to cook vegetables because there is no fat added and all of the health benefits of the vegetables are retained. Set aside.

5. Heat a large nonstick wok or large nonstick sauté pan over high heat. Drain the chicken (this is important, because if you don't drain the chicken properly and add it with the marinade, you'll get a big sticky mess) and toss with 1 tablespoon cornstarch. When the pan is hot, add 1 tablespoon of peanut oil and swirl to coat the sides of the pan. As soon as the oil is shimmering on the surface of the pan, drop a handful of the marinated chicken (about a third) into the wok and and stir-fry until all sides of the chicken strips are nicely browned and the chicken is cooked through, 3 to 5 minutes. Remove from the pan with a stir-fry spatula or skimmer and transfer to a bowl. Repeat with the remaining two batches of chicken and set aside.

6. When all of the chicken has been cooked, turn the heat down to medium and add the sauce to the pan. Bring to a simmer, and simmer until it thickens (this happens quickly). Add salt and pepper, taste, and adjust seasonings. Add the noodles and the vegetables to the sauce and toss to warm through. Stir in the chicken, toss together, and transfer to a large platter. Garnish with the sliced green onions, and serve at once.

Nutritional Analysis per serving ▪ Calories 508 ▪ Fat (g) 8 ▪ Saturated Fat (g) 2 ▪ Carbohydrate (g) 72 ▪ Protein (g) 36 ▪ Cholesterol (mg) 66 ▪ Fiber (g) 6

OVEN-FRIED CHICKEN BREASTS

Anyone who likes chicken nuggets will appreciate these. You can achieve a crispy crust without using oil if you elevate the chicken breasts on a rack above a baking sheet. The dish is easy, doesn't make a mess, and will give you all the flavor of fried chicken without slamming your arteries shut.

SERVES 4

4 boneless, skinless chicken breasts

⅓ cup buttermilk

¼ cup seasoned bread crumbs

1 tablespoon freshly grated Parmesan

1 teaspoon paprika

1 teaspoon dried thyme

½ teaspoon garlic salt

¼ teaspoon cayenne

1. Place the chicken breasts in a resealable plastic bag and add the buttermilk. Seal the bag and lay flat to soak the chicken breasts evenly. Refrigerate for 1 to 4 hours.

2. Preheat the oven to 425°F. Place a wire rack above a sheet pan.

3. Combine the bread crumbs, Parmesan, paprika, thyme, garlic salt, and cayenne in a shallow dish. Dredge each chicken breast in this mixture, and place on the rack-lined sheet pan. Bake 20 minutes (15 for the thinner tenders), or until the bread crumb mixture is nicely browned and the chicken breasts are cooked through.

ALTERNATIVE METHOD Substitute 1 cup egg substitute for the buttermilk. Do not marinate the chicken breasts. If you wish, cut them in half lengthwise (butterfly them) for a very thin piece of meat. Dip the chicken breasts in the egg substitute, then dredge them in the bread crumb mix. Place on the rack and cook as directed.

Nutritional Analysis per serving ▪ Calories 175 ▪ Fat (g) 3 ▪ Saturated Fat (g) 1 ▪ Carbohydrate (g) 7 ▪ Protein (g) 30 ▪ Cholesterol (mg) 70 ▪ Fiber (g) 1

NOTE This is a nice recipe to do for one person. Marinate 1 chicken breast, in a plastic zipper bag, with 1½ tablespoons buttermilk. For each chicken breast, use 1 tablespoon bread crumbs, ¾ teaspoon Parmesan, ¼ teaspoon paprika, ¼ teaspoon thyme, ⅛ teaspoon garlic salt, and a pinch of cayenne.

PORK FRIED RICE

I love fatty Chinese take-out food, so I'm always looking for ways to rework my favorite dishes. Here I use a lean cut of pork instead of the traditional pork butt, which is not at all lean. I reduce the amount of oil that a Chinese recipe usually calls for, and replace whole eggs with egg substitute, so you don't get the cholesterol from egg yolks. Texture is very important in my cuisine, and brown rice has more of that—and more nutrients—than white rice.

SERVES 4

¾ pound center cut pork loin, cut into bite-size pieces

2 tablespoons hoisin sauce

1 tablespoon low-sodium soy sauce

2 tablespoon grated or minced fresh ginger

1 tablespoon minced garlic

1 tablespoon canola oil

5 green onions, sliced

1 tablespoon sesame oil

1 carrot, shredded

½ cup frozen peas, thawed

1 cup brown rice, cooked and cooled

½ cup egg substitute, such as Egg Beaters

1. Toss the pork with 1 tablespoon of the hoisin sauce, 1 teaspoon of the soy sauce, 1 tablespoon of the ginger and 2 teaspoons of the garlic. Mix well.

2. Heat a heavy nonstick wok or large nonstick sauté pan over medium-high heat and add ½ teaspoon of the canola oil. Add the pork and stir-fry until cooked through, 2 to 3 minutes. Remove from the wok, set aside, and keep warm.

3. Add the remaining canola oil to the wok and turn the heat to medium. Add the green onions and stir-fry until crisp-tender, about 1 minute. Add the remaining ginger and garlic and stir-fry for about 30 seconds, then stir in the remaining hoisin and soy sauces and the sesame oil, and stir together. Add the carrots, peas, and rice, and stir-fry until heated through, about 2 minutes. Add the egg substitute and stir constantly until scrambled. Stir the pork back into the wok, toss together, and serve.

Nutritional Analysis per serving ▪ Calories 411 ▪ Fat (g) 14 ▪ Saturated Fat (g) 3 ▪ Carbohydrate (g) 47 ▪ Protein (g) 23 ▪ Cholesterol (mg) 43 ▪ Fiber (g) 4

ROAST BEEF WITH ROOT VEGGIE GRAVY

I first came up with this variation on gravy when my father-in-law was put on a very fat-restricted diet. It was Thanksgiving, and I knew how much he loves gravy. In my book, gravy meant lots of roux, which meant lots of butter. So I thought of using root vegetables as a thickener instead of roux. I know some of you will be asking, "But what about the carbs in the root vegetables?" Yes, there are some, but the main one I use is sweet potato, which has a low glycemic index. And it's worth the tradeoff in fat. Remember, fat makes fat. I also use a sirlon tip roast rather than a standing rib, cutting out some of the saturated fat in standing rib. And by the way, this gravy is so good that I eat the leftovers as a soup!

SERVES 8

3-pound sirloin tip roast, trimmed of fat

2 tablespoons cracked black pepper

1 tablespoon kosher or sea salt, plus additional for the gravy

10 cloves garlic, minced

Olive oil or canola cooking spray

1 cup peeled, diced sweet potato

½ cup peeled, sliced parsnip

½ large or 1 small onion, diced

½ cup peeled, sliced carrot

A few dashes nutmeg

1 teaspoon fresh thyme

2 to 3 cups beef stock, as needed

1. Preheat the oven to 400°F. Trim all of the visible fat from the sirloin. Mix together the pepper, salt, and garlic and spread all over the roast. Cover with plastic wrap and refrigerate while you roast the vegetables.

2. Spray a sheet pan or baking pan with olive oil or canola cooking spray. Toss the sweet potatoes, parsnip, onion, and carrot together with the nutmeg and thyme. Spray with the cooking spray and toss again. Spray one more time and toss together again. Spread on the baking sheet in an even layer. Cover with foil. Place in the oven and roast for 30 to 40 minutes, stirring every 10 to 15 minutes, until browned and tender. Meanwhile, heat 2 cups of the beef stock to a simmer in a medium saucepan.

3. When the vegetables are tender, remove from the heat and scrape into a bowl. Ladle a little bit of the hot stock into the baking pan and scrape up any tasty vegetable bits that are sticking to the bottom of the pan. Add to the bowl with the vegetables. Set aside.

4. Place a rack on the roasting pan or sheet pan, unwrap the meat, and place on the rack. Roast for 15 minutes. Insert a meat thermometer and turn the heat down to 325°F. Roast until the meat reaches an internal temperature of 125°F for rare, 130°F for medium rare; about 30 more minutes. Remove from the oven, tent with a sheet of aluminum foil, and allow to rest for 15 minutes.

3. Meanwhile, make the gravy. Add the remaining warm broth to the vegetables and puree until smooth, either with a hand blender or in a regular blender, in batches. Transfer to the saucepan and heat through. Thin out with additional broth. Taste and add salt as desired.

4. Slice the meat and arrange on a platter. Pour any remaining juices from the meat into the gravy and mix well. Pour some of the gravy over the meat and serve, passing additional gravy in a bowl.

> **VARIATIONS** For the truly fat observant, I recommend buffalo meat. It's increasingly available online and at specialty butchers, and it's very tasty and low in fat.
>
> You can also use this for turkey, substituting chicken stock for the beef stock.

Nutritional Analysis per serving ▪ Calories 289 ▪ Fat (g) 7 ▪ Saturated Fat (g) 3 ▪ Carbohydrate (g) 15 ▪ Protein (g) 39 ▪ Cholesterol (mg) 63 ▪ Fiber (g) 3

QUICK SHOYU CHICKEN

This flavorful dish makes a great party recipe. It's easy to increase the recipe, and can be cooked ahead, reheated, and garnished just before serving. It also packs nicely in a lunchbox, and kids like it (maybe without the garnishes for the little ones).

SERVES 8

2 pounds boneless, skinless chicken breast, diced

¼ cup low-sodium soy sauce

3 tablespoons honey

1½ teaspoons hoisin sauce

1 star anise

1 tablespoon minced fresh ginger

5 green onions, thinly sliced

½ cup chopped cilantro

1. Preheat the oven to 375°F. In a large baking dish, toss together the chicken, soy sauce, honey, hoisin sauce, star anise, and ginger. Bake for 25 to 35 miutes, until the chicken is cooked through.

2. Remove from the heat, garnish with green onions and cilantro, and serve.

Nutritional Analysis per serving ▪ Calories 162 ▪ Fat (g) 1 ▪ Saturated Fat (g) 0 ▪ Carbohydrate (g) 9 ▪ Protein (g) 27 ▪ Cholesterol (mg) 66 ▪ Fiber (g) 1

SLOW-BRAISED CARNITAS

When I worked in a Mexican restaurant I had carnitas and flan every night for dinner. I love carnitas, but unless I figured out a way to make them without all the lard, I'd have to give them up. Impossible! These are made with pork loin, a much leaner cut of pork than the pork butt that is traditionally used. I threw in lots of flavor to make up for the fat, and gave everything a long, slow cook in a slow cooker.

SERVES 6

1 pound, 2 ounces boneless lean pork loin, cut in large dice

1 (28-ounce) can red enchilada sauce

1 (14-ounce) can beef stock

Salt

1 Anaheim chili, cut in large dice

1 green bell pepper, cut in large dice

1 yellow bell pepper, cut in large dice

4 Roma tomatoes, cut in large dice

½ bunch cilantro, chopped

6 whole-wheat pita breads

1. Combine the pork, enchilada sauce, beef stock, salt to taste, and Anaheim chili in a slow cooker and simmer on low for 3 hours, until the meat is falling apart. If you don't have a slow cooker, use a heavy Dutch oven. Simmer over low heat for 2 hours, or until the meat is falling apart. Remove the meat from the sauce and shred.

2. Toss together the bell peppers, tomatoes, and cilantro to make a salsa. Season to taste with salt. Stuff the pitas with the shredded meat and the salsa, and serve.

Nutritional Analysis per serving ▪ Calories 362 ▪ Fat (g) 8 ▪ Saturated Fat (g) 2 ▪ Carbohydrate (g) 48 ▪ Protein (g) 26 ▪ Cholesterol (mg) 48 ▪ Fiber (g) 8

SPICY KOREAN RICE WITH FLANK STEAK

Fat isn't the only nutrient that leaves you with a full feeling; fiber does too. And this dish is full of fiber, flavor, color, and crunch.

SERVES 6

1 tablespoon soy sauce

1 tablespoon garlic chili sauce, such as Lee Kum Kee

6 ounces trimmed flank steak, thinly sliced

½ cup broccoli florets

½ cup sugar snap peas

½ cup sliced carrots

½ cup sliced cucumbers

½ teaspoon sesame oil

1 teaspoon toasted sesame seeds

1 tablespoon canola oil

2 cups cooked rice

1 cup thinly sliced mushrooms

1 cup baby spinach

1. Stir together the soy sauce and 2½ teaspoons of the chili sauce. Toss with the steak and marinate in the refrigerator for 1 hour, stirring occasionally.

2. Place the broccoli, snap peas, and carrots in a microwave-safe dish. Add 2 tablespoons water, cover with plastic, and microwave at 100% power for 2 minutes, until crisp-tender. Rinse with cold water and drain.

3. Mix the microwaved vegetables with the cucumbers, sesame oil, remaining chili sauce, and the sesame seeds. Cover and set aside.

4. Heat a large nonstick skillet over high heat and add the canola oil. As soon as it shimmers, add the beef. Cook for 2 to 3 minutes, stirring constantly. Scoop the beef out of the pan and transfer to a bowl. Add the rice to the pan and heat through, stirring constantly.

5. Divide the rice evenly among 6 plates or wide bowls. Top with the vegetables, then the beef. Garnish with mushrooms and spinach.

Nutritional Analysis per serving ▪ Calories 152 ▪ Fat (g) 5 ▪ Saturated Fat (g) 1 ▪ Carbohydrate (g) 18 ▪ Protein (g) 8 ▪ Cholesterol (mg) 11 ▪ Fiber (g) 1

SWEET POTATO SHEPHERD'S PIE

Sometimes you just crave something big, meaty, and comforting. This dish fits that definition, but I've made some Calorie Countdown changes to the traditional dish. Sweet potatoes may be sweet, but they have more fiber and fewer carbohydrates than the starchy potatoes traditionally used in shepherd's pie, and I mash them up with buttermilk, not cream. I substitute turkey for the beef, so the saturated fats are also way down.

SERVES 6

2½ pounds sweet potatoes, scrubbed

Pan spray

Salt and freshly ground black pepper

1 cup buttermilk

2 teaspoons ground cinnamon

1 tablespoon light butter, melted

1 tablespoon olive oil

2 cloves garlic, minced

2 cups chopped mushrooms

1 large carrot, diced

2 tablespoons tomato paste

2 tablespoons steak sauce

1 tablespoon all-purpose flour

1 cup beef broth

1 pound turkey thighs or chicken thighs, roasted and shredded (see page 210)

1 tablespoon light butter for topping

1. Preheat the oven to 425°F. Cover a baking sheet with foil. Pierce the sweet potatoes in a few places with a knife, and place on the foil. Bake until tender and beginning to ooze, about 45 minutes. Remove from the heat and allow to cool until you can handle them. Turn the oven down to 375°F. Lightly oil a 2-quart casserole with pan spray.

2. Cut the sweet potatoes in half and scoop the flesh out from the skins. Transfer to a bowl and mash with a potato masher. Add the salt and pepper, buttermilk, cinnamon, and light butter and mix in until well blended (you can do this in a mixer fitted with the paddle attachment). Taste, adjust seasoning, and set aside.

3. Heat the olive oil over medium heat in a large nonstick skillet. Add the garlic and sauté for 30 seconds, until fragrant. Add the mushrooms and carrots and cook, stirring, until the mushrooms are soft, 5 to 10 minutes. Add the tomato paste and steak sauce and stir together to coat all of the vegetables. Sprinkle the flour over the vegetables and cook, stirring, until the flour begins to smell a little toasty, about 2 minutes. Slowly pour in the stock, stirring constantly with a wooden spoon. Add the shredded turkey and season with salt and pepper. Simmer the mixture until the sauce is thick, 5 to 10 minutes. Taste and adjust seasoning.

4. Transfer the turkey mixture to the 2-quart casserole. Top with the sweet potatoes and smooth them over to form a layer that covers the turkey mixture completely. Dot with little pieces of light butter. Place in the oven and bake 45 to 50 minutes, or until the top is nicely browned. Serve hot.

Nutritional Analysis per serving ▪ Calories 365 ▪ Fat (g) 8 ▪ Saturated Fat (g) 3 ▪ Carbohydrate (g) 55 ▪ Protein (g) 18 ▪ Cholesterol (mg) 40 ▪ Fiber (g) 7

ROASTED TURKEY OR CHICKEN THIGHS

CHICKEN THIGHS

Preheat the oven to 350°F. Cover a baking sheet with foil and lightly oil the foil. Season the thighs generously with salt and pepper on both sides. Place skin side down on the foil. Bake chicken thighs for 20 minutes, turn over and bake for another 20 minutes, until the juice runs clear when pierced with a knife. Remove the skin and proceed as directed.

TURKEY THIGHS

These will take longer, and it's best if you use a meat thermometer. Roast until the meat reaches an internal temperature of 170°F, about 1 hour.

LIGHT BEEF TACO WRAPS

In these light tacos, I replace the crunchiness of a deep-fried taco shell with a crisp iceberg let-tuce leaf and with the jicama in the filling. That saves a ton of calories, but you have to replace the satisfaction you get from fats with something else. So I pack in a lot of flavor with the spices.

SERVES 4

1 pound eye of round beef, trimmed of all visible fat and sliced into thin 1-inch strips

1 teaspoon ground cumin

1 teaspoon chipotle chili powder

½ teaspoon ground cinnamon

Salt and freshly ground black pepper

1½ tablespoons canola oil

1 large tomato, diced

½ cup diced jicama

Juice of 1 lime

¼ to ½ cup chopped cilantro

12 large iceberg lettuce leaves

1 cup shredded low-fat Cheddar cheese

1. In a medium bowl, toss together the beef strips, cumin, chipotle chili powder, cinna-mon, and salt and pepper to taste.

2. Heat a heavy medium nonstick skillet over medium heat and add the canola oil. When the oil is hot, add the beef strips. Sauté until the beef strips are thoroughly cooked, about 2 minutes. Add the tomatoes, jicama, and lime juice. Cook for another minute. Remove from the heat and stir in cilantro to taste. Taste and adjust seasonings.

3. Place ½ cup of the beef mixture on each lettuce leaf. Top each with 1½ tablespoons of the shredded cheese, and serve.

Nutritional Analysis per serving ▪ Calories 260 ▪ Fat (g) 11 ▪ Saturated Fat (g) 3 ▪ Carbohy-drate (g) 7 ▪ Protein (g) 33 ▪ Cholesterol (mg) 53 ▪ Fiber (g) 2

TEA-SMOKED CHICKEN

This dish never ceases to surprise people. How can it be so juicy and so low in fat? Whenever you smoke foods—and it's easy to do—make sure to open your kitchen window and that you know how to shut off your smoke alarm. It's not dangerous to do the dish, but the smoke alarm may not know that. You can also use this method for trout or salmon.

SERVES 4

2 whole chicken breasts, split and skinned

Salt

1 teaspoon Szechuan peppercorns, crushed

1 teaspoon five-spice powder

½ cup black Chinese tea leaves

½ cup brown sugar

½ cup uncooked rice

¼ cup minced fresh ginger

2 teaspoons sesame oil

1. Rinse the chicken breasts and pat dry. Season with salt. Mix together the peppercorns and five-spice powder and rub over the chicken breasts. Set aside.

2. Line a wok with aluminum foil. Mix together the tea, brown sugar, rice, and ginger and place in the wok. Place the wok over medium heat and heat until the mixture begins to smoke. Place the chicken on a rack three inches over the mixture, rounded side up. Cover with a lid and seal the edges with aluminum foil.

3. Smoke for 20 minutes. Check for doneness (there should be no traces of pink in the chicken). If the chicken is not done, smoke for 5 minutes more. When the chicken is done, transfer to plates and brush with sesame oil. Serve with steamed vegetables and rice.

Nutritional Analysis per serving ■ Calories 285 ■ Fat (g) 5 ■ Saturated Fat (g) 1 ■ Carbohydrate (g) 1 ■ Protein (g) 55 ■ Cholesterol (mg) 137 ■ Fiber (g) 0

TEQUILA CHICKEN FAJITAS

I was tired of the same old boring chicken fajitas, so I came up with this zesty tequila marinade. Tequila adds a unique flavor and not much in the way of calories, since it's used as a marinade. There's lots of vitamin C and crunch here, and of course, being my food, spice. Pull back on the heat if you want to.

SERVES 4

¾ pound boneless, skinless chicken breasts, cut across the grain in thin strips

¼ cup tequila

¼ cup fresh lime juice

1 tablespoon Worcestershire sauce

½ teaspoon red pepper flakes

1 teaspoon chili powder

½ teaspoon salt

¼ teaspoon freshly ground black pepper

4 cloves garlic, minced

2 teaspoons canola oil

1 red bell pepper, sliced in strips

1 yellow bell pepper, sliced in strips

½ medium red onion, sliced in strips

4 (6-inch) corn tortillas

¼ cup chopped cilantro

1. Place the chicken breasts in a heavy-duty resealable plastic bag. Mix together the tequila, lime juice, Worcestershire sauce, red pepper flakes, chili powder, salt, pepper, and garlic in a bowl. Pour into the bag with the chicken breasts and place in the refrigerator for 45 minutes or longer.

2. Heat a large nonstick skillet over medium-high heat and add the canola oil. When it's hot, sauté the bell peppers and onion until crisp-tender, 3 to 5 minutes. Remove from the pan and keep warm.

3. Remove the chicken breast strips from the marinade and discard the marinade. Cook in the same pan in which you cooked the vegetables for about 6 minutes, or until there is no trace of pink left. Return the onions and bell peppers to the pan and heat through for about 1 minute. Season with salt and pepper to taste.

4. Warm the tortillas and place on plates. Divide the chicken mixture evenly among the tortillas, sprinkle with cilantro, and serve.

> **VARIATIONS** Tequila Steak Fajitas: Substitute ¾ pound flank steak for the chicken breasts.
>
> Tequila Shrimp Fajitas: Substitute ¾ pound shrimp for the chicken. Cook the shrimp for 2 minutes, or just until pink.

Nutritional Analysis per serving ▪ Calories 168 ▪ Fat (g) 4 ▪ Saturated Fat (g) 1 ▪ Carbohydrate (g) 12 ▪ Protein (g) 21 ▪ Cholesterol (mg) 49 ▪ Fiber (g) 2

MY MOM'S TORTILLA CASSEROLE

This comforting dish is a family favorite, but the authentic recipe is made with cream of mushroom soup, sour cream, and lots of fatty cheese. This low-fat version fools me into thinking I'm eating the original.

SERVES 6 TO 8

Canola oil spray

1½ cups chicken stock

1 tablespoon cornstarch

1 cup nonfat milk

½ cup drained nonfat plain yogurt (see page 215)

1 (14-ounce) can chopped tomatoes, with juice

1 (4-ounce) can chopped mild green chiles, drained

¼ cup chopped cilantro

1 tablespoon chili powder

1 teaspoon oregano

1½ teaspoons ground cumin

Salt and freshly ground black pepper

1½ teaspoons vegetable or canola oil

1 large onion, chopped

1 red bell pepper, diced

2 garlic cloves, minced

12 corn tortillas, quartered

1 whole boneless, skinless chicken breast, poached (see page 215) and shredded or diced (2 cups)

½ cup shredded reduced-fat Cheddar cheese

½ cup chopped green bell pepper

1. Preheat the oven to 375°F. Spray a 2-quart baking dish with oil spray. Bring the chicken stock to a simmer in a medium saucepan. Blend the cornstarch with 2 tablespoons of the milk and whisk it in along with the rest of the milk. Stir until the mixture is thick and smooth. Remove from the heat.

2. Whisk the yogurt, tomatoes, chiles, cilantro, chili powder, oregano, and cumin into the thickened stock. Season to taste with salt and pepper.

3. Heat a large nonstick skillet over medium heat and add the oil and the onions. Stir together for a few minutes, until the onions begin to wilt, and add the red bell pepper and salt to taste. Cook, stirring, until tender, about 5 minutes. Add the garlic and cook for another minute, until fragrant. Remove from the heat.

4. Line the bottom of your prepared baking dish with half the tortillas. Top with half the chicken and half the vegetables. Pour on half the sauce and repeat the layers. Top with the cheese. Spray the cheese lightly with canola oil spray.

5. Place in the oven and bake for 30 minutes, until bubbly. Sprinkle the chopped green peppers over the top and serve.

Nutritional Analysis per serving ▪ Calories 221 ▪ Fat (g) 5 ▪ Saturated Fat (g) 2 ▪ Carbohydrate (g) 28 ▪ Protein (g) 18 ▪ Cholesterol (mg) 29 ▪ Fiber (g) 5

Poached Chicken Breasts

5 cups water

1 onion, quartered

2 garlic cloves, peeled and crushed

1 whole chicken breast, skinned and split, or 2 boneless, skinless chicken breast halves

1 teaspoon salt

Combine the water, onion, and garlic in a 2-quart saucepan and bring to a simmer over medium heat. Add the chicken breasts and salt, and bring back to a simmer (not a boil). Cover partially, reduce the heat to low, and poach for 12 to 15 minutes, until the chicken is cooked through. Remove from the heat. Allow the chicken breasts to cool in the broth if there is time. Remove from the broth and when cool enough to handle, shred or dice.

DRAINED YOGURT

Drained yogurt, sometimes called yogurt cheese, is yogurt that has been thickened by draining out much of its water content. It tastes like thick, full-fat yogurt. Line a strainer with cheesecloth and place over a bowl. Place a cup of nonfat yogurt in the strainer and refrigerate for several hours or overnight. In the morning your bowl will be full of water, and your yogurt will be thick. 1 cup yogurt will make ½ cup thickened yogurt.

TURKEY OR CHICKEN FOR ONE

I call this "toaster oven turkey." To ensure quick, healthy dinners throughout the week, on Monday I take turkey or chicken cutlets and bag them up in plastic zipper bags with this combination of barbecue and chili sauce. When I'm ready for dinner I pull one out and cook it in my toaster oven. This takes all of 10 minutes. While the meat is cooking I thaw some frozen veggies and do a quick sauté with my favorite salad dressing. It makes a quick, light meal that always satisfies.

SERVES 1

½ cup barbecue sauce

1 teaspoon Southeast Asian chili sauce (to taste)

2 turkey or chicken breast cutlets, about 3 ounces each

Cooking spray

1. Stir together the barbecue sauce and the chili sauce, and place in a plastic zipper bag. Place the turkey or chicken breast cutlets in the bag, seal, and turn it over a few times to coat the cutlets. Refrigerate until ready to use.

2. Preheat the toaster oven to 350°F (or use your regular oven). Remove the cutlets from the bag and place on a lightly oiled baking sheet. Bake 10 minutes, or until cooked through. Serve with vegetables and/or a salad.

Nutritional Analysis per serving ▪ Calories 125 ▪ Fat (g) 1 ▪ Saturated Fat (g) 0 ▪ Carbohydrate (g) 7 ▪ Protein (g) 20 ▪ Cholesterol (mg) 58 ▪ Fiber (g) 0

TURKEY MEATLOAF

Meatloaf calls for dark meat. So how do you achieve a meatloaf if you're substituting lean ground turkey for the beef? I do it by adding very finely chopped mushrooms and eggplant to the mix. The vegetables give it a meatier texture, and also add lots of moisture and flavor.

SERVES 6

1 portobello mushroom, stem trimmed, coarsely chopped

1 eggplant, peeled and coarsely chopped

1 tablespoon canola oil

½ medium or ¼ large red onion, finely chopped

2 cloves garlic, minced

Salt and freshly ground black pepper to taste (be generous)

Cooking spray

1 pound lean ground turkey

¼ cup tomato paste

2 teaspoons chopped fresh oregano or 1 teaspoon dried

1 tablespoon chopped fresh basil

1 tablespoon oyster sauce or hoisin sauce

1 large egg

1 tablespoon Worcestershire sauce

1 teaspoon paprika

1. Combine the mushroom and eggplant in a food processor fitted with the steel blade and chop very fine.

2. Heat the oil over medium heat in a large nonstick skillet and add the onion. Cook, stirring, until translucent, 3 to 5 minutes, and add the garlic, mushrooms, and eggplant. Add about 1 teaspoon salt, and pepper to taste, and cook, stirring, until the vegetables are tender, 5 to 10 minutes. Return to the food processor and process to a puree.

3. Preheat the oven to 350°F. Spray a loaf pan with pan spray and line the bottom with parchment. Spray the parchment. In a large bowl, combine the mushroom mixture with the turkey and the remaining ingredients. Season generously with salt and pepper. Spoon into the loaf pan and smooth the top.

4. Bake 45 to 50 minutes, until the loaf reaches an internal temperature of 160°F. Let cool in the pan until the moisture is reabsorbed, at least 15 minutes.

Nutritional Analysis per serving ▪ Calories 236 ▪ Fat (g) 6 ▪ Saturated Fat (g) 1 ▪ Carbohydrate (g) 13 ▪ Protein (g) 31 ▪ Cholesterol (mg) 130 ▪ Fiber (g) 5

TURKEY TACOS FIESTA

Sometimes you just want the crunch of tortilla chips. So I air-bake the tortillas to get the crunch without the fat. It takes a while, but it's worth it. Have a party with these low-fat tacos. Present the crispy air-baked tortillas on a tray, the ground turkey topping and garnishes in bowls, and let guests assemble their own tacos.

SERVES 4

8 corn tortillas

2 teaspoons canola oil

½ medium red onion, finely chopped

½ teaspoon ground cumin

½ teaspoon paprika

½ teaspoon ground cinnamon

1 pound lean ground turkey

Salt and freshly ground black pepper

½ cup prepared salsa

⅓ cup chopped cilantro

¾ avocado, diced

¼ cup nonfat sour cream

1 cup shredded nonfat Cheddar cheese

1 lime, cut in wedges

1. Preheat the oven to 350°F. Place the tortillas on the middle rack and bake until crispy, about 10 minutes. Remove from the heat and set out on a tray or plate.

2. Heat the canola oil over medium heat in a nonstick skillet and add the onion. Cook, stirring, until translucent and tender, 3 to 5 minutes. Add the cumin, paprika, and cinnamon and stir to blend. Then add the ground turkey, season with salt and pepper, and cook, stirring and breaking up with a wooden spoon, until all of the pink is gone, about 10 minutes.

3. If any fat has rendered out of the meat, drain it out of the pan. Add the salsa to the pan and stir together. Taste and adjust seasoning. Sprinkle with cilantro. Transfer to a serving bowl. Place on a buffet next to the tortillas, with the avocado, the sour cream, the cheese, and the lime wedges, each in their own bowls.

4. Top the crisp tortillas with a spoonful of the turkey and salsa mixture and a spoonful each of avocado and sour cream. Sprinkle on the cheese, squeeze on some fresh lime juice, and serve.

Nutritional Analysis per serving ▪ Calories 345 ▪ Fat (g) 10 ▪ Saturated Fat (g) 1 ▪ Carbohydrate (g) 24 ▪ Protein (g) 40 ▪ Cholesterol (mg) 84 ▪ Fiber (g) 5

BRAISED SHRIMP

This is an easy one-pan meal, with lots of flavor and texture and lean protein. You could double the recipe easily and serve it for a dinner party. As long as everybody eats shrimp, they'll love it.

SERVES 4

12 jumbo shrimp or 16 large shrimp (1 pound), shelled and deveined

Salt and freshly ground black pepper

2 tablespoons olive oil

1 medium onion, diced

1 green bell pepper, diced

4 cloves garlic, minced

4 ounces Canadian bacon, diced

1 large tomato, chopped

1 (15-ounce) can crushed tomatoes, with juice

2 teaspoons chopped fresh oregano, or 1 teaspoon dried

1 tablespoon chopped cilantro (optional)

1 to 2 tablespoons fresh lemon juice

1. Season the shrimp with salt and pepper and let sit in the refrigerator while you prepare the remaining ingredients.

2. Heat the oil over medium heat in a 12-inch nonstick skillet. Add the onions and bell peppers, and sauté until crisp-tender, about 5 minutes. Add the garlic and stir for another minute, until fragrant. Add the Canadian bacon, tomato, crushed tomatoes, oregano, and salt and pepper, and bring to a simmer. Reduce the heat and simmer 10 to 15 minutes, until the tomatoes have cooked down somewhat. Add the cilantro and lemon juice to taste, stir together, taste, and adjust seasonings.

3. Add the shrimp and continue to simmer for 5 to 10 minutes, turning them over once or until the shrimp are cooked through. Serve warm.

Nutritional Analysis per serving ▪ Calories 246 ▪ Fat (g) 9 ▪ Saturated Fat (g) 2 ▪ Carbohydrate (g) 15 ▪ Protein (g) 26 ▪ Cholesterol (mg) 183 ▪ Fiber (g) 4

BROCCOLI-HALIBUT STIR-FRY

Here's a great dinner when you want something quick and easy, with lots of light protein. I developed it for a guy who loved Chinese food, to prove that you could actually make a Chinese meal in less time than it would take to order and receive Chinese take-out.

SERVES 4

2 tablespoons teriyaki sauce

2 tablespoons oyster sauce

1 tablespoon plus 1 teaspoon cornstarch

2 teaspoons seasoned rice wine vinegar

1 teaspoon sesame oil

1 tablespoon canola oil

1 pound halibut fillet, cubed

1 cup broccoli florets

1 cup snow peas

1 red bell pepper, sliced in strips

1 teaspoon grated fresh ginger

1. In a small bowl, mix the teriyaki sauce, oyster sauce, 1 teaspoon cornstarch, the rice vinegar, and sesame oil until well blended. Set aside.

2. Heat the canola oil in a nonstick wok or large nonstick sauté pan over medium-high heat. Toss the halibut in the remaining cornstarch and add to hot oil. Sear quickly on all sides, about 3 minutes total. Remove halibut from the wok and set aside. Add the broccoli, snow peas, bell pepper, and ginger to the wok with ¼ cup of water and cover. Steam vegetables until crisp-tender, about 3 minutes. Add the teriyaki sauce mixture and stir until the vegetables are well coated. Simmer over low heat until the sauce thickens. Once the sauce has thickened, return the halibut to the wok and cook until warmed through. Serve immediately.

Nutritional Analysis per serving ▪ Calories 221 ▪ Fat (g) 7 ▪ Saturated Fat (g) 1 ▪ Carbohydrate (g) 12 ▪ Protein (g) 26 ▪ Cholesterol (mg) 36 ▪ Fiber (g) 2

CRAB AND AVOCADO QUESADILLAS

In this dish we save a lot of fat by not deep-frying the tortillas, and by using low-fat cheese instead of regular cheese. Avocados give us the satisfaction we like to get from fat, but the fats in avocados are good fats.

SERVES 4

4 ounces lump crabmeat, drained

1 (4-ounce) can chopped green chiles, drained

1 ripe avocado, diced small

Salt

Fresh lime juice

8 (6-inch) corn tortillas

1½ cups shredded low-fat Monterey Jack cheese

½ cup fat-free sour cream

¼ teaspoon chili powder

1. Heat a sturdy cast-iron pan or griddle over medium-high heat while you prepare the ingredients. Mix together the crab, canned chiles, and avocado. Season to taste with salt and lime juice.

2. When the griddle is hot, place up to 4 tortillas on it (or however many will fit) and warm until they begin to puff and the edges begin to brown. Flip the tortillas over and sprinkle with half the cheese. Top with the crab mixture and sprinkle on the remaining cheese. Top with the remaining tortillas, press down lightly, and flip the quesadillas over.

3. Heat through on the other side for 2 to 3 minutes, until the cheese melts. Transfer to plates and using a pair of kitchen scissors, quarter the quesadillas. Top with fat-free sour cream and dust with chili powder.

Nutritional Analysis per serving ▪ Calories 263 ▪ Fat (g) 10 ▪ Saturated Fat (g) 3 ▪ Carbohydrate (g) 23 ▪ Protein (g) 21 ▪ Cholesterol (mg) 35 ▪ Fiber (g) 5

FENNEL-ROASTED SEA BASS

Fennel is a traditional Mediterranean ingredient used to accompany sea bass. In addition to the fennel we have other typical Mediterranean ingredients here, like zucchini, fresh oregano, thyme, dill, and lots of garlic. Then, just to confuse you, I've thrown some green tomatillos into the mix. Olive oil is a healthy fat, and adds richness to the dish.

SERVES 6

Olive oil or cooking spray

¼ cup olive oil

4 medium-size fennel bulbs, trimmed, quartered, cored, and sliced

Salt and freshly ground black pepper

1 whole sea bass, about 2½ pounds, cleaned and scaled

2 bunches fresh oregano

1 bunch fresh thyme

1 bunch fresh dill

3 heads garlic, sliced in half

5 medium zucchini, sliced into ½-inch rounds

5 medium tomatillos, cut in half

½ cup green olives

1 cup water

1. Preheat the oven to 425°F. Spray a large roasting pan, large enough to accommodate the fish, with olive oil or cooking spray. Heat 2 tablespoons of the olive oil over medium heat in a large nonstick skillet. Add the fennel and cook, stirring often, until crisp-tender, about 5 minutes. Season to taste with salt and pepper, and transfer to the roasting pan.

2. Season the sea bass on both sides with salt and pepper. Make three 3-inch-long incisions on each side of the fish. Insert a slice of fennel into each incision. Lay fish on top of the fennel. Drizzle the remaining olive oil over the fish. Surround and cover the fish with the herbs, garlic, zucchini, tomatillos, and olives. Pour the water into the roasting pan and cover tightly.

3. Place in the oven and bake 30 to 40 minutes, until the fish is opaque and pulls apart easily when poked with a fork.

4. To serve, transfer the fish to a platter. Discard the herbs. Taste the vegetables and adjust seasonings, then arrange on the platter around the fish. Cut 3 pieces of fish from each side and serve with the vegetables.

Nutritional Analysis per serving (for 6 servings) ▪ Calories 406 ▪ Fat (g) 16 ▪ Saturated Fat (g) 3 ▪ Carbohydrate (g) 27 ▪ Protein (g) 43 ▪ Cholesterol (mg) 82 ▪ Fiber (g) 8

GARLIC SHRIMP SCAMPI

You don't need a lot of cream for shrimp scampi. What you need is a bunch of shrimp and a lot of flavor. We're also saving calories by using tofu noodles, one of my favorite new discoveries. They take on all the flavors of the scampi. Just don't tell your friends they're tofu. You'll find them in the tofu section of the supermarket.

SERVES 4

1 tablespoon olive oil

4 to 6 cloves garlic, minced

½ to 1 teaspoon red pepper flakes (more to taste)

2 Roma tomatoes, peeled, seeded, and chopped

2 tablespoons chopped fresh basil leaves

Salt and freshly ground pepper

1½ pounds medium or large shrimp, peeled and deveined

3 tablespoons chopped fresh parsley

Juice of ½ lemon

1 tablespoon finely chopped lemon zest

1 (8-ounce) package soy noodles, cooked and drained

Heat the oil over medium heat in a 12-inch nonstick skillet and add the garlic and red pepper flakes to taste. Cook, stirring, until fragrant, about 1 minute. Stir in the tomatoes, basil, salt, and pepper. Sauté for 5–10 minutes, until the tomatoes begin to cook down, and add the shrimp. Season with salt and pepper. Sauté the shrimp for 2 to 3 minutes, until cooked through, and stir in the parsley, lemon juice, and lemon zest. Taste and adjust seasonings. Add the soy noodles and toss together to warm. Serve immediately.

Nutritional Analysis per serving ▪ Calories 359 ▪ Fat (g) 5 ▪ Saturated Fat (g) 1 ▪ Carbohydrate (g) 50 ▪ Protein (g) 28 ▪ Cholesterol (mg) 252 ▪ Fiber (g) 3

GINGER-LIME SNAPPER

This is a bachelor-friendly, slam-dunk easy dish. It's high in light protein with the great tangy flavors of cilantro, lime juice, and ginger.

SERVES 4

Pan spray

1 (2-pound) whole red snapper or other firm-fleshed white fish

Salt and freshly ground black pepper

2 cups chopped cilantro

½ sweet onion, chopped

3 tablespoons minced fresh ginger

1 cup fresh lime juice, preferably from Key limes (the small ones)

1. Lightly oil with pan spray a baking dish large enough to accommodate the fish. Make three 3-inch-long slashes on both sides of the fish. Season the fish generously with salt and pepper.

2. Place the fish in the baking dish and top with half the cilantro, onion, and ginger. Turn the fish over and cover the other side with the remaining cilantro, onion, and ginger. Pour on the lime juice. Cover the dish tightly with foil and marinate in the refrigerator for 30 minutes. Meanwhile, preheat the oven to 375°F.

3. Remove the fish from the refrigerator and place in the oven. Bake 35 minutes. Check doneness. It should be opaque and pull apart easily when poked with a fork. Return to the oven for 5 minutes if not quite done. Serve with rice.

Nutritional Analysis per serving ▪ Calories 246 ▪ Fat (g) 3 ▪ Saturated Fat (g) 1 ▪ Carbohydrate (g) 8 ▪ Protein (g) 46 ▪ Cholesterol (mg) 80 ▪ Fiber (g) 1

GINGER PACKET SALMON, TOASTER STYLE

This dish is so easy it's almost ridiculous. I made it for a guy who bet me that it was impossible to make a romantic, healthy dinner in a toaster oven. I won the bet. Since then I've made up many a salmon packet and taken them to family barbecues, ready to throw on the grill.

SERVES 2

3 or 4 heads baby bok choy, quartered and rinsed

8 spears asparagus, trimmed

2 tablespoons low-sodium soy sauce

1 tablespoon minced ginger

1 tablespoon seasoned rice wine vinegar

1 tablespoon thinly sliced green onions

Pan spray

2 (4-ounce) salmon fillets

Salt and freshly ground black pepper

1. Preheat your toaster oven to 450°F. Place the bok choy and asparagus in a microwave-safe bowl, cover tightly with plastic, pierce the plastic, and microwave for 2½ to 3 minutes on high, until crisp-tender. Remove from the microwave and carefully peel back the plastic. Set aside.

2. Mix together the soy sauce, ginger, vinegar, and green onions in a bowl. Spray a double sheet of aluminum foil large enough to make a packet around the fish with pan spray. Place the salmon fillets in the middle of the foil. Salt and pepper lightly. Arrange the bok choy and the asparagus on top of the fish, and pour on the marinade. Fold the edges of the foil up toward each other and crimp together tightly to form a packet.

3. Place in the toaster oven and bake 15 to 20 minutes, until the fish is cooked through. Carefully remove from the packet and transfer the fish and vegetables to plates. Pour the juices that remain in the foil over the fish and vegetables, and serve.

VARIATION Grilled Ginger Packet Salmon: Make up the packets as directed and cook on a hot grill for 10 minutes.

Nutritional Analysis per serving ▪ Calories 195 ▪ Fat (g) 5 ▪ Saturated Fat (g) 1 ▪ Carbohydrate (g) 9 ▪ Protein (g) 30 ▪ Cholesterol (mg) 65 ▪ Fiber (g) 3

KALAMATA HALIBUT

This is a meal that you can pack up in a microwave-safe container, take to work, and zap for lunch. Accompany the Greek-style fish with a steamed bright green vegetable, like broccoli, and rice, for soaking up the sauce.

SERVES 4

4 (6-ounce) halibut fillets

Salt and freshly ground black pepper

1 (14-ounce) can stewed tomatoes with garlic and herbs, with juice

¼ cup pitted Kalamata olives, cut in half lengthwise

1. In a microwave-safe dish, arrange the halibut in a single layer. Season with salt and pepper. In a bowl, mix together the tomatoes and olives. Season to taste with salt and pepper. Pour over the fish.

2. Loosely cover the dish with plastic wrap or a lid. Pierce the plastic in a few places with the tip of a knife if not using a lid.

3. Microwave on high for 2 minutes. If your microwave doesn't have a turntable, then turn the dish 180 degrees. Cook on high for another 3 minutes. Allow to stand, covered, for 2 minutes. Carefully peel back the plastic and serve.

Nutritional Analysis per serving ▪ Calories 238 ▪ Fat (g) 6 ▪ Saturated Fat (g) 1 ▪ Carbohydrate (g) 6 ▪ Protein (g) 36 ▪ Cholesterol (mg) 54 ▪ Fiber (g) 2

NEW ENGLAND CLAM CHOWDER

Traditional clam chowder has lots of cream, and salt pork or bacon. We pulled all but ¼ cup of the cream and added a little flour to thicken this one, and we used Canadian bacon instead of the higher-calorie regular bacon. People never believe that you can crisp Canadian bacon without oil, but you can.

SERVES 6 TO 8

1 tablespoon butter

1 cup cleaned, thinly sliced leeks (white and light green parts only)

1 cup diced celery

½ teaspoon dried thyme

2 tablespoons all-purpose flour

¾ pound potatoes, scrubbed and diced small

2 (14-ounce) cans chicken broth

1 (10-ounce) can chopped sea clams, with liquid

2 (8-ounce) bottles clam juice

½ teaspoon freshly ground black pepper

1 bay leaf

2 ounces Canadian bacon, diced

Salt and pepper

¼ cup heavy cream

½ cup sliced green onions

1. Heat a heavy nonstick casserole or Dutch oven over medium heat and add the butter. When it begins to foam, add the leeks, celery, and thyme, and cook, stirring, for 1 to 3 minutes, until the leeks are just tender. Sprinkle on the flour and stir together until the vegetables are well coated.

2. Add the potatoes, chicken broth, liquid from the canned clams, clam juice, pepper, and bay leaf. Bring to a simmer, stirring with a wooden spoon, cover, and simmer over medium-low heat, stirring from time to time, until the potatoes are tender and the soup thick, about 35 minutes. Stir in the clams and heat through.

3. Meanwhile, heat a medium nonstick skillet over high heat and add the Canadian bacon. Sauté, stirring, until crisped. Remove from the heat and set aside.

4. When the soup has thickened, taste and add salt and pepper as desired. Remove the bay leaf, stir in the cream, and stir until well blended. Do not boil. Taste and adjust seasonings, and serve, garnished with green onions and the crisped Canadian bacon.

Nutritional Analysis per serving ▪ Calories 165 ▪ Fat (g) 6 ▪ Saturated Fat (g) 4 ▪ Carbohydrate (g) 19 ▪ Protein (g) 9 ▪ Cholesterol (mg) 40 ▪ Fiber (g) 2

SPICY GARLIC SHRIMP WITH BELL PEPPERS

This is one of the most popular recipes in my Countdown arsenal. The peppers add lots of color, crunch, and vitamin C, and the chili sauce makes it hot and highly flavorful. If your palate isn't as hot as mine, use less chili sauce.

SERVES 6

1 pound large shrimp, shelled and deveined

1 to 2 tablespoons garlic chili sauce

1 tablespoon canola oil

1 onion, thinly sliced

1 red bell pepper, seeded, and sliced

1 green bell pepper, seeded and sliced

1 yellow bell pepper, seeded and sliced

Salt and freshly ground black pepper

1. Toss the shrimp with the garlic chili sauce and refrigerate for 1 hour.

2. Heat the canola oil over medium heat in a nonstick wok or large nonstick skillet and add the onion and peppers. Cook, stirring, until tender, 5 to 8 minutes. Add the shrimp, season with salt and pepper, and cook, stirring, until the shrimp are bright pink and cooked through, about 4 minutes. Taste, adjust seasonings and serve, with rice or soy noodles.

Nutritional Analysis per serving ▪ Calories 101 ▪ Fat (g) 3 ▪ Saturated Fat (g) 0 ▪ Carbohydrate (g) 5 ▪ Protein (g) 13 ▪ Cholesterol (mg) 112 ▪ Fiber (g) 2

SPICY SEARED SCALLOPS

I usually season the hell out of light proteins like scallops. The seasonings make me forget that the fat isn't there, and contribute to the satisfaction you get from this dish.

SERVES 4

1½ pounds large scallops, cleaned

2 teaspoons paprika

1 teaspoon dried oregano

1 to 2 teaspoons Cajun seasoning

¼ teaspoon salt

¼ teaspoon freshly ground black pepper

1 tablespoon canola oil

Canola oil cooking spray

1. Combine all of the ingredients except the cooking spray in a large resealable bag. Marinate in the refrigerate for 30 minutes to an hour, but no longer than an hour.

2. Heat a heavy nonstick griddle until very hot. Lightly spray with the canola-oil cooking spray. Remove the scallops from the marinade and arrange them on the hot griddle, being careful not to crowd the griddle. Cook 2 minutes on each side. Serve with sautéed vegetables and rice.

Nutritional Analysis per serving ▪ Calories 187 ▪ Fat (g) 5 ▪ Saturated Fat (g) 0 ▪ Carbohydrate (g) 5 ▪ Protein (g) 29 ▪ Cholesterol (mg) 56 ▪ Fiber (g) 1

SUNSET FISH SKEWERS

The marinade for these fish kebabs has the color and the fire of a spectacular sunset, making it perfect for a dockside grilled dinner.

SERVES 4

FOR THE SUNSET MARINADE

2 tablespoons pineapple juice

2 tablespoons orange juice

4 tablespoons low-sodium soy sauce

1 tablespoon garlic chili sauce (to taste)

2 tablespoons minced fresh ginger

FOR THE FISH SKEWERS

1 pound firm-fleshed white fish, such as shark, swordfish, halibut, mahi mahi, or ono, cut into large cubes

1 bunch green onions, cut into 1-inch lengths

2 red bell peppers, cut into 1-inch squares

8 large shrimp, peeled and deveined

8 medium scallops

4 9-inch wooden skewers, soaked for 30 minutes in water, or 4 metal skewers

1. Mix together the ingredients for the marinade and place in a bowl. Add the fish, shrimp, and scallops, toss together, and marinate for 15 to 30 minutes.

2. Prepare a medium-hot grill. Assemble the skewers, beginning with a piece of fish, then a piece of onion, then red pepper, followed by shrimp, onion, red pepper, and finally scallop, onion, red pepper. Leave an inch clear at each end of the skewer.

3. Grill for 6–12 minutes, turning every three minutes. Serve with rice.

Nutritional Analysis per serving ▪ Calories 243 ▪ Fat (g) 4 ▪ Saturated Fat (g) 1 ▪ Carbohydrate (g) 8 ▪ Protein (g) 41 ▪ Cholesterol (mg) 157 ▪ Fiber (g) 3

CALZONES

These are really low-cal Hot Pockets®. Low-cal because I use phyllo instead of bread dough. You can freeze them and transfer them directly to the oven for a quick meal.

SERVES 4

1 tablespoon olive oil

4 cloves garlic, minced

¼ to ½ teaspoon red pepper flakes

1 (28-ounce) can chopped tomatoes with liquid

Salt

1 tablespoon slivered fresh basil leaves

Freshly ground black pepper

½ pound spicy chicken sausage (uncooked)

½ cup diced Canadian bacon

¾ cup shredded part-skim mozzarella

16 (9 × 14-inch) sheets phyllo dough

Olive oil cooking spray

Kosher salt

2 teaspoons Italian seasoning

1. Heat the olive oil over medium heat in a nonstick 10- or 12-inch skillet. Add the garlic and sauté until just fragrant, 30 seconds to 1 minute. Add red pepper flakes to taste and sauté for 30 seconds more. Add the tomatoes and salt to taste, bring to a simmer, and simmer over medium heat until thick, about 15 minutes. Remove from the heat and stir in the basil (adding the basil after the cooking will keep the basil flavor fresh). Taste and adjust seasonings.

2. Remove the casings from the sausage and discard. Cook the sausage over medium-high heat in a nonstick 10-inch sauté pan, stirring to break the sausage into small pieces. Continue to sauté until completely cooked through, about 4 minutes. Drain and discard any grease and liquid remaining in the pan.

3. In a medium bowl, mix the sausage, bacon, and mozzarella until well blended. Add ½ cup of the tomato sauce and stir to blend. Divide the filling into 4 portions.

4. Preheat the oven to 350°F. Place 1 sheet of phyllo dough on a clean work surface, with the short end closest to you. Keep the remaining sheets covered with a slightly damp kitchen towel. Spray once lightly with the olive oil cooking spray and then lightly sprinkle with kosher salt and Italian seasoning. Top with another sheet of dough. Repeat the spray, seasoning, and laying process 2 more times for a total of 4 sheets.

5. Place one-quarter of the sausage mixture (1 portion) on the upper right-hand corner of the prepared sheets, about an inch down from the end. Lift the upper left-hand corner of the pastry and fold it over the filling diagonally until the shorter edge of the phyllo meets the longer edge. Now fold the triangle of covered filling towards you, and continue folding over and down at right angles, to completely enclose the filling. Repeat the process 3 more times with the remaining dough and filling.

6. Set a wire rack on top of a baking sheet and then spray the rack once lightly with olive oil cooking spray. Place the triangular packets on the wire rack. With a paring knife, make a single ½-inch slit in the top of each of the packets. Lightly spray each packet once with olive oil cooking spray. Bake for 35 minutes or until golden brown. Let set for 5 minutes and serve with the remaining warm tomato sauce.

Nutritional Analysis per serving ▪ Calories 403 ▪ Fat (g) 14 ▪ Saturated Fat (g) 5 ▪ Carbohydrate (g) 47 ▪ Protein (g) 22 ▪ Cholesterol (mg) 71 ▪ Fiber (g) 3

CREAMY FOUR-CHEESE MACARONI WITH BROCCOLI

Adding broccoli to this low-fat version of a traditionally calorie-packed dish makes it an easy one-dish meal, and it's also a great way to sneak vegetables into your kids' dinner. If your whole family is participating in the Calorie Countdown diet, this one will be a winner.

SERVES 6

1½ cups broccoli florets

Cooking spray

3 tablespoons all-purpose flour

2⅓ cups 1% milk

½ cup shredded fontina cheese

½ cup freshly grated Parmesan cheese

½ cup shredded nonfat Cheddar cheese

3 ounces Velveeta Light, cubed

6 cups cooked elbow macaroni (3 cups uncooked)

Salt

3 tablespoons seasoned bread crumbs

1. Steam the broccoli florets for 4 minutes, rinse with cold water, and set aside. Preheat the oven to 375°F. Spray a 2-quart casserole or baking dish with cooking spray. Place the flour and milk in a large saucepan and whisk until well blended. Bring to a simmer over medium heat and cook, stirring constantly, until thick, about 10 minutes.

2. Add the cheeses and stir until all the cheese melts.

3. Remove from the heat and stir in the macaroni, the broccoli, and salt. Taste and adjust seasonings. Scrape into the baking dish and top with the bread crumbs.

4. Place in the oven and bake for 30 minutes, until bubbly.

> **VARIATION** You can omit the broccoli for just plain light macaroni and cheese. It's good without the Velveeta, too.

Nutritional Analysis per serving ▪ Calories 408 ▪ Fat (g) 9 ▪ Saturated Fat (g) 5 ▪ Carbohydrate (g) 57 ▪ Protein (g) 24 ▪ Cholesterol (mg) 30 ▪ Fiber (g) 3

CURRIED EGGPLANT

Eggplant will suck up as much oil as you give it. The key to a light eggplant dish like this is not to give it a lot. 2 tablespoons is sufficient here, as long as you have a good, heavy nonstick pan. This dish is even better if it's refrigerated overnight and reheated the next day. Serve this with the Cucumber-Dill Salad on page 177.

SERVES 4

2 tablespoons canola oil

1 small onion, diced

2 medium potatoes, peeled and diced

2 medium eggplants, diced

1 tablespoon curry powder

1 teaspoon salt

2 medium tomatoes, peeled, seeded, and diced

¼ cup water

Heat the canola oil over medium heat in a large, heavy nonstick or cast-iron skillet. Add the onion and potatoes and cook, stirring, until the onion is tender, 3 to 5 minutes. Add the eggplant, curry powder, and salt, and stir together for a couple of minutes to coat the eggplant. Add the tomatoes, turn the heat to medium-high, and cook, stirring, for a few minutes, until the vegetables smell fragrant and are beginning to soften. Add the water, stir together, cover, reduce the heat to low, and cook, stirring often, until the potatoes and eggplant are thoroughly cooked and the mixture has thickened, about 30 minutes. Stir often and add a little water if the vegetables are sticking to the pan (they won't burn if you have a good nonstick one). Taste and adjust seasoning. This dish needs a generous amount of salt. Remove from the heat and serve hot.

Nutritional Analysis per serving ▪ Calories 239 ▪ Fat (g) 8 ▪ Saturated Fat (g) 1 ▪ Carbohydrate (g) 41 ▪ Protein (g) 6 ▪ Cholesterol (mg) 0 ▪ Fiber (g) 14

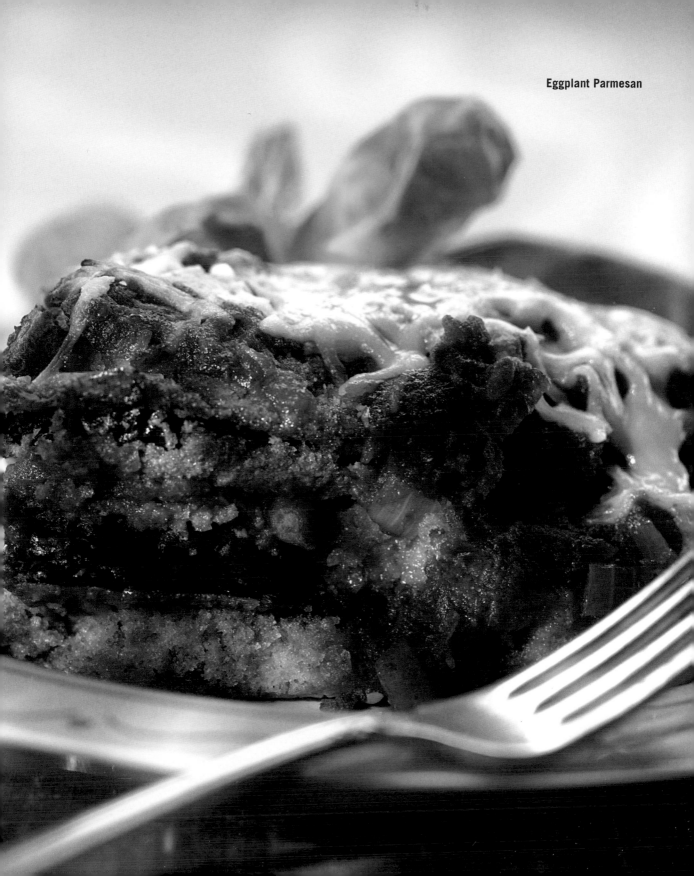

Eggplant Parmesan

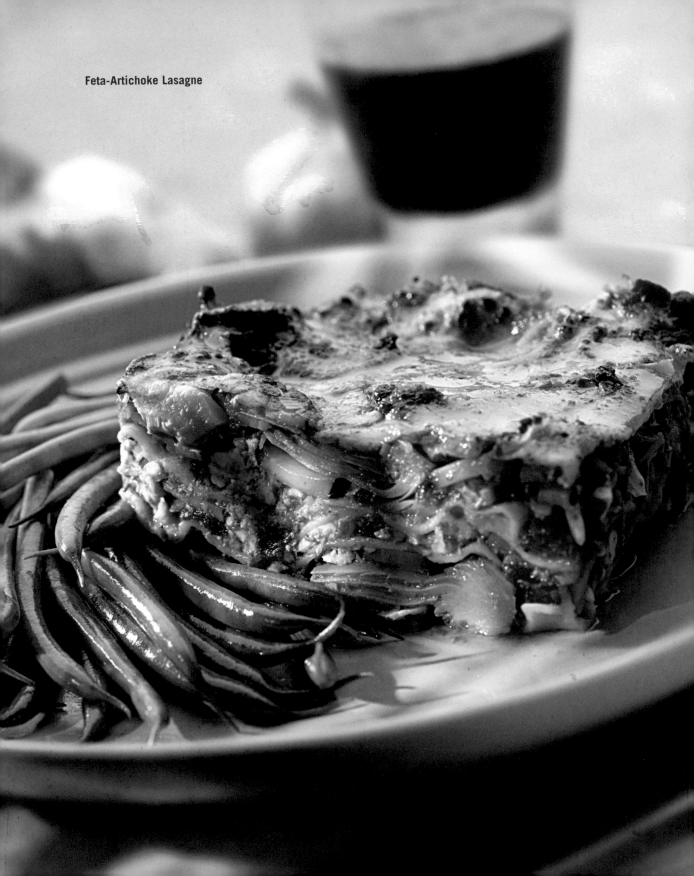

Feta-Artichoke Lasagne

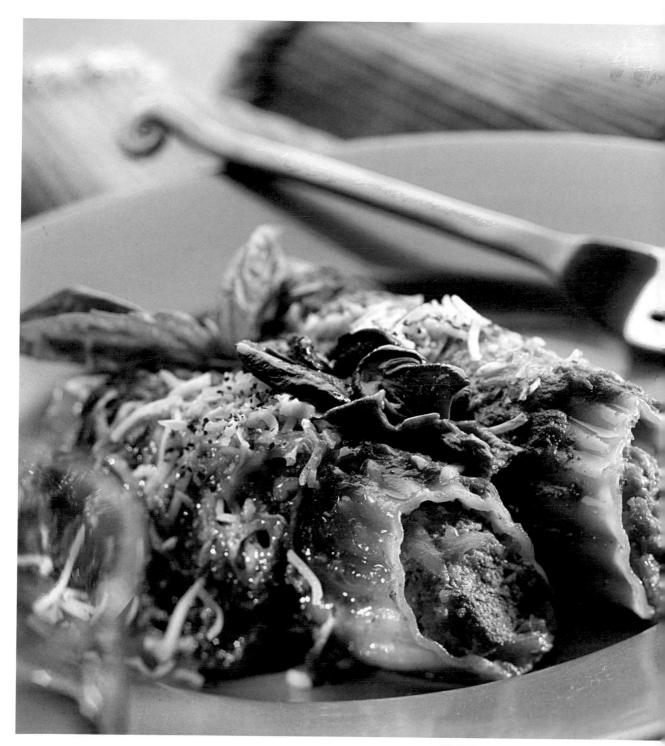

Wild Mushroom Manicotti

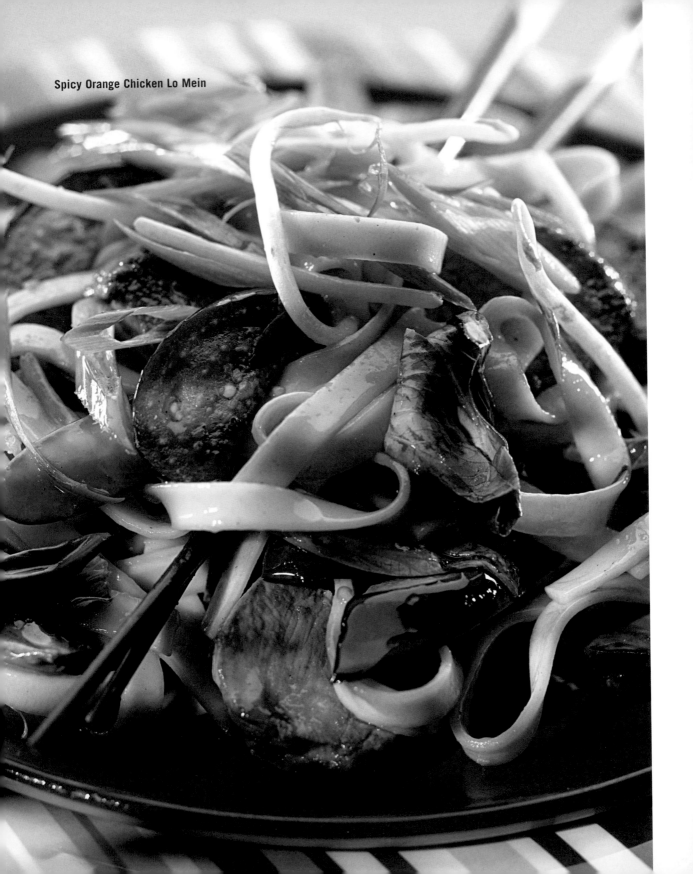

Spicy Orange Chicken Lo Mein

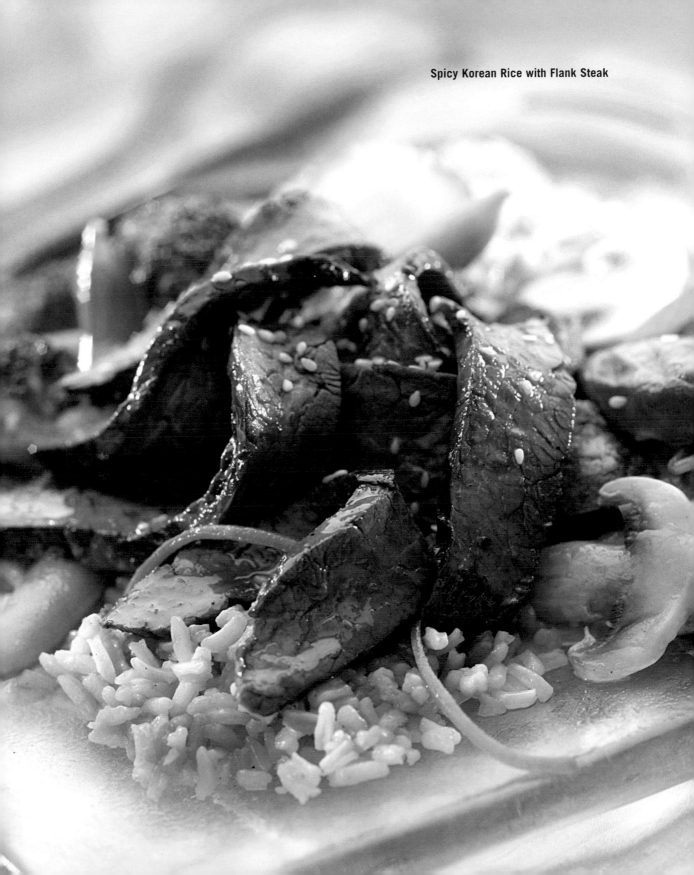

Spicy Korean Rice with Flank Steak

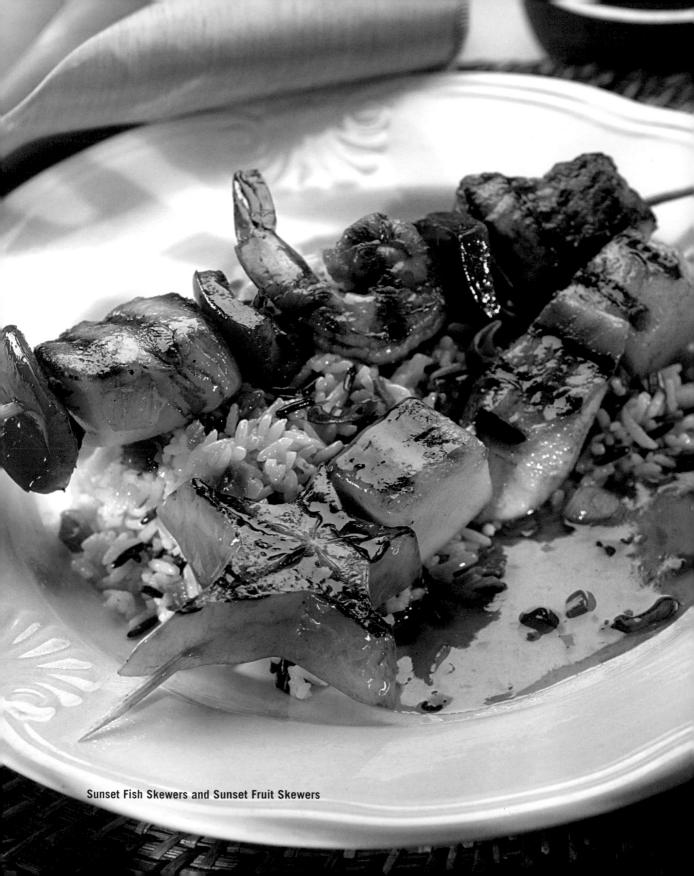

Sunset Fish Skewers and Sunset Fruit Skewers

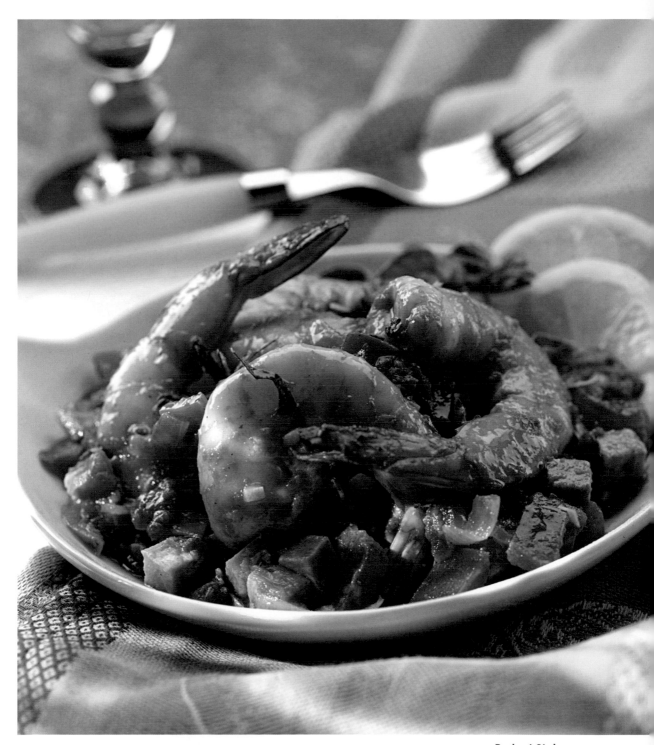

Braised Shrimp

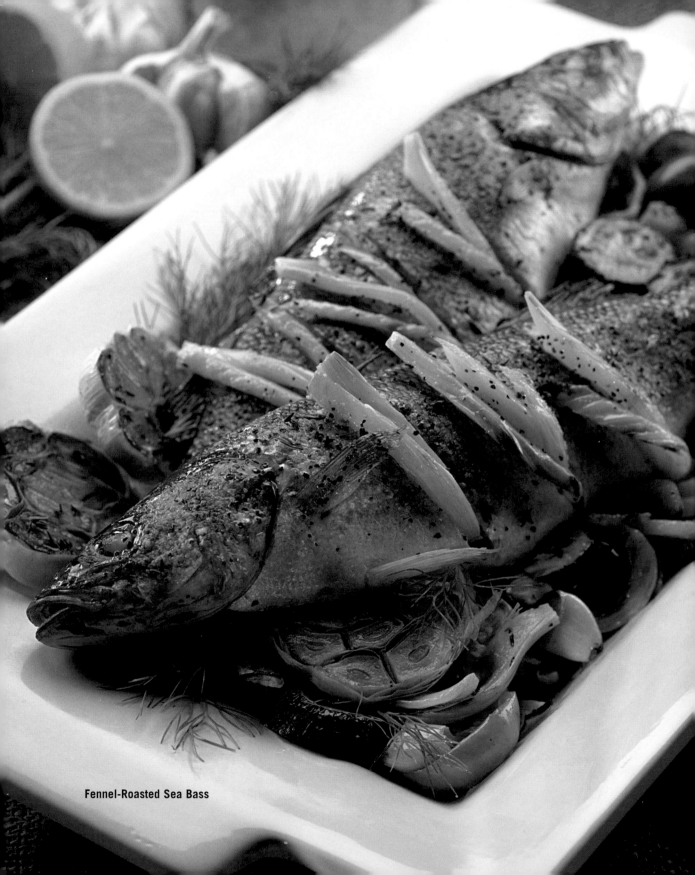

Fennel-Roasted Sea Bass

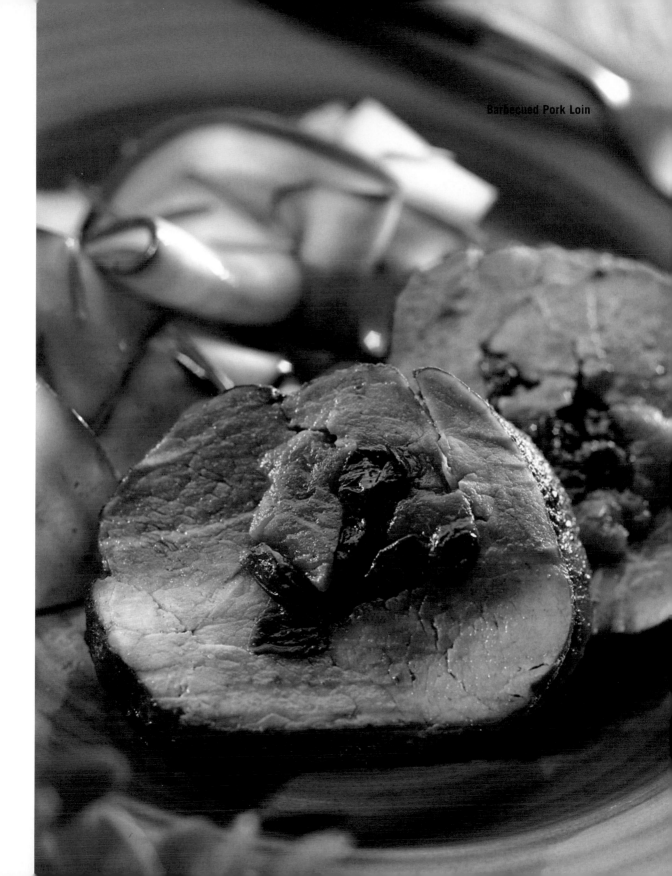

Barbecued Pork Loin

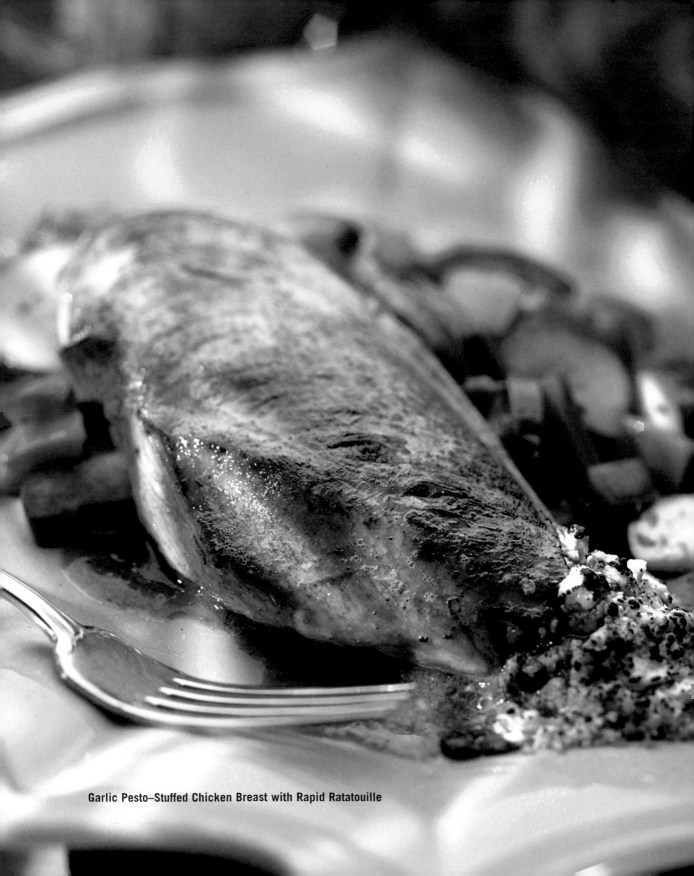

Garlic Pesto–Stuffed Chicken Breast with Rapid Ratatouille

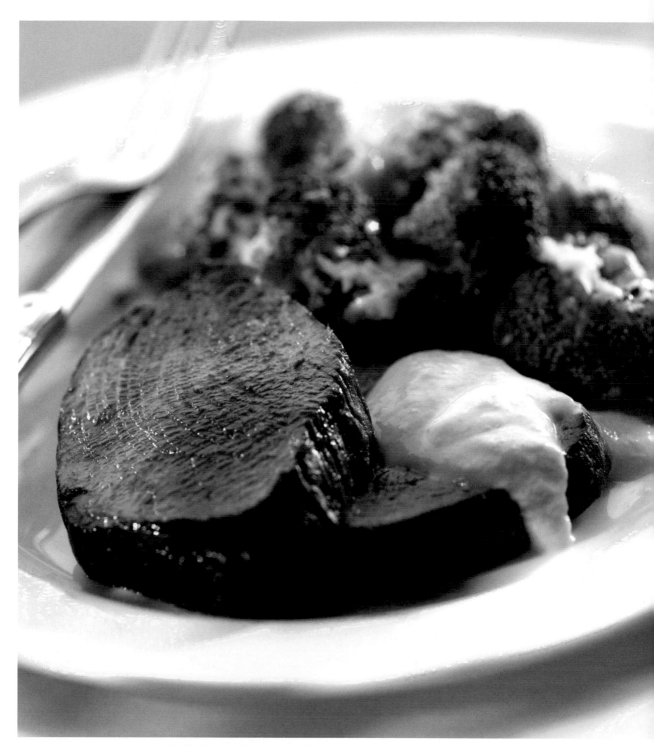

Garlic-Roasted Tenderloin with Horseradish Cream and Cheese-Roasted Broccoli

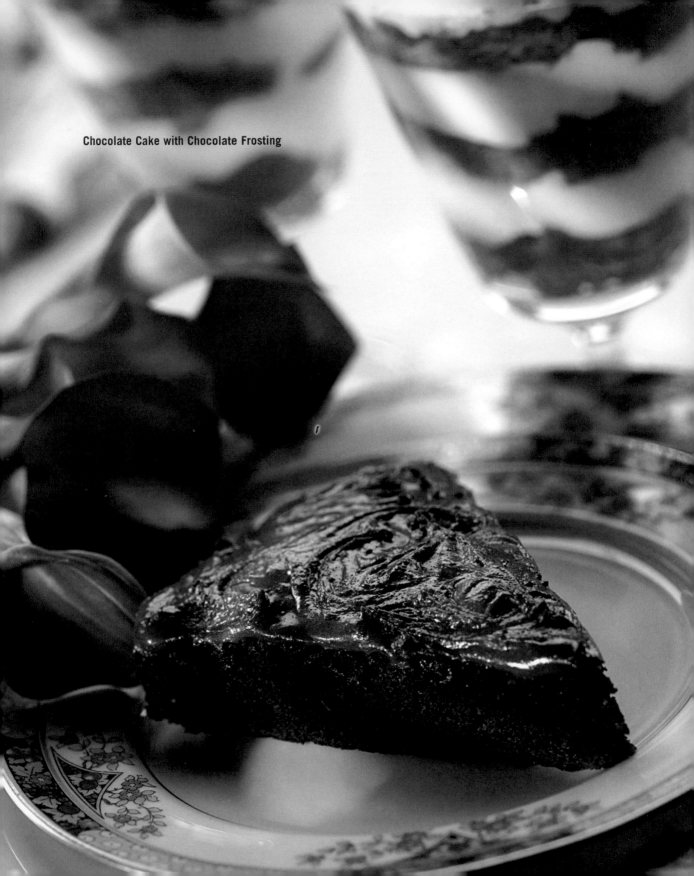

Chocolate Cake with Chocolate Frosting

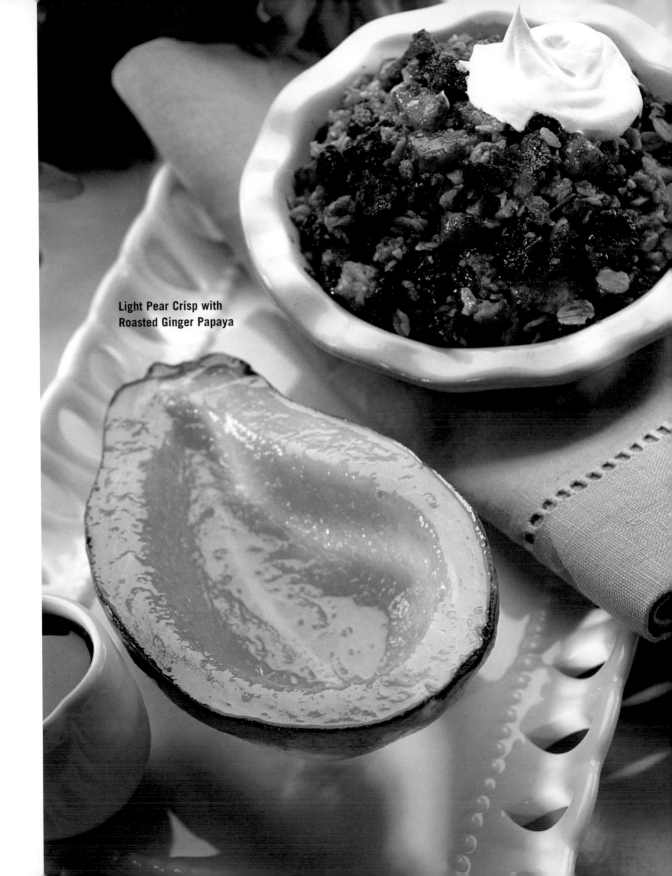

**Light Pear Crisp with
Roasted Ginger Papaya**

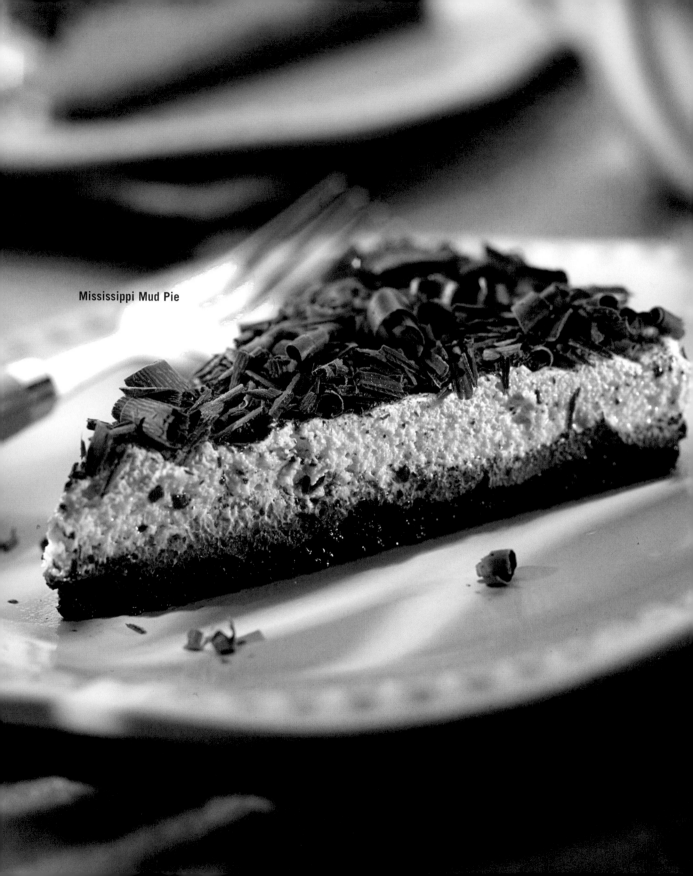

Mississippi Mud Pie

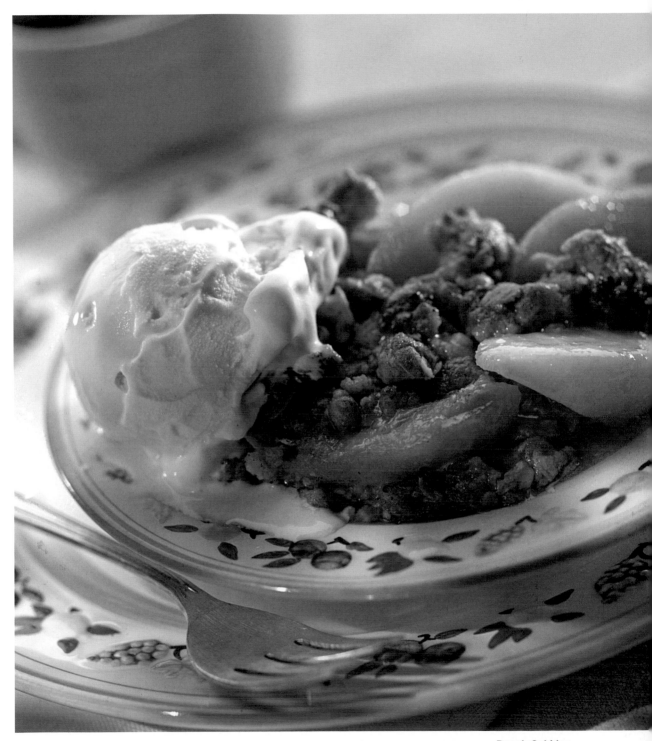

Peach Cobbler

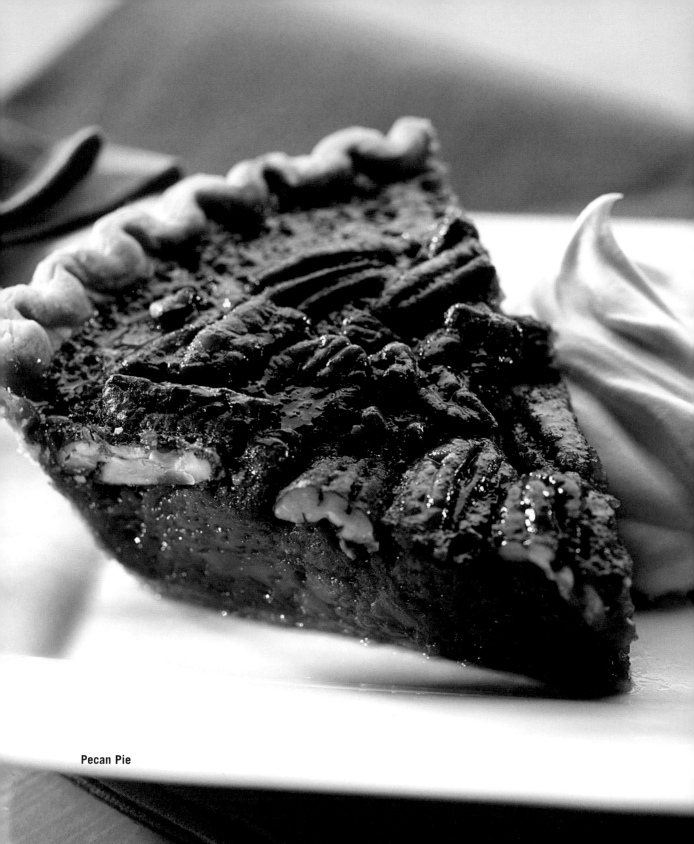

Pecan Pie

DENVER QUICHE

This is my version of a Denver omelet, inside a light crust.

SERVES 6

FOR THE CRUST

1 cup sifted cake flour

½ teaspoon sugar

¼ teaspoon salt

3 tablespoons ice-cold butter, cut in ½-inch pieces

3 tablespoons ice water

FOR THE FILLING

Cooking spray

1¾ cups shredded Yukon Gold potatoes (½ pound potatoes)

½ cup chopped green onions

4 ounces Canadian bacon or turkey bacon, chopped

½ cup grated low-fat Swiss cheese

½ teaspoon dry mustard

¼ teaspoon salt (to taste)

⅛ teaspoon cayenne pepper

1¼ cups nonfat milk

1¼ cups egg substitute

Chopped green onions and cherry tomatoes for garnish

1. Make the crust: Combine the flour, sugar, and salt in the bowl of a food processor fitted with the steel blade and pulse to combine. Add the butter and cut into the flour using the pulse action, until the mixture resembles coarse meal. With the machine running, add the ice water and process until the dough comes together on the blades of the processor. Immediately turn off the processor, scrape out the dough, and gently press into a 4-inch circle. Lightly flour your work surface, and with plastic wrap over the dough, or between pieces of plastic wrap, whichever is easiest, roll out the dough to a 12-inch circle. Refrigerate between pieces of plastic wrap, for 20 minutes.

2. Preheat the oven to 400°F. Spray a 9-inch pie dish with cooking spray and line with the crust. Pinch a lip around the rim. Prick the bottom in several places with a fork, and bake 7 minutes. Remove from the heat and allow to cool completely. Turn the oven down to 350°F.

3. Heat a large nonstick skillet over medium heat and spray with cooking spray. Add the potatoes, onions, and Canadian bacon, and cook, stirring, until the potatoes are lightly browned and tender, about 10 minutes. Remove from the heat, add the cheese, and mix together. Spoon into the pastry shell.

4. In a medium bowl, combine the dry mustard, salt, and cayenne. Whisk in the milk and the egg substitute and whisk until smooth. Pour over the potato mixture.

5. Bake at 350°F for 45 minutes, or until lightly browned and set. Let stand 15 minutes before serving. Garnish with chopped green onions and cherry tomatoes.

Nutritional Analysis per serving ▪ Calories 252 ▪ Fat (g) 7 ▪ Saturated Fat (g) 4 ▪ Carbohydrate (g) 30 ▪ Protein (g) 15 ▪ Cholesterol (mg) 29 ▪ Fiber (g) 2

EGGPLANT PARMESAN

I get more fan mail for this than for any other dish I make. People are just amazed by how well it works. The Calorie Countdown trick is air-frying the eggplant, using only a few sprays of olive oil.

SERVES 6

Olive oil cooking spray

1 cup regular or Italian-flavor bread crumbs

½ cup egg substitute

¼ teaspoon salt

1 large eggplant, sliced in ½-inch thick rounds

1 tablespoon olive oil

1 small yellow onion, chopped

3 garlic cloves, minced

½ teaspoon red pepper flakes (to taste)

1 (28-ounce) can crushed tomatoes

1 tablespoon tomato paste

Freshly ground black pepper

2 tablespoons chopped fresh basil leaves

1 cup shredded low-fat mozzarella cheese

½ cup freshly grated Parmesan

1. Preheat the oven to 375°F. Spray a 2-quart baking dish with olive oil cooking spray. Fit a cookie sheet with a wire rack.

2. Place the bread crumbs in a shallow bowl and the egg substitute in another shallow bowl. Beat about ¼ teaspoon salt into the egg substitute. One by one, dip the eggplant rounds into the egg substitute, making sure to cover them completely. Dredge in the bread crumbs until completely coated and place on the wire rack. When all of the eggplant slices have been coated, spray them lightly with olive oil spray. Turn them over and spray the other side. Place in the oven and bake for 30 minutes, or until the eggplant is tender and the bread crumbs browned. The eggplant slices will look dry on the surface; test them with a skewer or toothpick to make sure they are tender in the middle.

3. While the eggplant rounds are baking, make the sauce. Heat the olive oil over medium heat in a large nonstick saucepan or frying pan and add the onions. Sauté until tender, 3 to 5 minutes. Add the garlic and red pepper flakes and cook, stirring, for 1 minute. Add the crushed tomatoes and tomato paste and blend completely. Bring to a simmer, add salt and pepper, and simmer for 20 minutes, until thick and fragrant. Stir in the basil. Taste and adjust seasoning.

4. Layer the eggplant rounds in the baking dish, overlapping them slightly. Cover with the sauce. Mix together the cheeses and sprinkle over the top. Bake 25 to 30 minutes, until the cheese has melted and begun to color and the Eggplant Parmesan is bubbly. Remove from the oven and allow to sit for 5 minutes before serving.

An alternative method for browning the eggplant slices is to use an indoor panini grill. Preheat the grill while you coat the slices as directed. Place as many as will fit in a layer in the grill, and grill 2 minutes, or until the eggplant is cooked through and browned. Proceed as directed.

Nutritional Analysis per serving ▪ Calories 246 ▪ Fat (g) 7 ▪ Saturated Fat (g) 2 ▪ Carbohydrate (g) 32 ▪ Protein (g) 15 ▪ Cholesterol (mg) 13 ▪ Fiber (g) 8

FETA-ARTICHOKE LASAGNE

Lasagne can be luscious and satisfying, even if it isn't a traditional lasagne loaded with cheese and béchamel sauce. This one is heavy on the vegetables and light on the fat.

SERVES 8

Olive oil cooking spray

2 tablespoons olive oil

1 leek, white and light green parts, cleaned and sliced ¼ inch thick

4 cloves garlic, minced

1 medium zucchini, chopped

½ cup sliced bulb fennel (1 medium bulb)

1 (14-ounce) can water-packed artichoke hearts, drained and cut in quarters

1 (28-ounce) can crushed tomatoes

Salt and freshly ground black pepper to taste

1 tablespoon chopped fresh oregano, or 1 teaspoon dried

6 no-boil lasagna noodles

4 ounces feta cheese, crumbled (about 1 cup)

¾ cup shredded part-skim mozzarella

1. Preheat the oven to 350°F. Lightly coat a lasagne pan with olive-oil cooking spray.

2. Heat the olive oil over medium heat in a medium saucepan. Add the leek and sauté until translucent, about 3 minutes. Add the garlic and sauté for another minute, then add the zucchini and the fennel and sauté until they begin to wilt, about 3 to 5 minutes. Stir in the artichoke hearts and crushed tomatoes. Bring to a simmer, season generously with salt and pepper, and add the oregano. Bring to a simmer and cook, stirring occasionally, for 15 minutes, until thick and fragrant.

3. Spread 1 cup of the tomato mixture over the bottom of your lasagna pan. Place three lasagna noodles in a single layer on top of the tomato mixture. Dot with half the feta cheese. Top with half the remaining tomato sauce and spread in an even layer. Sprinkle on half the mozzarella. Add the remaining 3 lasagna noodles and dot with the remaining feta. Top with the remaining tomato mixture. Sprinkle the remaining mozzarella over the top. Spray the mozzarella lightly with olive-oil spray. Cover tightly with foil.

4. Bake for 30 minutes in the preheated oven, until the cheese is bubbly. Remove the foil and bake another 10 to 15 minutes, until lightly browned. Remove from the oven, allow to sit for 5 to 10 minutes, and serve hot.

Nutritional Analysis per serving ▪ Calories 190 ▪ Fat (g) 8 ▪ Saturated Fat (g) 4 ▪ Carbohydrate (g) 20 ▪ Protein (g) 9 ▪ Cholesterol (mg) 19 ▪ Fiber (g) 2

FETTUCINE ALFREDO

Fettucine Alfredo is the richest pasta dish in the world. It's made by sautéing garlic in butter (wow, what a combo), then adding cream and cheese. All fat! Yum! The challenge here is keeping the flavor and the texture while reducing fat. So I roast lots of garlic and make a flavorful paste, then thin the paste out with stock. You can now get fat-free half-and-half (I didn't believe it was real, but hey, this is America!). I also use whole-wheat pasta. So have your decadent pasta and eat it too!

SERVES 4

2 heads garlic, roasted (see page 180) and cooled

1 cup chicken stock

1 cup nonfat half-and-half

½ cup freshly grated Parmesan, plus additional for passing at the table

Salt and freshly ground black pepper to taste

½ pound whole-wheat fettucine

1. Bring a large pot of water to a boil. Meanwhile, squeeze the cooled roasted garlic into a small saucepan. Add the chicken stock and warm over medium heat. Using an immersion blender, blend the mixture until well mixed. (Be sure to immerse the blender all the way or the stock will splutter all over you.) Bring to a boil and reduce the heat. Simmer until half the stock has evaporated.

2. Whisk in the half-and-half, and bring back to a simmer. Don't let it boil, or it will curdle. Simmer gently until thick. Add the cheese and blend again with the hand blender. Season to taste with salt and pepper.

3. When the pasta water comes to a rolling boil, add a tablespoon of salt and the pasta. Cook until al dente, just firm to the bite, and drain. Toss with the sauce and serve, passing additional Parmesan at the table.

Nutritional Analysis per serving ▪ Calories 312 ▪ Fat (g) 4 ▪ Saturated Fat (g) 2 ▪ Carbohydrate (g) 53 ▪ Protein (g) 18 ▪ Cholesterol (mg) 9 ▪ Fiber (g) 9

SPAGHETTI SQUASH WITH ROASTED GARLIC PESTO

Using spaghetti squash instead of spaghetti reduces calories and carbs, and it also adds lots of fiber and nutritional value. And hey, it tastes good too! Serve this as a main dish, a side dish, or a starter. This is one of my favorite ways to get my pesto fix.

SERVES 2 AS A MAIN DISH, 4 AS A SIDE

Cooking spray

1 (2-pound) spaghetti squash, halved, seeds removed

Salt and freshly ground black pepper

1 batch Roasted Garlic Pesto (page 179)

¼ cup freshly grated Parmesan

1. Preheat the oven to 350°F. Spray a baking sheet with cooking spray and place the spaghetti squash on it, cut side down. Roast for 45 minutes, until easily pierced with a fork. Remove from the heat.

2. Hold onto the hot squash with a towel. Using a fork, scrape the squash out from the skin into a bowl. Season with salt and pepper. Toss with the Roasted Garlic Pesto, taste, and adjust seasonings. Serve, topping each serving with grated Parmesan.

Nutritional Analysis per serving ▪ Calories 240 ▪ Fat (g) 3 ▪ Saturated Fat (g) 1 ▪ Carbohydrate (g) 51 ▪ Protein (g) 9 ▪ Cholesterol (mg) 2 ▪ Fiber (g) 9

PORTOBELLO PIZZA

Here's a way to have pizza with no crust at all. Use a flat, wide portobello mushroom as a base, and top with the usual pizza toppings. You can make this in a toaster oven for an incredibly fast and memorable meal.

1 OR 2 SERVINGS

2 large portobello mushrooms

Olive oil cooking spray

Salt and freshly ground black pepper

½ cup shredded low-fat Cheddar or mozzarella cheese

¼ cup oil-packed sun-dried tomatoes, drained and chopped, or marinara sauce

2 tablespoons pine nuts

10 basil leaves, slivered

Preheat a toaster oven to 400°F. Stem the mushrooms and mist with olive oil cooking spray. Season generously with salt and pepper. Place in the toaster oven and bake for 10 minutes, until soft. Remove from the oven and top with the cheese, sun-dried tomatoes or marinara sauce, and the pine nuts. Bake for another 5 minutes, until the cheese melts. Remove from the heat, sprinkle with the slivered basil, and serve.

Nutritional Analysis per serving ▪ Calories 264 ▪ Fat (g) 16 ▪ Saturated Fat (g) 4 ▪ Carbohydrate (g) 15 ▪ Protein (g) 21 ▪ Cholesterol (mg) 12 ▪ Fiber (g) 4

QUICK TIPS

To get that nonfat cheese to melt on your pizza or grilled cheese sandwich, after topping the pizza or sandwich, spray the cheese lightly— and I do mean *lightly*—with cooking spray.

PORTOBELLO MUSHROOM–PHYLLO PACKETS

I developed these for a vegetarian who still longed for the texture and flavor of meat. He had a hard time believing that I hadn't slipped some in here. But portobellos are meaty mushrooms. When I made the dish on *Calorie Commando*, the oven door kept opening and hitting my shins; maybe that oven didn't want me to eat healthy.

SERVES 4

1 medium tomato, diced

1 ounce feta cheese, crumbled (about ¼ cup)

2 tablespoons chopped fresh oregano leaves

¼ of a 14-ounce can water-packed hearts of palm, drained and diced (about ¼ cup)

1 large portobello mushroom, stemmed and diced

Salt and freshly ground black pepper

12 (9 × 14-inch) sheets phyllo dough

2 tablespoons tomato paste

Olive oil cooking spray

1. Preheat the oven to 400°F. Place a wire rack over a cookie sheet.

2. In a large bowl, mix the tomato, feta cheese, oregano, hearts of palm, and portobello mushroom. Season with salt and pepper and toss well.

3. Lay 1 sheet of the phyllo dough on a clean work surface and brush lightly with the tomato paste. Top with another sheet of the phyllo dough. Spray lightly with olive oil and top with another sheet of phyllo. Take one-quarter of the mushroom mixture and place it in the center of the phyllo dough, leaving a border at the bottom and the top of the prepared sheets of phyllo dough. Fold the bottom of the sheet up over the filling, then fold in the sides. Now roll the packet up, so you have what looks like a rectangular burrito. Spray lightly with olive oil spray and set, seam side down, on the wire rack. Repeat the process, three more times. Once all packets are made and placed on the wire rack, lightly spray once with the olive oil cooking spray. Bake for 15 to 20 minutes, until golden brown.

Nutritional Analysis per serving ▪ Calories 221 ▪ Fat (g) 3 ▪ Saturated Fat (g) 1 ▪ Carbohydrate (g) 41 ▪ Protein (g) 5 ▪ Cholesterol (mg) 6 ▪ Fiber (g) 2

SPAGHETTI SQUASH SPAGHETTI AND MEATBALLS

This dish made a believer out of an Italian nonbeliever, an actor who always plays the heavy, but wanted to do it without being so heavy. By substituting spaghetti squash for pasta in this family favorite, I've reduced the calories considerably, so I can allow myself the tasty turkey sausage, which I use for the meatballs. Turkey sausage is far lower in fat than its pork equivalent.

SERVES 4

Cooking spray

1 large (3-pound) spaghetti squash

½ pound hot or mild turkey Italian sausage links

2 tablespoons olive oil

3 cloves garlic, minced

1 pound plum tomatoes, peeled, seeded, and diced, or 1 (14-ounce) can

¼ cup kalamata olives, pitted and halved

1 tablespoon capers, drained and rinsed

Salt and freshly ground black pepper

2 tablespoons chopped fresh basil

⅓ cup freshly grated Parmesan

1. Preheat the oven to 350°F. Spray a baking sheet with cooking spray. Cut the squash in half lengthwise, remove the seeds, and place, cut side down, on the baking sheet. Bake 30 to 40 minutes, until the flesh can be easily pierced with a knife.

2. Take the sausage out of its casings and form small balls, about the diameter of a quarter. Heat a large, heavy nonstick pan over medium heat and add the olive oil. When the oil is hot, add the meatballs and brown on all sides, about 10 minutes. Transfer to a bowl. Add the garlic to the pan and cook just until fragrant, about 30 seconds. Add the tomatoes, olives, and capers and bring to a simmer. Cook, stirring often, until the tomatoes cook down somewhat and smell fragrant, 5 to 10 minutes. Add salt and pepper to taste (remember that the olives and capers are salty). Stir the meatballs back into the sauce, along with the basil.

3. While the sauce is simmering, scrape the squash out from its skin with a fork, into a wide serving bowl. Top with the sauce and the Parmesan, and serve.

Nutritional Analysis per serving ▪ Calories 306 ▪ Fat (g) 17 ▪ Saturated Fat (g) 4 ▪ Carbohydrate (g) 25 ▪ Protein (g) 14 ▪ Cholesterol (mg) 54 ▪ Fiber (g) 6

TUNA NOODLE CASSEROLE

Lots of families rely on this simple, friendly standby. A low-fat version was requested by one of our *Weighing In* people. I did it with reduced-fat cheese and bulked it up by using whole-wheat macaroni. With the vegetables, this makes a perfect one-dish meal.

SERVES 8

Olive oil spray or butter-flavored cooking spray

2 cups whole-wheat macaroni, cooked

½ cup lowfat sour cream

¾ cup shredded reduced-fat Cheddar cheese

1 cup frozen peas

1 (7-ounce) can sliced mushrooms, drained

2 6-ounce cans water-packed tuna, drained

¼ cup chopped pimiento, drained

2 teaspoons paprika

2 teaspoons chopped fresh dill

1 teaspoon salt

¼ teaspoon freshly ground black pepper

½ cup sliced green onions

1. Preheat the oven to 350°F. Spray a 2-quart casserole or baking dish with cooking spray.

2. In a large bowl, combine the macaroni, sour cream, ½ cup of the Cheddar cheese, the peas, mushrooms, tuna, pimiento, paprika, dill, salt, and pepper. Stir until well blended. Scrape into the baking dish.

3. Bake for 30 minutes, or until bubbly. Remove from the oven and sprinkle with the green onions and remaining Cheddar cheese. Serve hot.

Nutritional Analysis per serving ▪ Calories 218 ▪ Fat (g) 5 ▪ Saturated Fat (g) 3 ▪ Carbohydrate (g) 26 ▪ Protein (g) 19 ▪ Cholesterol (mg) 28 ▪ Fiber (g) 4

WHOLE-WHEAT PIZZA WITH ASSORTED TOPPINGS

Everybody loves pizza, and there's no reason you can't have it on this diet, as long as you don't load it up with high-fat cheese. I use whole-wheat flour in the crust to add some fiber and protein.

MAKES TWO 12-INCH PIZZAS

FOR THE CRUST

1 cup lukewarm water

2 teaspoons active dry yeast

½ teaspoon honey

1 tablespoon olive oil

1 cup whole-wheat flour

1¾ cups all-purpose flour, plus extra for kneading

¾ teaspoon salt

Olive oil spray

FOR EACH PIZZA

1 (15-ounce) can crushed tomatoes, drained

3 tablespoons chopped fresh basil leaves

1 tablespoon chopped fresh oregano or 1 teaspoon dried

2 tablespoons pine nuts

Salt and freshly ground black pepper

1½ cups shredded low-fat mozzarella cheese

4 tablespoons shredded Asiago cheese

1. In a 2-cup measure, combine the water and yeast and stir to dissolve. Stir in the honey and olive oil. Set aside.

2. In the bowl of a food processor fitted with the steel blade, combine the whole-wheat flour, all-purpose flour, and salt. Pulse a few times to mix. Turn on the machine and pour in the yeast mixture with the machine running. Process until the dough gathers on the blades. If it is too wet, add all-purpose flour a teaspoon at a time, until the dough comes together.

3. Scrape out of the food processor and knead for a couple of minutes on a lightly floured surface, until the dough is smooth. Lightly spray a bowl with olive oil spray. Shape into a ball and place in the oiled bowl, rounded side down first, then rounded side up. Cover with plastic and let rise until doubled in bulk, about 1 hour.

4. Preheat the oven to 425°F. Punch down the dough and knead for a few minutes. Divide in two and shape each half into a ball. Cover with plastic and allow to rest for 15 minutes. Roll out each piece of dough and line a 12-inch pizza pan or a baking sheet covered with parchment. Pinch a lip around the edge. Freeze one of the crusts if not using.

5. In a bowl, mix the crushed tomatoes, basil, oregano, pine nuts, and salt and pepper. Spread over the dough. Top with the cheeses.

6. Bake for 20 to 30 minutes, until the cheese is melted and bubbly and the edges of the crust are nicely browned.

OTHER TOPPING SUGGESTIONS

Soy chorizo

Turkey pepperoni

Fresh sliced or chopped tomatoes

Low-fat marinara sauce

Sautéed chicken breast with teriyaki sauce and pineapple

Sautéed chicken breast with barbecue sauce

Nutritional Analysis per slice with sauce but without toppings (8 slices per pizza): ▪ Calories 168 ▪ Fat (g) 5 ▪ Saturated Fat (g) 2 ▪ Carbohydrate (g) 21 ▪ Protein (g) 10 ▪ Cholesterol (mg) 11 ▪ Fiber (g) 3

Nutritional Analysis for 1 whole pizza crust: ▪ Calories 681 ▪ Fat (g) 9 ▪ Saturated Fat (g) 1 ▪ Carbohydrate (g) 130 ▪ Protein (g) 21 ▪ Cholesterol (mg) 0 ▪ Fiber (g) 11

WILD MUSHROOM MANICOTTI

This is one of those rich Italian dishes that you think you're going to have to give up when you diet. I swapped out beef for porcini mushrooms and turkey. The low-fat ricotta adds creaminess.

SERVES 6

Olive oil cooking spray

½ ounce dried porcini mushrooms

½ pound lean ground turkey

Salt and freshly ground black pepper

1 small onion, sliced thin

4 cloves garlic, minced

1¼ cups jarred roasted red bell pepper, chopped

½ cup low-fat ricotta

6 large manicotti shells

2 cups tomato or marinara sauce for topping

¼ cup freshly grated Parmesan

1. Preheat the oven to 350°F. Lightly coat an 8 × 8-inch baking pan with olive oil spray.

2. Place the mushrooms in a bowl and cover with boiling water. Soak for 30 minutes. Drain and rinse in several changes of water to rid the mushrooms of sand. Set aside.

3. Heat a medium nonstick pan over medium-high heat and spray with olive oil spray. Add the ground turkey and brown, breaking it up with your spoon so that it cooks evenly. Season with salt and pepper. Transfer the browned turkey to a bowl and drain excess fat from the pan.

4. Return the pan to the heat and spray again with olive oil. Add the onion and cook, stirring, until translucent, about 5 minutes. Add the garlic and cook, stirring, until fragrant, about 30 seconds. Add the mushrooms and chopped red pepper and stir together for a couple of minutes. Return the browned turkey to the pan, stir everything together and remove from the heat. Stir in the ricotta. Season generously with salt and freshly ground pepper.

5. Cook the shells as directed on the package. Drain, rinse with cold water, and pat dry. Fill with the turkey mixture and place in the baking pan. Spread any unused filling over the top, as well as marinara sauce, and sprinkle on the Parmesan. Place in the oven and bake 25 minutes, or until bubbling. Serve hot.

VARIATION Use lean ground beef in place of the turkey.

Nutritional Analysis per serving ▪ Calories 193 ▪ Fat (g) 3 ▪ Saturated Fat (g) 1 ▪ Carbohydrate (g) 25 ▪ Protein (g) 17 ▪ Cholesterol (mg) 34 ▪ Fiber (g) 1

Side Dishes

Air Fries

Air Fries with Nacho Cheese

Air-Fried Okra

Air-Fried Zucchini Sticks

Broccoli with Garlic Chili Sauce

Calorie Countdown Baked Beans

Cheese Fries

Cheese-Roasted Broccoli

Herbed Zucchini Noodles

Maple-Roasted Butternut Squash

Mashed Cauliflower

Mashed Potatoes with Horseradish

Quick Vegetable Skewers

Rapid Ratatouille

Stir-Fried Asparagus and Peppers

Sunset Fruit Skewers

Toasted Almond Green Beans

Wilted Garlic Spinach

Zucchini Latkes

Sweet Potato Casserole with Caramelized Bananas

AIR FRIES

What chronic dieter doesn't love fries? These oven-baked potatoes will make fries a possibility for you. The recipe works best if you use a convection oven.

SERVES 4

½ pound starchy or waxy potatoes, peeled

½ pound sweet potatoes, peeled

Olive oil cooking spray

Salt and freshly ground black pepper

Fat-free ranch dressing, low-fat blue cheese dressing, or ketchup for serving

1. Preheat the oven to 400°F. Place a rack on top of a baking sheet.

2. Cut the potatoes into large matchsticks. Place in a large bowl and spray with olive oil spray for 2 seconds. Toss and spray again, sprinkle generously with salt and pepper, and toss again.

3. Transfer the potatoes to the wire rack, in an even layer (you may have to do this in batches). Roast for 30 to 35 minutes, or until crunchy on the outside and soft in the middle. Serve hot, with the condiment of your choice.

VARIATION Don't peel the potatoes. Quarter them, spray with the olive oil spray, toss with salt and pepper, and roast in a baking dish, turning every 10 minutes, until browned and tender, about 30 minutes.

Nutritional analysis per serving (without condiments): ▪ Calories 92 ▪ Fat (g) 0 ▪ Saturated Fat (g) 0 ▪ Carbohydrate (g) 21 ▪ Protein (g) 2 ▪ Cholesterol (mg) 0 ▪ Fiber (g) 3

AIR FRIES WITH NACHO CHEESE

What's more decadent than French fries? French fries with nacho cheese. Here's the Calorie Countdown version. You see, all things are possible!

SERVES 4

1 recipe Air Fries (page 250)   1 recipe Nacho Cheese (page 163)

Make the air fries as instructed. Make the nacho cheese as instructed. Pour the nacho cheese over the air fries and serve.

Nutritional Analysis per serving ▪ Calories 228 ▪ Fat (g) 6 ▪ Saturated Fat (g) 4 ▪ Carbohydrate (g) 30 ▪ Protein (g) 13 ▪ Cholesterol (mg) 24 ▪ Fiber (g) 3

AIR-FRIED OKRA

This low-cal version of a New Orleans favorite is great with Air-Fried Pork Chops (page 184). It's best done in a convection oven. I had one of the best compliments in my life for this dish: I had just finished my workout at the gym, and an elegant young man in a beautiful suit came up to me (sweaty from my workout, unshaved), his 2-year-old on his hip, and told me he tried the Air-Fried Okra and that his son eats it like candy.

SERVES 4

½ cup egg substitute

½ teaspoon Tabasco sauce

1 teaspoon ground white pepper

½ teaspoon salt

1 cup panko (Japanese bread crumbs, found in most supermarkets)

½ pound okra, stems trimmed about ¼ inch down from the end

1. Preheat the oven to 450°F. Place a rack over a 12 × 15-inch cookie sheet.

2. Mix together the egg substitute and Tabasco sauce. Toss together the white pepper, salt, and panko and place in a 1-gallon plastic freezer bag.

3. Roll the okra in the egg substitute mixture. Place in the plastic bag with the panko and shake the bag to coat the okra. Transfer okra to the rack-lined baking sheet.

4. Place in the oven and bake 10 to 15 minutes, until crisp on the outside and tender in the middle.

NOTE This works best in a convection oven. It will take less time—5 to 10 minutes.

Nutritional Analysis per serving ▪ Calories 84 ▪ Fat (g) 0 ▪ Saturated Fat (g) 0 ▪ Carbohydrate (g) 15 ▪ Protein (g) 6 ▪ Cholesterol (mg) 0 ▪ Fiber (g) 2

AIR-FRIED ZUCCHINI STICKS

These are like healthy French fries. Everybody loves the crunchy exterior with the tender middle. They go well with anything you'd serve a fry with.

SERVES 4

3 large zucchini (about 1½ pounds)

½ cup Italian-flavor bread crumbs

¼ cup finely grated Parmesan cheese

2 teaspoons dried oregano

1 teaspoon dried basil

½ teaspoon kosher salt

½ teaspoon freshly cracked black pepper

¼ teaspoon cayenne pepper (to taste)

2 large egg whites

Olive oil cooking spray

1. Preheat the oven to 450°F.

2. Cut each zucchini into 3-inch-long pieces, then cut the pieces lengthwise into quarters. Set aside.

3. In a shallow dish, mix together the bread crumbs, Parmesan, oregano, basil, salt, and black and cayenne peppers.

4. Whisk the egg whites in a medium bowl just until frothy. Coat zucchini sticks with egg white and then roll in bread crumb mixture until completely covered.

5. Place a wire rack on top of a baking sheet. Arrange the coated zucchini on the wire rack, about ½ inch apart from each other. Spray lightly with cooking spray. Bake for 10 to 15 minutes or until crispy. Serve immediately.

NOTE: This works best in a convection oven. It will take about 7 minutes.

Nutritional Analysis per serving ▪ Calories 127 ▪ Fat (g) 2 ▪ Saturated Fat (g) 1 ▪ Carbohydrate (g) 19 ▪ Protein (g) 9 ▪ Cholesterol (mg) 5 ▪ Fiber (g) 4

BROCCOLI WITH GARLIC CHILI SAUCE

This dish is strangely addictive, especially if you like spicy, crunchy dishes.

SERVES 4 TO 6

1 medium head broccoli, broken into florets, the stems chopped

2 to 3 teaspoons garlic chili sauce, to taste

2 teaspoons Chinese sesame oil

Soy sauce or salt to taste

2 teaspoons toasted sesame seeds

1. Steam the broccoli for 3 minutes, until crisp-tender. Drain and rinse with cold water. Toss with the garlic chili sauce.

2. Heat a nonstick wok or skillet over medium-high heat and coat with the sesame oil. Add the broccoli and stir-fry until heated through, about 1 minute. Season with soy sauce or salt. Taste and adjust seasonings. Sprinkle with the toasted sesame seeds and serve.

Nutritional Analysis per serving ▪ Calories 48 ▪ Fat (g) 3 ▪ Saturated Fat (g) 0 ▪ Carbohydrate (g) 3 ▪ Protein (g) 2 ▪ Cholesterol (mg) 0 ▪ Fiber (g) 2

CALORIE COUNTDOWN BAKED BEANS

Baked beans traditionally have salt pork and fat. Instead, I use turkey bacon, another important ingredient in my Calorie Countdown arsenal for flavor.

3 cups Great Northern beans, rinsed, picked over, and soaked overnight or for 6 hours

Vegetable cooking spray

1 medium onion, chopped

1 green bell pepper, seeded and chopped

5 cups chicken stock

¼ cup ketchup

¼ cup sugar-free maple syrup

2 tablespoons Dijon mustard

1 teaspoon paprika

Salt to taste (at least 1 teaspoon)

Freshly ground black pepper to taste

5 slices turkey bacon, cut crosswise into ¼-inch strips

1. Drain the soaked beans. Place the beans in a large ovenproof pot or Dutch oven. Add enough water to cover by 2 inches. Bring to a boil, reduce the heat, and simmer gently for 45 minutes to an hour, until just tender. Drain.

2. Preheat the oven to 325°F. Wipe the Dutch oven dry and heat over medium heat. Coat with cooking spray and add the onion and bell pepper. Sauté, stirring, until tender, about 5 minutes. Add the beans, chicken stock, and remaining ingredients, stir together, and bring to a simmer. Cover and place in the oven for 2 hours. Check from time to time and add water as needed. Uncover, and bake for another 45 minutes to an hour, stirring every 15 minutes, until the sauce is thick. Taste and adjust seasonings. Serve hot.

Nutritional Analysis per serving ▪ Calories 255 ▪ Fat (g) 3 ▪ Saturated Fat (g) 1 ▪ Carbohydrate (g) 43 ▪ Protein (g) 17 ▪ Cholesterol (mg) 8 ▪ Fiber (g) 13

CHEESE FRIES

How can you possibly make low-fat, low-calorie fries? My first decision was to bake—what I call air-fry—rather than deep-fry the fries, drastically reducing the amount of oil I would need. A convection oven is ideal for this. I can get the same crisp outside if I spray them with a little oil and bake them on a rack, so that the air circulates. Instead of using regular baking potatoes, I use sweet potatoes, which are naturally sweet and full of fiber and vitamins. The cheese is Parmesan; with its strong, salty flavor, you don't need much to get a cheesy bang. If you don't have a convection oven, the outside won't be as crisp, but they'll still be fries.

SERVES 4

2 pounds sweet potatoes, well-scrubbed and cut into ¼ × 2½-inch sticks

Olive oil cooking spray

1 teaspoon seasoned salt or kosher salt

1 tablespoon paprika

½ cup finely grated Parmesan cheese

1. Preheat the oven to 400°F. Place a rack on top of a baking sheet.

2. Place the sweet potatoes in a large bowl. Spray for 2 seconds with olive oil spray, toss, and spray for another 2 seconds. Sprinkle with the salt and paprika and toss until well coated.

3. Transfer the sweet potatoes to the wire rack, in an even layer (you may have to do this in batches). Roast for 30 to 35 minutes, or until crunchy on the outside and soft in the middle.

4. Remove from the oven and transfer to a bowl. Toss immediately with the Parmesan cheese until well coated. Return to the wire rack and place back in the oven for 5 minutes, or until the cheese is lightly browned. Remove from the heat and serve warm.

Nutritional Analysis per serving ▪ Calories 292 ▪ Fat (g) 3 ▪ Saturated Fat (g) 2 ▪ Carbohydrate (g) 57 ▪ Protein (g) 8 ▪ Cholesterol (mg) 9 ▪ Fiber (g) 8

CHEESE-ROASTED BROCCOLI

There are lots of ways to pep up broccoli. It loves spice, and it loves cheese. This makes a great side dish with just about anything.

SERVES 4

Olive oil cooking spray

1 large head broccoli, cut into florets, the stalks and stems chopped

½ teaspoon red pepper flakes (to taste)

Salt

2 cloves garlic, minced (to taste)

½ cup shredded Asiago cheese

1. Preheat the oven to 400°F. Spray a 2-quart baking dish with olive oil cooking spray.

2. Steam the broccoli florets until tender, about 5 minutes. Transfer to a large bowl and spray once with the olive oil cooking spray. Toss the florets and spray again with the cooking spray. Add the red pepper flakes, salt to taste, garlic, and half the cheese, and stir until well distributed. Transfer the mixture to the baking dish and top with the remaining cheese. Place in the oven and roast for 10 to 15 minutes, until the cheese has melted and is just beginning to brown. Serve warm.

Nutritional Analysis per serving ▪ Calories 87 ▪ Fat (g) 5 ▪ Saturated Fat (g) 3 ▪ Carbohydrate (g) 7 ▪ Protein (g) 6 ▪ Cholesterol (mg) 13 ▪ Fiber (g) 2

HERBED ZUCCHINI NOODLES

You can eat noodles on this diet, but here we swapped out half of them for zucchini strands, cutting the calories considerably and adding lots of additional texture and flavor to the dish. This will feel like a pasta side dish, not a vegetable side.

SERVES 4

2 large zucchini, about 1 pound

2 teaspoons unsalted butter

1 tablespoon chopped flat-leaf parsley

1 teaspoon chopped fresh thyme leaves

1 teaspoon chopped fresh oregano leaves

½ teaspoon lemon pepper (to taste)

½ teaspoon salt (to taste)

4 ounces egg noodles, cooked and drained

Freshly ground black pepper

1 to 2 tablespoons freshly grated Parmesan cheese

1. Carefully drag a vegetable peeler the length of the zucchini to create long ribbons. Discard centers with the seeds.

2. Heat a large nonstick sauté pan over medium heat and add the butter. Add the zucchini and quickly toss to coat with the butter. Add the parsley, thyme, oregano, lemon pepper, and salt. Toss again and warm through, about 1 minute. Add the egg noodles. Toss once again until pasta is warmed through but the zucchini remains crisp-tender. Taste and adjust the flavor with salt and pepper. Sprinkle with Parmesan to taste, toss again, and serve warm.

Nutritional Analysis per serving ▪ Calories 160 ▪ Fat (g) 4 ▪ Saturated Fat (g) 2 ▪ Carbohydrate (g) 26 ▪ Protein (g) 7 ▪ Cholesterol (mg) 33 ▪ Fiber (g) 3

MAPLE-ROASTED BUTTERNUT SQUASH

This is a perfect holiday dish. Butternut squash has a rich, buttery texture and flavor. There's just enough maple syrup here to sweeten the squash and add lots of flavor without adding a ton of calories to the dish.

SERVES 4

1 large butternut squash (about 1 pound), quartered lengthwise and seeded

¼ cup pure maple syrup

1. Preheat the broiler. Cover a baking sheet with foil.

2. Place the squash on a plate in the microwave and microwave for 10 minutes, until tender. You may have to do this in batches. Alternatively, place on a foil-covered baking sheet, cover, and roast in a 400°F oven until tender, about 45 minutes.

3. If you microwaved, transfer to the foil-covered baking sheet. Brush the cooked squash with the maple syrup and place under the broiler for 1 to 2 minutes (watch carefully!), until golden brown. Serve warm.

> **VARIATION** Substitute 2 acorn squash, halved and seeded, for the butternut squash. Follow the directions above.

Nutritional Analysis per serving ▪ Calories 159 ▪ Fat (g) 0 ▪ Saturated Fat (g) 0 ▪ Carbohydrate (g) 41 ▪ Protein (g) 2 ▪ Cholesterol (mg) 0 ▪ Fiber (g) 5

MASHED CAULIFLOWER

This makes a great substitute for mashed potatoes. You should try it even if you think you don't like cauliflower. When I made it the first time, I thought it still needed the buttery flavor of mashed potatoes, so I introduced some Molly McButter, one of my many dieter's secret weapons.

SERVES 4

1 medium head cauliflower, broken into florets, or 1 pound frozen cauliflower

1½ tablespoons Molly McButter

1 head roasted garlic (see page 180)

Salt and freshly ground black pepper

¼ cup fat-free half-and-half

1. Place fresh or frozen cauliflower in a microwave-safe bowl. Add a couple of tablespoons of water if using fresh cauliflower. Cover and microwave for 5 to 7 minutes on high, or until tender (depending on your microwave). You can also steam the fresh cauliflower until tender, 5 to 8 minutes. Drain and transfer to the bowl of a food processor fitted with the steel blade. Add the Molly McButter, the roasted garlic, about ½ teaspoon salt, and pepper to taste.

2. Process the cauliflower while gradually adding the half-and-half, until the mixture has a smooth texture. Taste and adjust seasoning. Serve warm. If not serving right away, transfer to a lightly oiled baking dish and reheat either in a microwave or a 325°F oven before serving.

Nutritional Analysis per serving ▪ Calories 65 ▪ Fat (g) 0 ▪ Saturated Fat (g) 0 ▪ Carbohydrate (g) 14 ▪ Protein (g) 4 ▪ Cholesterol (mg) 0 ▪ Fiber (g) 4

MASHED POTATOES WITH HORSERADISH

Some meals just need mashed potatoes, that's all there is to it. But there's only so many times you can use Molly McButter to lighten mashed potatoes before you get bored. So I made a completely new version of mashed potatoes, with light cream cheese, buttermilk, and horseradish for lots of body and flavor.

SERVES 4

2½ pounds baking potatoes, well washed, and quartered (skin-on)

1 teaspoon salt

½ cup buttermilk

¼ cup light cream cheese

2 tablespoons chives

2 tablespoons prepared horseradish, drained

1. Place the potatoes in a 5-quart saucepan and cover with water. Add a teaspoon of salt. Bring to boil over medium-high heat, then simmer until the potatoes are tender to the tip of a knife, about 20 minutes. Drain and return to the pot. Cover tightly and allow the potatoes to steam for 5 minutes.

2. Transfer to the bowl of an electric mixer fitted with the paddle attachment, or to a large bowl. Add the buttermilk and cream cheese and mash or mix until smooth. Add salt to taste (it will take a lot). Stir in the chives and the horseradish, and serve.

Nutritional Analysis per serving ▪ Calories 275 ▪ Fat (g) 3 ▪ Saturated Fat (g) 2 ▪ Carbohydrate (g) 55 ▪ Protein (g) 9 ▪ Cholesterol (mg) 9 ▪ Fiber (g) 4

QUICK VEGETABLE SKEWERS

Whenever my family has a cookout there's always plenty of protein, but aside from potato salad I always felt that we lacked side dishes—until I began to bring these vegetable skewers. These make an easy complement to any barbecue, and they also make vegetarians very happy.

SERVES 4

¼ cup balsamic vinegar

½ teaspoon salt

¼ cup extra virgin olive oil

1 tablespoon chopped fresh dill

Freshly ground black pepper

8 large cloves garlic

8 button mushrooms

2 medium zucchini, cut into 1-inch lengths

1 small red onion, cut into 1-inch squares

4 Roma tomatoes, cut in half crosswise

4 9-inch wooden skewers, soaked in water for 30 minutes, or 4 metal skewers

1. Prepare a medium-hot grill. Stir together the balsamic vinegar, salt, olive oil, dill, and pepper to taste. Toss with the vegetables in a large bowl.

2. Arrange the vegetables on skewers in this order: garlic, mushroom, zucchini, onion, tomato. Repeat until the skewer is full, leaving one inch clear on each end. Brush the vegetables with any marinade that remains in the bowl.

3. Grill for about 10 minutes, or until charred and tender, turning halfway through.

Nutritional Analysis per serving ▪ Calories 96 ▪ Fat (g) 4 ▪ Saturated Fat (g) 1 ▪ Carbohydrate (g) 14 ▪ Protein (g) 4 ▪ Cholesterol (mg) 0 ▪ Fiber (g) 4

RAPID RATATOUILLE

Ratatouille is a wonderful Mediterranean vegetable stew, whose only drawback is the time that it takes to prepare it. By using the microwave, I've cut down on cooking time by more than an hour, and also reduced the need for so much oil.

SERVES 4

1 cup diced eggplant (¾ inch)

1 cup diced roasted red bell pepper (¾ inch)

1 cup diced zucchini (¾ inch)

1 cup diced yellow squash (¾ inch)

1 cup peeled, seeded, and diced Roma tomatoes (½ inch)

3 garlic cloves, minced

1 teaspoon salt

Freshly ground black pepper

1 tablespoon balsamic vinegar

1 tablespoon olive oil

2 tablespoons chopped or slivered fresh basil

Toss all of the ingredients except the basil together with 1 teaspoon salt and pepper to taste in a large microwave-safe bowl. Cover with plastic wrap, pierce the plastic in a couple of places, and microwave on high for 2 minutes. Stir, cover again, and microwave for another 3 minutes. Stir, cover again, and microwave for another 5 minutes, or until the vegetables are tender. Stir in the basil. Taste and adjust seasonings.

Nutritional Analysis per serving ▪ Calories 59 ▪ Fat (g) 4 ▪ Saturated Fat (g) 1 ▪ Carbohydrate (g) 7 ▪ Protein (g) 1 ▪ Cholesterol (mg) 0 ▪ Fiber (g) 2

STIR-FRIED ASPARAGUS AND PEPPERS

If you're dieting, your food's gotta look good, and this one is incredibly colorful and tasty. The peppers are packed with vitamin C, which helps metabolize the food you're eating, particularly iron.

SERVES 4

2 teaspoons canola oil

⅛ teaspoon red pepper flakes

1 red bell pepper, thinly sliced

1 green bell pepper, thinly sliced

1 yellow bell pepper, thinly sliced

10 spears asparagus, trimmed and cut into 2-inch lengths

¼ teaspoon salt (or to taste)

¼ teaspoon freshly ground black pepper (or to taste)

Heat the canola oil with the red pepper flakes in a wok over medium-high heat until hot. Add the bell peppers and asparagus and stir-fry until crisp-tender, about 5 minutes. Season with salt and pepper, and remove from the heat. Serve warm.

Nutritional Analysis per serving ▪ Calories 49 ▪ Fat (g) 2 ▪ Saturated Fat (g) 0 ▪ Carbohydrate (g) 6 ▪ Protein (g) 2 ▪ Cholesterol (mg) 0 ▪ Fiber (g) 3

SUNSET FRUIT SKEWERS

Meat isn't the only food that can go on a barbecue! I created this as a side dish for a family occasion. It would also make a good dessert.

SERVES 4

2 cups diced pineapple (1-inch dice)

2 large, firm bananas, cut into 1-inch lengths

1 large mango, cut into 1-inch cubes

4 star fruits, cut into ½-inch slices

1 recipe (about ⅓ cup) Sunset Marinade (see page 230)

4 (9-inch) wooden skewers, soaked in water for 30 minutes, or 4 metal skewers

Combine the fruit and toss with the marinade. Let sit for about 15 minutes. Arrange the fruit on skewers, in this order: pineapple, banana, mango, star fruit. Repeat until the skewer is full, leaving 1 inch clear on each end of the skewer. Place the skewer on the grill and grill for about 5 minutes, turning halfway through.

Nutritional Analysis per serving ▪ Calories 164 ▪ Fat (g) 1 ▪ Saturated Fat (g) 0 ▪ Carbohydrate (g) 41 ▪ Protein (g) 3 ▪ Cholesterol (mg) 0 ▪ Fiber (g) 6

TOASTED ALMOND GREEN BEANS

This classic combination is usually quite buttery. But the butter isn't necessary; it's the beans and the almonds that really matter here. If using lemon juice, add it just before serving so the bright green color of the beans doesn't fade.

SERVES 4

¾ **pound green beans, trimmed**

½ **cup sliced almonds**

Salt and freshly ground black pepper

1 tablespoon lemon juice (optional)

1. Steam the green beans until crisp-tender, about 5 minutes. Remove from the heat and rinse briefly with cold water.

2. Heat a small skillet over medium-high heat and add the sliced almonds. Toss constantly in the pan until they are brown and toasty.

3. Transfer to a serving bowl. Add the green beans, season with salt, pepper, and lemon juice (if using), and toss together until the beans and almonds are well mixed. Serve.

Nutritional Analysis per serving ▪ Calories 89 ▪ Fat (g) 6 ▪ Saturated Fat (g) 0 ▪ Carbohydrate (g) 7 ▪ Protein (g) 4 ▪ Cholesterol (mg) 0 ▪ Fiber (g) 4

WILTED GARLIC SPINACH

Spinach goes with just about everything, and this dish is quick and easy, especially if you get spinach that's already stemmed and washed.

SERVES 2

4 cups (tightly packed) stemmed spinach leaves

1 tablespoon olive oil

2 or 3 cloves garlic, minced

Salt and freshly ground black pepper

1. Wash the spinach leaves in two changes of water, until there is no trace of sand. Do not spin dry.

2. Heat a large heavy nonstick pan over medium-high heat. Add the olive oil and the garlic, and as soon as the garlic sizzles and smells fragrant, after about 30 seconds, add the spinach. Cook, stirring, until the spinach wilts, about 2 minutes. Season to taste with salt and pepper, and serve.

Nutritional Analysis per serving ▪ Calories 78 ▪ Fat (g) 7 ▪ Saturated Fat (g) 1 ▪ Carbohydrate (g) 3 ▪ Protein (g) 2 ▪ Cholesterol (mg) 0 ▪ Fiber (g) 1

ZUCCHINI LATKES

Here's one way to have latkes and not pack on the pounds. Substitute shredded zucchini for the potatoes and use olive oil for frying. You save lots of calories when you swap out the zucchini for potatoes.

SERVES 6

2 pounds summer squash (such as zucchini), grated

Salt

1 medium onion, grated

¼ cup matzo meal

½ cup egg substitute

½ teaspoon freshly ground black pepper

¼ cup olive oil

1. Place the squash in a colander and sprinkle liberally with salt. Let sit 30 minutes, then squeeze out moisture from the squash. Get as much out as you can.

2. Combine the squash, onion, matzo meal, egg substitute, ½ teaspoon additional salt, and pepper in a bowl and stir together until well blended.

3. Heat a large nonstick skillet over medium-high heat and add a tablespoon of the olive oil. When the oil shimmers, it is hot enough. Drop ¼ cup of the squash mixture into the skillet and flatten with a spatula to form a pancake. Cook until golden brown on each side and transfer to a rack. Taste the first one and adjust seasonings if necessary. Continue to cook until the batter is used up, adding oil to the pan as necessary.

>   **VARIATION** For an even lower-fat version, use canola oil spray in a nonstick pan instead of the olive oil.

Nutritional Analysis per serving ▪ Calories 124 ▪ Fat (g) 9 ▪ Saturated Fat (g) 1 ▪ Carbohydrate (g) 8 ▪ Protein (g) 4 ▪ Cholesterol (mg) 0 ▪ Fiber (g) 2

SWEET POTATO CASSEROLE WITH CARAMELIZED BANANAS

This dish stands in for candied yams at Thanksgiving. You save so many empty calories by using bananas to top the casserole instead of marshmallows. They caramelize beautifully under the broiler. I also use chicken stock instead of cream, and with all the flavor here, you don't miss the cream at all.

SERVES 8

Butter-flavored cooking spray

3½ pounds sweet potatoes

2 teaspoons butter

1 cup chicken stock

Salt and freshly ground black pepper

1 teaspoon ground cinnamon

2 large bananas, thinly sliced on an angle

¼ cup dark brown sugar, tightly packed

1. Preheat the oven to 400°F. Spray a 2-quart baking dish with butter-flavored cooking spray.

2. Cover a baking sheet with foil. Place the sweet potatoes on the baking sheet and and pierce in a few places with the tip of a knife. Roast until tender, 40 minutes to an hour, depending on the size. Remove from the heat and let cool until cool enough to handle. Turn the oven down to 350°F.

3. Peel and mash the sweet potatoes in a bowl until smooth. Stir in the butter, stock, salt and pepper to taste, and the cinnamon. Transfer to the prepared baking dish. Cover the surface of the potatoes with the banana slices by laying them on top, slightly overlapping in concentric circles. Sprinkle the brown sugar evenly over the top. Bake for 20 minutes, until bubbly. Preheat the broiler and place the casserole underneath for 2 to 3 minutes, until the bananas caramelize.

Nutritional Analysis per serving ▪ Calories 176 ▪ Fat (g) 1 ▪ Saturated Fat (g) 1 ▪ Carbohydrate (g) 40 ▪ Protein (g) 3 ▪ Cholesterol (mg) 3 ▪ Fiber (g) 5

Snacks

BARBECUED POPCORN

Popcorn can be a real bugaboo for the person who loves to snack. How does the dieter achieve something so salty, greasy, and crunchy? I did it by using butter-flavored cooking spray. There are 20 calories in 3 seconds' worth of the cooking spray, compared to 240 calories in 2 tablespoons melted butter.

6 CUPS, SERVING 10

6 cups air-popped popcorn

Butter-flavored cooking spray

2 teaspoons dried parsley

½ teaspoon hickory-smoked salt

½ teaspoon onion powder

¼ teaspoon garlic powder

2 tablespoons freshly grated Parmesan cheese

1. Spread the popcorn on a baking pan and lightly spray with cooking spray. Mix together the dried parsley, hickory-smoked salt, onion powder, garlic powder, and Parmesan.

2. Transfer the popcorn to a large bowl and toss with the seasoning mix. Serve.

Nutritional Analysis per serving ▪ Calories 24 ▪ Fat (g) 1 ▪ Saturated Fat (g) 0 ▪ Carbohydrate (g) 4 ▪ Protein (g) 1 ▪ Cholesterol (mg) 1 ▪ Fiber (g) 1

QUICK TIP

Juice is really a calorie delivery system. The container may say "Made with 100% fruit," but it is also 100 percent sugar. If you have to have your juice, dilute it with water first. This is an important point if you are concerned about your children, especially babies and toddlers.

COTTAGE CHEESE, WALNUTS, AND FRUIT

This is a high-protein, power-packed pick-me-up snack. It's simple and quick to throw together.

SERVES 4

2 cups cottage cheese

1 cup chopped fresh pineapple

1 cup grapes, halved

½ cup chopped walnuts

In a small bowl, combine all ingredients until well mixed. Divide into 4 equal portions and serve chilled.

Nutritional Analysis per serving ▪ Calories 226 ▪ Fat (g) 11 ▪ Saturated Fat (g) 2 ▪ Carbohydrate (g) 17 ▪ Protein (g) 17 ▪ Cholesterol (mg) 5 ▪ Fiber (g) 2

CRUNCHY PEANUT GRANOLA

Who doesn't love crunchy peanut granola? This is an energy food, and portion control is essential or you'll be back to Square One. Still, as a post-workout snack it's hard to beat this.

`10 CUPS, SERVING 30`

1½ cups light brown sugar

½ cup water

¼ cup chunky peanut butter

1 teaspoon salt

4 teaspoons vanilla extract

8 cups rolled oats

2 cups pecans

1. Preheat the oven to 300°F. Line 1 or 2 baking sheets with parchment. Combine the brown sugar and water in a saucepan and bring to a simmer. Simmer until all the sugar has dissolved. Stir in the peanut butter, salt, and vanilla extract and combine well.

2. In a large bowl, combine the oats and nuts. Stir in the brown sugar mixture and combine thoroughly. Spread on the baking sheets and bake 45 minutes to an hour, until crunchy, stirring every 10 minutes. Remove from the oven and allow to cool completely on the baking sheets, then store in an airtight container.

Nutritional Analysis per ⅓ cup serving ▪ Calories 188 ▪ Fat (g) 8 ▪ Saturated Fat (g) 1 ▪ Carbohydrate (g) 26 ▪ Protein (g) 5 ▪ Cholesterol (mg) 0 ▪ Fiber (g) 3

PINEAPPLE-PEANUT SALAD

A nutritionist helped me develop this quick energy salad. It's got lots of potassium, lots of texture, and a ton of flavor.

SERVES 4

2 cups diced fresh pineapple

¼ cup coarsely chopped peanuts

2 ripe bananas

2 tablespoons honey

¼ cup shredded coconut

1. Toss together the pineapple and peanuts in a bowl.

2. Mash the bananas with the honey and toss with the pineapple-peanut mixture. Sprinkle the coconut over the top and serve.

Nutritional Analysis per serving ▪ Calories 188 ▪ Fat (g) 6 ▪ Saturated Fat (g) 2 ▪ Carbohydrate (g) 34 ▪ Protein (g) 3 ▪ Cholesterol (mg) 0 ▪ Fiber (g) 4

POST-WORKOUT SHAKE

You can get shakes like this in yuppie chains for about $7. You'll get lots of protein, potassium, and natural sugars here but the cost in calories and fat—as well as the actual cost—is low. Egg Beaters are pasteurized, so don't worry about the fact that they aren't cooked here.

SERVES 2

1 cup unsweetened frozen strawberries

½ cup frozen blueberries

½ cup sliced banana

½ cup orange juice

¾ cup Egg Beaters

¾ cup soy milk or nonfat milk

Place all of the ingredients in a blender and blend until smooth. Serve cold.

Nutritional Analysis per serving ▪ Calories 200 ▪ Fat (g) 2 ▪ Saturated Fat (g) 0 ▪ Carbohydrate (g) 33 ▪ Protein (g) 14 ▪ Cholesterol (mg) 0 ▪ Fiber (g) 5

QUICK TIP

Calcium may aid in the breakdown of body fat. It's not just for strong bones.

ALMONDS AND YOGURT SNACK

This makes a great snack either before or after a workout. Almonds are a super-food, with lots of good oils and protein. And you get lots of good protein and calcium from the yogurt.

SERVES 6

1 cup chopped almonds

3 cups nonfat plain yogurt

2 tablespoons honey

Mix together all of the ingredients. Divide among 6 containers, chill, and enjoy.

Nutritional Analysis per serving ▪ Calories 194 ▪ Fat (g) 9 ▪ Saturated Fat (g) 1 ▪ Carbohydrate (g) 19 ▪ Protein (g) 11 ▪ Cholesterol (mg) 2 ▪ Fiber (g) 2

Desserts

Banana Cream Pie

Bread Pudding

Brownies

Chocolate Angel Food Cake with
Strawberries

Chocolate-Banana Milkshake

Chocolate Cake with Chocolate Frosting

Chocolate-Chip Cookies

Chocolate Tofu Cheesecake

Lemon Squares

Light Pear Crisp

Light Pie Shell

Mississippi Mud Pie

Oatmeal-Craisin Cookies

Peach Cobbler

Peanut Butter–Banana Cookies

Pear-Walnut Blintzes

Pecan Pie

Pound Cake

Pumpkin Pie

Raspberry Frozen Yogurt

Roasted Ginger Papaya

Roasted Pineapple

Tiramisu

Zinfandel-Poached Pears

BANANA CREAM PIE

A bit of an indulgence, but occasional indulgences will help keep you on the diet. Here's an example of making a trade-off of sugar for fat. Puffed marshmallow cream isn't an everyday ingredient, but I chose to use it here to get lots of sweet sugary flavor and fluffy texture with no fat. And to throw some fun into dieting.

MAKES ONE 9-INCH PIE, SERVING 8 TO 10

1 cup chocolate wafer cookie crumbs (made from about 1⅔ cups cookies; use no-carb cookies if possible)

1 tablespoon light brown sugar

1 teaspoon canola oil

1 teaspoon instant espresso powder dissolved in 1 teaspoon water

2 ripe but firm bananas, sliced

¼ to ½ cup banana liqueur (to taste)

1 cup puffed marshmallow cream

1 cup frozen nonfat whipped topping, thawed

2 tablespoons chocolate shavings

1. In the bowl of a food processor fitted with the steel blade, pulse together the chocolate wafer cookies and the brown sugar until blended. With the machine running, add the canola oil and the espresso and blend together.

2. Sprinkle the cookie mixture over the bottom of a 9-inch pie pan in an even layer. Set aside.

3. In a medium bowl, combine the bananas and the banana liqueur and toss together.

4. Place the marshmallow cream in a bowl and fold in the thawed whipped topping. Drain the booze-soaked bananas and fold into the cream. Scrape into the prepared pie pan. Chill in the refrigerator for 1 hour or longer, and top with a layer of chocolate shavings. Serve cold.

Nutritional Analysis per serving ▪ Calories 197 ▪ Fat (g) 4 ▪ Saturated Fat (g) 1 ▪ Carbohydrate (g) 38 ▪ Protein (g) 2 ▪ Cholesterol (mg) 3 ▪ Fiber (g) 3

VARIATION Banana Chiffon Cream Meringue Pie

To the above recipe add:

3 egg whites

⅓ cup Splenda

Make the pie as directed. Preheat the oven to 350°F. Place the egg whites in a clean mixing bowl or the bowl of a standing mixer fitted with a whip attachment. Whip at high speed until foamy, then turn speed to low and continue to beat while you slowly add the Splenda, a tablespoon at a time. Beat until the egg whites reach firm, shiny peaks. Spread in an even layer over the chilled pie. Bake for 10 minutes, just until the meringue is set and beginning to brown. (If you have a kitchen blowtorch and want to have fun, you can use the blowtorch to brown the meringue.)

BREAD PUDDING

When I worked as a hotel pastry chef I used to make bread pudding with Danish left over from Sunday brunch, whole eggs, and cream. Condensed milk stands in for cream here, so you do get a nice rich mouthfeel with less fat. Instead of real eggs I cut way down on cholesterol by using egg substitute, and low-carb bread stands in for the Danish, making this Calorie Countdown bread pudding a real departure from the classic.

SERVES 8

Cooking spray

4 cups cubed low-carb cinnamon-raisin bread, preferably stale

1 (14-ounce) can fat-free sweetened condensed milk

1 cup egg substitute

1 teaspoon vanilla extract

1 teaspoon ground cinnamon

½ cup raisins

½ cup pecans

¼ to ½ cup bourbon, to taste (optional for adults only)

2 tablespoons Splenda

1½ teaspoons cornstarch

1. Preheat the oven to 350°F. Spray a 2-quart casserole with cooking spray.

2. Place the raisin bread cubes in a baking dish and dry out in the oven for 10 to 15 minutes. Remove.

3. In a large bowl, whisk together the sweetened condensed milk, the egg substitute, vanilla, and cinnamon. Add the bread, raisins, and pecans and toss together. Scrape into the prepared casserole. Place in the oven and bake 45 minutes, or until a knife comes out clean. Remove from the oven and douse with the bourbon, if desired. Allow to soak in.

4. Mix together the Splenda and cornstarch and pulverize in a spice mill or a food processor fitted with the steel blade. Dust the bread pudding, and serve warm.

Nutritional Analysis per serving ▪ Calories 281 ▪ Fat (g) 6 ▪ Saturated Fat (g) 1 ▪ Carbohydrate (g) 47 ▪ Protein (g) 10 ▪ Cholesterol (mg) 5 ▪ Fiber (g) 2

BROWNIES

Here I'm using apple butter in place of real butter or oil. You can use applesauce if you can't find apple butter. I even used peach baby food once and it worked! These brownies are more cake-like than fudgy.

MAKES 12 BROWNIES

Cooking spray

½ cup all-purpose flour

¼ teaspoon baking soda

¾ cup sugar

⅛ teaspoon salt

¼ cup unsweetened cocoa powder

¼ cup boiling water

⅓ cup apple butter or applesauce

¼ cup egg substitute

1 teaspoon vanilla extract

1. Preheat the oven to 350°F. Spray an 8 × 8-inch pan with cooking spray.

2. In a medium bowl, sift together the flour, baking soda, sugar, and salt.

3. In another bowl mix together the cocoa powder and boiling water and stir to dissolve. Mix in the apple butter or applesauce, egg substitute, and vanilla. Stir in the flour mixture and combine thoroughly. Scrape into the prepared pan.

4. Bake 25 to 30 minutes, until the top is firm when gently pressed and a toothpick comes out not quite clean when inserted.

Nutritional Analysis per serving ▪ Calories 92 ▪ Fat (g) 0 ▪ Saturated Fat (g) 0 ▪ Carbohydrate (g) 21 ▪ Protein (g) 1 ▪ Cholesterol (mg) 0 ▪ Fiber (g) 1

CHOCOLATE ANGEL FOOD CAKE WITH STRAWBERRIES

Angel food cake is a dieter's dream, because it's virtually fat-free. I substitute baking sugar replacement for sugar, so this one is also low-carb.

SERVES 8

⅔ cup cake flour

⅓ cup cocoa powder

¼ teaspoon salt

12 large egg whites

½ cup baking sugar replacement (such as Splenda Sugar Blend for Baking)

1½ teaspoons vanilla extract

1 cup nonfat vanilla yogurt

1 tablespoon honey

1 pint fresh ripe strawberries, hulled and quartered

8 sprigs mint for garnish

1. Preheat the oven to 350°F. Line a 10-inch tube pan (also known as an angel food cake pan) with parchment. Sift together the cake flour, cocoa powder, and salt, and set aside.

2. In the bowl of a stand mixer fitted with the whip attachment, or in a large bowl using electric beaters, beat the egg whites on medium speed until they form soft peaks. Turn the speed to medium-high and gradually add the baking sugar replacement, a tablespoon at a time. Continue to beat until the whites have formed medium-stiff peaks. Beat in the vanilla.

3. Gently fold in the flour mixture with a rubber spatula, 2 tablespoons at a time. When all of the flour has been folded in, carefully scoop the batter into the prepared pan. Bake in the middle of the preheated oven for 35 minutes, or until the cake springs back when lightly touched. Remove from the oven and invert the pan on a rack. Allow the cake to cool in the pan.

4. Meanwhile, combine the yogurt and honey in a medium bowl. Add the strawberries and fold together. Refrigerate until ready to serve.

5. When the cake has cooled, remove from the pan and slice into 8 wedges and place on plates. Top with the strawberry mixture, garnish with a mint sprig, and serve.

Nutritional Analysis per serving ▪ Calories 136 ▪ Fat (g) 1 ▪ Saturated Fat (g) 0 ▪ Carbohydrate (g) 22 ▪ Protein (g) 9 ▪ Cholesterol (mg) 2 ▪ Fiber (g) 2

CHOCOLATE-BANANA MILKSHAKE

This high-potassium drink is a great dessert for kids. Nobody needs to know it's low in fat. Keep a few bananas on hand in the freezer for an even icier drink.

SERVES 4

1 large banana, peeled and cut up

1½ cups nonfat vanilla frozen yogurt

2 tablespoons skimmed malted milk powder

¼ cup chocolate syrup

1. Place the banana in the freezer for 1 hour if you have time.

2. Combine the frozen yogurt and the skimmed malted milk powder in the jar of a blender and blend until smooth. With the machine running, drop in the banana chunks and syrup, and blend until smooth.

Nutritional Analysis per serving ▪ Calories 167 ▪ Fat (g) 1 ▪ Saturated Fat (g) 0 ▪ Carbohydrate (g) 37 ▪ Protein (g) 5 ▪ Cholesterol (mg) 2 ▪ Fiber (g) 2

CHOCOLATE CAKE WITH CHOCOLATE FROSTING

When I made this on my television show, the guests couldn't believe that it was low-fat. I use regular sugar in the cake, because you need it for moisture. But you can use sugar replacement in the frosting. As far as saturated fat and cholesterol go, applesauce and egg substitute stand in for butter and eggs.

MAKES ONE 9-INCH 1-LAYER CAKE, SERVING 10

Cooking spray

¼ teaspoon baking soda

¾ cup sugar

½ cup all-purpose flour

⅛ teaspoon salt

¼ cup unsweetened cocoa powder

¼ cup boiling water

⅓ cup unsweetened applesauce

¼ cup egg substitute

1 teaspoon vanilla extract

Chocolate Frosting (recipe follows)

1. Preheat the oven to 350°F. Spray a 9-inch cake pan with cooking spray and cut a circle of parchment paper to fit the bottom. Spray the parchment.

2. Sift the baking soda, sugar, flour, and salt into a large bowl. Combine the cocoa powder and hot water and stir until smooth. Stir in the applesauce, egg substitute, and vanilla, and combine with the dry ingredients. Scrape the batter into the prepared pan. Bake on the middle rack of the oven for 35 minutes, or until the cake bounces back when lightly pressed with a finger, and the sides begin to pull away from the pan. Cool the cake for 10 minutes in the pan, then remove from the pan and cool completely on a rack before frosting.

Chocolate Frosting

8 ounces light cream cheese

1 tablespoon light butter

2 cups sugar substitute, such as Splenda

½ cup unsweetened cocoa powder

⅛ teaspoon salt

1 teaspoon vanilla extract

3 tablespoons skim milk, or as needed

In the bowl of an electric mixer, beat the cream cheese and butter together until smooth. Add the sugar substitute and beat until incorporated. Add the cocoa powder, salt, and vanilla and beat until blended. If the frosting is too thick to spread, add the milk, 1 tablespoon at a time, with the mixer on low, until spreading consistency is achieved.

Nutritional Analysis per serving ▪ Calories 191 ▪ Fat (g) 5 ▪ Saturated Fat (g) 3 ▪ Carbohydrate (g) 31 ▪ Protein (g) 5 ▪ Cholesterol (mg) 12 ▪ Fiber (g) 2

CHOCOLATE-CHIP COOKIES

Remember my chocolate-chip cookie theory? You could begin substituting these chocolate-chip cookies for your higher-fat, higher-carb brand. I use Splenda instead of real sugar, and light butter and drained yogurt instead of butter. I knew I was on to something good when I was developing this, because I kept snacking on the dough.

MAKES 3 DOZEN COOKIES

2 cups all-purpose flour

1 teaspoon baking soda

¼ teaspoon salt

4 tablespoons light butter

½ cup firm drained yogurt (see page 215)

1¾ cups Splenda

¼ cup sugar-free maple syrup

2 large eggs

2 large egg whites

2 teaspoons vanilla

1 cup mini chocolate chips

1. Preheat the oven to 350ºF with the rack adjusted to the lower third of the oven. Line baking sheets with parchment, or preferably with a silicone mat.

2. Sift together the flour, baking soda, and salt. Set aside.

3. In the bowl of a stand mixer fitted with the paddle, or in a bowl with electric beaters, cream the butter until fluffy. Add the yogurt and cream together until fluffy and smooth. Add the Splenda and the maple syrup and continue to cream on medium speed until smooth. Add the eggs and egg whites, one at a time, scraping down the bowl and beaters after each addition. Add the vanilla and blend in. With the machine on low, slowly add the flour mixture and beat until blended. Add the chocolate chips and beat to blend. The dough will be runny.

4. Drop by tablespoons onto the lined baking sheet, leaving a good 2 inches between each cookie. Bake 10 to 15 minutes, turning the baking sheet front to back halfway through, until the cookies are lightly browned. Remove from the heat and allow to cool on a rack.

Nutritional Analysis per serving ▪ Calories 68 ▪ Fat (g) 3 ▪ Saturated Fat (g) 1 ▪ Carbohydrate (g) 16 ▪ Protein (g) 2 ▪ Cholesterol (mg) 13 ▪ Fiber (g) 1

CHOCOLATE TOFU CHEESECAKE

You'd never know that this was tofu. It really does have the taste and texture of a cheesecake, with a fraction of the fat.

SERVES 10

Cooking spray

1½ cups chocolate graham cracker crumbs (made from about 2½ cups broken-up chocolate graham crackers)

2 tablespoons canola oil

¼ cup coffee liqueur, such as Kahlua

½ pound firm tofu

½ cup part-skim ricotta

2 tablespoons light cream cheese

⅓ cup pure maple syrup

½ cup Splenda Sugar Blend for Baking

2 large egg whites

1 large egg

¼ cup cocoa powder

1. Preheat the oven to 350°F. Spray a 9-inch springform pan with cooking spray and line with parchment. Spray the parchment.

2. Mix the graham cracker crumbs with the canola oil and 1 tablespoon of the coffee liqueur. Press into the prepared pan in a single layer.

3. In a food processor fitted with the steel blade, blend together the tofu, remaining 3 tablespoons of coffee liqueur, the ricotta, cream cheese, maple syrup, Splenda, egg whites, egg, and cocoa powder until smooth. Pour into the pan.

4. Bake 1 hour, or until set. Turn off the heat and allow to sit in the oven for 30 minutes. Remove from the oven and allow to cool on a rack, then refrigerate overnight.

Nutritional Analysis per serving ▪ Calories 185 ▪ Fat (g) 6 ▪ Saturated Fat (g) 2 ▪ Carbohydrate (g) 23 ▪ Protein (g) 6 ▪ Cholesterol (mg) 28 ▪ Fiber (g) 1

LEMON SQUARES

Okay, sometimes you just have to indulge, and these make a good splurge. They're still a lot lighter than the classic.

MAKES 16 SQUARES

Cooking spray

1 cup cake flour

1 cup plus 2 tablespoons confectioners' sugar

4 tablespoons low-fat cream cheese

3 tablespoons vegetable oil

3 large egg whites

¾ cup granulated sugar

2 tablespoons finely chopped lemon zest

2 tablespoons potato flour

½ teaspoon baking powder

¼ teaspoon salt

⅓ cup fresh lemon juice

1. Preheat the oven to 350°F. Spray an 8 × 8-inch baking pan with cooking spray. Line with parchment and spray the parchment.

2. Sift the cake flour and 1 cup of the confectioners' sugar into a medium bowl or the bowl of a stand mixer fitted with the paddle. Add the cream cheese and beat at low speed or rub between your hands until well combined. Add the oil and continue to beat until the dough comes together. It will still be crumbly. Transfer to the prepared baking pan and press into the pan in an even layer.

3. Bake 25 minutes, until golden brown. Remove from the oven and allow to cool completely.

4. Make the filling: Beat together the egg whites, granulated sugar, and lemon zest until smooth. Combine the potato flour, baking powder, and salt, and sift into the egg white mixture. Whisk together. Whisk in the lemon juice and beat until smooth. Pour over the crust and return to the oven.

5. Bake 20 to 25 minutes, until set. Remove from the heat and allow to cool. Dust with the remaining confectioners' sugar and cut in 2-inch squares.

Nutritional Analysis per serving (1 square) ▪ Calories 141 ▪ Fat (g) 3 ▪ Saturated Fat (g) 1 ▪ Carbohydrate (g) 26 ▪ Protein (g) 2 ▪ Cholesterol (mg) 2 ▪ Fiber (g) 0

LIGHT PEAR CRISP

This crisp has all of the yummy ingredients that go into a classic crisp or crumble topping. It's just that there's less topping here: just enough to satisfy your sweet tooth, at half the calorie and fat cost.

SERVES 6

Butter-flavored cooking spray

4 medium-ripe but firm pears, peeled, cored, and cut in ½-inch dices

¼ cup dried cranberries

1 ¼ teaspoons ground cinnamon

¼ cup all-purpose flour

½ cup rolled oats (not instant)

¼ teaspoon salt

¼ cup light brown sugar, tightly packed

3 tablespoons cold butter, cut in small pieces

1. Preheat the oven to 350°F. Spray a 2-quart baking dish or gratin with butter-flavored cooking spray. Toss together the pears, dried cranberries, and 1 teaspoon of the cinnamon in the baking dish. Set aside.

2. In a medium bowl, combine the flour, the remaining cinnamon, the oats, salt, and brown sugar. Add the butter and rub the mixture briskly between your hands until it has a crumbly consistency. Sprinkle over the pears in an even layer.

3. Place in the oven on the middle rack and bake 25 minutes, or until the top is golden brown.

Nutritional Analysis per serving ▪ Calories 211 ▪ Fat (g) 6 ▪ Saturated Fat (g) 4 ▪ Carbohydrate (g) 39 ▪ Protein (g) 2 ▪ Cholesterol (mg) 15 ▪ Fiber (g) 5

LIGHT PIE SHELL

This pie shell is crisp rather than crumbly, with much less fat and sugar than a traditional pie crust. I use replacement sugar to sweeten, which has some sugar in it, but isn't 100 percent sugar. You need a little bit for the texture and the browning.

MAKES ONE 9-INCH PIE CRUST

1 cup all-purpose flour plus 1 tablespoon for rolling

2 tablespoons baking sugar replacement

1 ½ teaspoons baking powder

¼ teaspoon salt

1 tablespoon cold butter

¼ cup cold nonfat milk

1. In a large bowl, or in the bowl of a food processor fitted with the steel blade, mix together 1 cup of the flour, the sugar replacement, baking powder, and salt. Cut the butter into small pieces and pulse to combine in the food processor, or cut in using forks.

2. With the machine running, slowly add the milk and process until the dough comes together. If using forks, add gradually and mix until the dough holds together.

3. Pat the dough into a disc and wrap in plastic wrap. Allow to rest in the refrigerator for at least 1 hour.

4. Remove from the refrigerator and roll out the dough on a lightly floured surface. Place in a pie tin. Fold in excess dough and crimp the edges. Cover tightly with plastic and refrigerate until ready to use.

Nutritional Analysis per serving ▪ Calories 77 ▪ Fat (g) 2 ▪ Saturated Fat (g) 1 ▪ Carbohydrate (g) 13 ▪ Protein (g) 2 ▪ Cholesterol (mg) 4 ▪ Fiber (g) 0

MISSISSIPPI MUD PIE

Even special occasion desserts can be light. Mississippi Mud Pie is usually made with ice cream. I wanted to make a Mississippi Mud Pie without the fat, so I use marshmallow cream and nonfat whipped cream topping instead. It works!

MAKES ONE 10-INCH PIE, SERVING 12

FOR THE CRUST

1 cup chocolate wafer cookie crumbs (preferably low-carb cookies)

1 teaspoon light brown sugar

1 teaspoon canola oil

1 teaspoon instant espresso powder dissolved in 1 tablespoon hot water

FOR THE FILLING

2 cups puffed marshmallow cream

1½ cups frozen nonfat whipped topping, thawed

1 (3⅓-ounce) package nonfat white chocolate pudding mix

1½ ounces bittersweet chocolate

Scant ¼ cup (1 ounce) cocoa powder

2 tablespoons nonfat milk

2 teaspoons instant espresso powder dissolved in 1 tablespoon hot water

1 ounce shaved chocolate

1. In a food processor fitted with the steel blade, pulse the cookie crumbs with the brown sugar, canola oil, and the dissolved espresso powder until the mixture is moist. Press into the bottom of a 10-inch springform pan and refrigerate while you prepare the filling.

2. Place the marshmallow cream in a large bowl and fold in the whipped topping and the nonfat white chocolate pudding mix. Divide the mixture between 2 bowls.

3. Cut the bittersweet chocolate into ¼-inch pieces. Place in a stainless steel bowl, and melt over a double boiler. Fold into one of the bowls, along with the cocoa powder and the milk. Spread over the prepared pan. Fold the dissolved espresso into the second bowl. Spread over the chocolate layer. Place the pan in the refrigerator for a minimum of 2 hours, until set.

4. Run a warm, wet knife between the edge of the pie and the ring of the springform pan and remove the ring. Slice the pie with a hot, wet knife, top each serving with shaved chocolate, and serve.

Nutritional Analysis per serving ■ Calories 203 ■ Fat (g) 6 ■ Saturated Fat (g) 2 ■ Carbohydrate (g) 38 ■ Protein (g) 2 ■ Cholesterol (mg) 2 ■ Fiber (g) 2

OATMEAL-CRAISIN COOKIES

These bake up beautifully, despite the fact that applesauce replaces butter in this dough. I've made ice cream sandwiches using vanilla frozen yogurt with these, and they rocked!

MAKES 3 DOZEN COOKIES

1 cup whole-wheat flour

1½ cups quick-cooking oats

½ cup light brown sugar

1½ teaspoons baking soda

1 teaspoon ground cinnamon

½ teaspoon nutmeg

½ teaspoon ground ginger

⅔ cup unsweetened applesauce

1 teaspoon vanilla extract

1 large egg

1 tablespoon butter, softened

½ cup Craisins® (dried cranberries)

1. Preheat the oven to 350°F. Line baking sheets with parchment. Adjust the oven rack to the lower third of the oven.

2. In a medium bowl, combine the flour, oats, brown sugar, baking soda, cinnamon, nutmeg, and ginger.

3. In another bowl, beat together the applesauce, vanilla, egg, and butter. Stir into the dry ingredients, along with the Craisins.

4. Scoop out 2 teaspoons of the dough and drop onto cookie sheets. Fill the sheets, leaving 2 inches between each cookie. Flatten each cookie with the back of a spoon.

5. Bake 12 to 16 minutes, until nicely browned, turning the baking sheets front to back halfway through. Remove from the heat and slide the parchment off the baking sheets. Cool on a rack. When completely cool, store in an airtight container.

Nutritional Analysis per serving ▪ Calories 49 ▪ Fat (g) 1 ▪ Saturated Fat (g) 0 ▪ Carbohydrate (g) 10 ▪ Protein (g) 1 ▪ Cholesterol (mg) 7 ▪ Fiber (g) 1

PEACH COBBLER

This classic American dessert can be tinkered with so that you can have it when you're on the Calorie Countdown. I use low-fat Bisquick® in the topping, and replace some of the sugar with Splenda in the filling. It's fine to use frozen peaches.

SERVES 6

FOR THE FILLING
Butter-flavored cooking spray

2 pounds peaches, peeled and sliced

¼ cup light brown sugar

¼ cup Splenda

3 tablespoons all-purpose flour

½ teaspoon nutmeg

¼ cup finely chopped candied ginger

FOR THE TOPPING
½ cup reduced-fat Bisquick

½ cup quick or regular rolled oats

¼ cup light brown sugar

1 teaspoon ground cinnamon

4 tablespoons chilled butter, cut into small pieces

½ cup reduced-calorie whipped topping or nonfat ice cream for topping

1. Preheat the oven to 350°F. Lightly spray a 2-quart baking dish with butter-flavored cooking spray.

2. Toss together the peaches, brown sugar, Splenda, flour, nutmeg, and ginger in a large bowl, and scrape into the baking dish.

3. Combine the Bisquick, oats, brown sugar, and cinnamon. Cut in the butter until the mixture resembles coarse meal. Sprinkle on top of the filling.

4. Place in the oven and bake until golden brown, 40 to 50 minutes. Remove from the oven and allow to cool. Serve warm or at room temperature, with reduced-calorie whipped topping.

Nutritional Analysis per serving ▪ Calories 320 ▪ Fat (g) 10 ▪ Saturated Fat (g) 6 ▪ Carbohydrate (g) 60 ▪ Protein (g) 5 ▪ Cholesterol (mg) 20 ▪ Fiber (g) 4

VARIATION Serve with nonfat vanilla ice cream instead of the whipped topping.

PEANUT BUTTER–BANANA COOKIES

Peanut butter and bananas make a great combination in a cookie, and the banana stands in for some of the fat. Make sure to get a high-quality peanut butter for this. I haven't had much luck with generic brands. Also, it's very important to press the dough down with a fork once you spoon it onto the baking sheets, because it won't spread as it bakes.

MAKES 3 DOZEN COOKIES

2½ cups all-purpose flour

1 teaspoon baking powder

1½ teaspoons baking soda

½ cup (1 stick) butter, at room temperature

1 cup reduced-fat peanut butter

1 cup light brown sugar

1 cup Splenda

½ cup mashed banana (1 small banana)

½ cup egg substitute

1. Preheat the oven to 350°F with the rack adjusted to the lower third. Line baking sheets with parchment or silicone mats. Sift together the flour, baking powder, and baking soda, and set aside.

2. In a standing mixer fitted with the paddle attachment, or in a bowl with electric beaters, cream the butter and peanut butter together on low speed. Add the brown sugar and Splenda and cream together on medium speed until fluffy, about 2 minutes. Add the banana and mix in. Scrape down the bowl and beaters. Beat in the egg substitute. Stop the machine and scrape down the bowl and beaters. With the machine on low speed, add the flour mixture a cup at a time.

3. Spoon out the dough by tablespoons, shape them into balls, and place on the baking sheet. Press down with a fork, then place in the oven. Bake 16 minutes, or until lightly browned, turning the baking sheet front to back halfway through. Cool on racks before eating.

Nutritional Analysis per serving ▪ Calories 126 ▪ Fat (g) 6 ▪ Saturated Fat (g) 2 ▪ Carbohydrate (g) 18 ▪ Protein (g) 3 ▪ Cholesterol (mg) 9 ▪ Fiber (g) 1

PEAR-WALNUT BLINTZES

If the truth be known, I have always loved blintzes, and to this day that's what I order when we go to IHOP. I lightened up this version by substituting egg whites for eggs and nonfat milk for regular milk. I use a nonstick pan to cook the crêpes, which eliminates the need for a lot of butter, but I want some butter flavor so I use butter-flavored cooking spray. Anyone who has ever made crêpes knows that the first couple of crêpes you make, even in a nonstick pan—the only way to go, in my opinion—always come out less than perfect. So don't make yourself crazy when you begin. The filling can be varied; I love the pears and walnuts, but blueberries or caramelized apples also rock. You can make up these packets in advance and freeze them. Transfer directly from the freezer to the oven and bake 5 to 10 minutes to heat through.

SERVES 8

FOR THE CRÊPES
1 cup all-purpose flour, sifted

½ teaspoon baking powder

¼ teaspoon salt

1½ cups nonfat milk

2 tablespoons canola oil

2 large egg whites

1 large egg

2 teaspoons honey

1 teaspoon vanilla extract

Butter-flavored cooking spray

FOR THE FILLING
1 cup of low-fat cottage cheese

¼ cup walnuts, chopped

1 small pear, peeled and finely diced (½ cup)

1 teaspoon ground cinnamon

¼ teaspoon ground cardamom

1 teaspoon honey

Confectioners' sugar for dusting

1. Make the crêpe batter: Sift together the flour, baking powder, and salt. Place the milk, canola oil, egg whites, egg, honey, and vanilla in a blender jar and cover tightly. Turn on the blender, and when the mixture stops leaping around, slowly add the flour mixture with the machine running. Blend for 1 minute. Refrigerate for 1 hour.

2. Meanwhile, make the pear and cottage cheese filling: In a large bowl fold together the cottage cheese, walnuts, pears, cinnamon, cardamom, and honey until well mixed. Set aside.

3. Place a 6- to 8-inch nonstick crêpe pan (or other nonstick flat round pan) over medium heat until hot enough to make a test drop of water dance. Spray with butter-flavored cooking spray. Spoon 3 tablespoons of batter onto the pan and swirl until the batter is evenly distributed on the bottom of the pan. Cook until the edges of the crêpe are golden brown. Loosen with a spatula and turn the crêpe over. Cook for another minute. Remove from the pan and place on wax paper or parchment. Repeat with the remaining batter, placing a sheet of wax paper or parchment in between each crêpe.

4. When ready to assemble, preheat the oven to 350°F. Place a crêpe on a clean work surface and place 2 tablespoons of filling in the center. Fold two sides of the crêpe in toward the middle (so that the crêpe looks like the beginning of a burrito). Then, fold the remaining two sides in toward the middle to form a square package. Lightly spray a nonstick cookie sheet with the cooking spray and place the packages, seam side down, on the sheet. Leave about 1½ inches between each blintz.

5. Place in the oven and bake for 20 minutes or until completely warmed. Remove from the oven, dust with confectioners' sugar, and serve warm, with reduced-calorie or reduced-sugar jam.

Nutritional Analysis per serving ▪ Calories 178 ▪ Fat (g) 7 ▪ Saturated Fat (g) 1 ▪ Carbohydrate (g) 20 ▪ Protein (g) 9 ▪ Cholesterol (mg) 28 ▪ Fiber (g) 1

PECAN PIE

Here's another holiday pie that you don't have to give up if you do it my way. Use egg whites instead of whole eggs, baking sugar replacement instead of sugar, and then go ahead, use that corn syrup.

MAKES ONE 9-INCH PIE, SERVING 8

1 large egg

4 large egg whites

½ cup dark corn syrup

¼ cup baking sugar replacement

¼ cup pure maple syrup

¼ teaspoon salt

1 teaspoon vanilla extract

1 cup pecans

1 Light Pie Shell (page 289)

1 cup fat-free whipped topping

1 tablespoon bourbon

1. Preheat the oven to 350°F, preferably with a pizza stone* in it. In an electric mixer fitted with the paddle attachment, or in a food processor fitted with the steel blade, mix together the egg, egg whites, corn syrup, sugar replacement, maple syrup, salt, and vanilla. Sprinkle the pecans over the pie crust and scrape in the filling. Place in the oven and bake 45 to 50 minutes, until set. Remove from the oven and allow to cool.

2. Combine the whipped topping and the bourbon. Cut the pie into 8 servings and serve with a dollop of the bourbon cream.

* The pizza stone makes the crust crunchier.

Nutritional Analysis per serving ▪ Calories 271 ▪ Fat (g) 12 ▪ Saturated Fat (g) 2 ▪ Carbohydrate (g) 43 ▪ Protein (g) 6 ▪ Cholesterol (mg) 30 ▪ Fiber (g) 2

POUND CAKE

Applesauce replaces butter in this pound cake. You think it's not going to work, but it comes out of the oven looking and tasting like pound cake!

MAKES ONE 9 × 5-INCH LOAF

Cooking spray

1¾ cups all-purpose flour

2 teaspoons baking powder

¼ teaspoon salt

⅔ cup sugar

⅔ cup unsweetened applesauce

¼ cup light butter, at room temperature

2 large egg whites, at room temperature

1 large egg, at room temperature

½ teaspoon vanilla extract

½ teaspoon Butter Buds®

⅓ cup nonfat milk

1. Preheat the oven to 350°F. Spray a 9 × 5-inch loaf pan with cooking spray. Sift together the flour, baking powder, and salt, and set aside.

2. In the bowl of a standing mixer fitted with the paddle attachment, or in a bowl using electric beaters, combine the sugar, applesauce, and light butter, and beat at medium speed until light and fluffy, about 4 minutes. Add the egg whites and the egg, one at a time, scraping down the bowl after each addition. Add the vanilla extract and the Butter Buds and beat in.

3. At low speed, beat in one-third of the flour mixture, followed by 2 tablespoons of the milk. Add another third, then another 2 tablespoons milk and slowly beat together, then add the remaining flour and milk. Combine well.

4. Scrape into the prepared loaf pan and bake for 1 hour, or until a toothpick comes out clean. Remove from the oven and allow to cool in the pan for 10 minutes, then remove from the pan and cool on a rack.

Nutritional Analysis per serving ▪ Calories 216 ▪ Fat (g) 4 ▪ Saturated Fat (g) 2 ▪ Carbohydrate (g) 41 ▪ Protein (g) 5 ▪ Cholesterol (mg) 34 ▪ Fiber (g) 1

PUMPKIN PIE

Holidays can be lousy for dieters. But with this pie, dessert is a possibility. Egg whites replace some of the eggs, and baking sugar replacement stands in for sugar. Real maple syrup, however, is the real thing. There's a little of it, and the flavor is terrific. Make sure to use plain canned pumpkin and not pumpkin pie filling, which is full of sugar.

MAKES ONE 9-INCH PIE, SERVING 8

½ cup baking sugar replacement, such as Splenda Sugar Blend for Baking

2½ teaspoons pumpkin pie spice

1½ teaspoons ground ginger

¼ teaspoon ground allspice

¼ teaspoon salt

1 cup fat-free sour cream

2 tablespoons pure maple syrup

1 teaspoon vanilla extract

2 large egg whites

1 large egg

1 (15-ounce) can pureed pumpkin

1 Light Pie Shell (page 289)

1. Preheat the oven to 350°F, preferably with a pizza stone in it. In a large bowl, or in a food processor fitted with the steel blade, combine the sugar replacement, spices, and salt. Add the sour cream, maple syrup, vanilla, egg whites, and egg, and beat together. Beat in the pumpkin puree. Beat until the mixture is smooth.

2. Pour into the pie crust and bake for 1 hour, or until there is just a slight jiggle in the middle. Remove from the oven and cool on a wire rack before cutting.

Nutritional Analysis per serving ▪ Calories 164 ▪ Fat (g) 3 ▪ Saturated Fat (g) 1 ▪ Carbohydrate (g) 28 ▪ Protein (g) 7 ▪ Cholesterol (mg) 35 ▪ Fiber (g) 3

RASPBERRY FROZEN YOGURT

When you want ice cream without ice cream, try this. The recipe calls for powdered Splenda, which you can make by pulverizing Splenda in a spice mill.

SERVES 6

2 cups raspberries

½ cup confectioners' sugar or powdered Splenda

3 cups nonfat plain yogurt

Combine all of the ingredients in a blender and blend until smooth. Transfer to a 1½-quart freezer container, cover, and place in the coldest part of the freezer until set, at least 2 hours. Serve.

Nutritional Analysis per serving (using powdered Splenda) ■ Calories 129 ■ Fat (g) 0 ■ Saturated Fat (g) 0 ■ Carbohydrate (g) 24 ■ Protein (g) 8 ■ Cholesterol (mg) 2 ■ Fiber (g) 3

ROASTED GINGER PAPAYA

My family comes from the Caribbean, and we have a great love of roasted tropical fruit. I'll roast just about anything, but papaya is an absolute favorite. If you think papaya is bland, try this and think again. The ginger-honey glaze gives it a nice kick. You can roast this in an oven or in a toaster oven.

SERVES 4

Cooking spray

2 medium papayas

⅓ cup honey

1 tablespoon finely chopped or grated fresh ginger

1 lime, quartered

1. Preheat the oven to 350°F. Spray a baking sheet with cooking spray. Cut the papayas in half and scoop out the seeds.

2. Mix together the honey and ginger, and brush over the papayas. Place on the baking sheet, cut side up, and bake 15 minutes, or until nicely browned. Serve warm, with lime wedges.

Nutritional Analysis per serving ▪ Calories 146 ▪ Fat (g) 0 ▪ Saturated Fat (g) 0 ▪ Carbohydrate (g) 38 ▪ Protein (g) 1 ▪ Cholesterol (mg) 0 ▪ Fiber (g) 3

ROASTED PINEAPPLE

Here's another tropical fruit that I love to roast. Roasting brings out the sweetness of any fruit, and ginger adds spice. You could also use cinnamon. I used to make roasted pineapple when I was a pastry chef, always with lots of butter. But none of the flavor is lost when the butter is left out, so why keep it?

SERVES 8

1 large pineapple

½ cup light brown sugar

2 to 3 teaspoons ground ginger, to taste

1. Preheat the broiler. Cut the ends off the pineapple. Quarter it and cut away the core and skin from each quarter. Cut each quarter in half lengthwise.

2. Stir together the brown sugar and the ginger. Toss with the pineapple pieces. Place in a medium flameproof baking dish and broil for 10 minutes, turning the pieces over halfway through. Serve hot, warm, or at room temperature.

Nutritional Analysis per serving ▪ Calories 82 ▪ Fat (g) 0 ▪ Saturated Fat (g) 0 ▪ Carbohydrate (g) 21 ▪ Protein (g) 0 ▪ Cholesterol (mg) 0 ▪ Fiber (g) 1

TIRAMISU

This is a great "I'm bringing dessert" dessert. It's rich, but not nearly as rich as the traditional Italian dish. Ladyfingers stand in for cake, and these have virtually no fat. This looks great when prepared in a glass trifle bowl. You can also make it in individual bowls or sundae glasses.

SERVES 8

½ pound mascarpone

1 cup nonfat ricotta

1 (1-ounce) package sugar-free vanilla instant pudding mix

2 tablespoons Splenda

1 cup frozen reduced-calorie whipped topping, thawed

½ cup coffee liqueur, such as Kahlua

6 ounces ladyfingers

1 cup freshly brewed espresso

Cocoa powder for dusting

Chocolate-covered espresso beans for garnish (optional)

1. In a food processor fitted with the steel blade, blend together the mascarpone, ricotta, vanilla pudding mix, and Splenda until smooth. Scrape into a bowl and gently fold in the thawed whipped topping.

2. In a separate bowl, mix the liqueur and espresso. Dip half of the lady fingers into the mixture, just until moist, and line the bottom of a trifle bowl, 2-quart soufflé dish, or attractive serving bowl.

3. Gently spoon half of the cheese mixture over the lady fingers. Dip the remaining lady fingers in the espresso liqueur mix and layer over the cheese mixture. Top with the remaining cheese mixture and dust with cocoa powder. Cover tightly and refrigerate for at least 8 hours.

Nutritional Analysis per serving ▪ Calories 310 ▪ Fat (g) 15 ▪ Saturated Fat (g) 8 ▪ Carbohydrate (g) 31 ▪ Protein (g) 8 ▪ Cholesterol (mg) 42 ▪ Fiber (g) 0

ZINFANDEL-POACHED PEARS

This has so much flavor it's silly. It's a classic dessert that doesn't require a lot of sugar. Be careful not to overcook the pears. You can serve them warm or cold. If you don't have any zinfandel, use another fruity red wine, such as a syrah or a Beaujolais.

SERVES 4

2 cups red zinfandel

1 vanilla bean, split and scraped

½ cup light brown sugar

3 whole cloves

2 Bosc pears, peeled, halved, and cored

4 teaspoons low-fat sour cream

1. In a medium saucepan, combine the zinfandel, vanilla bean and seeds, brown sugar, and cloves, and bring to a simmer. Carefully add the pears. Turn the heat to low and simmer the pears uncovered for 30 minutes, or until the pears are tender when pricked with a paring knife.

2. Using tongs, remove the pears from the pan and transfer to a bowl. Allow to cool. Meanwhile, bring the wine to a boil, and boil until reduced to ½ cup. Remove from the heat. Spoon a tablespoon out onto each of 4 plates.

3. Cut each pear half lengthwise into thin slices and fan out on the plates. Pour the remaining sauce over the pears and top each with 1 teaspoon low-fat sour cream.

Nutritional Analysis per serving ▪ Calories 191 ▪ Fat (g) 1 ▪ Saturated Fat (g) 0 ▪ Carbohydrate (g) 39 ▪ Protein (g) 1 ▪ Cholesterol (mg) 3 ▪ Fiber (g) 2

ACKNOWLEDGMENTS

When I began to think of all the people whose help and support
made this book possible I began to worry that the Acknowledgments
page would be longer than the book itself. So many friends and col-
leagues have encouraged me that there is no way I can possibly include them all.

First and foremost I thank my beautiful wife for her belief in me
and encouragement to pursue my dreams. She encouraged me to
create a television show and take it all the way. But she still makes

me take the trash out. Thank you to my parents who let me experiment in the kitchen as a child.

To my editor, Lauren Marino, thank you for seeing the potential in this book, and thank you for your encouragement and guidance.

To my writer, Martha Rose Shulman. I'm amazed at how you can take my often disjointed manner of writing and rewrite it so that it still sounds like me.

To my food stylist, Denise Vivaldo. Your skill, patience, and artistry is amazing. Photographing food is an art unto itself, and my photographer, Ed Ouellette, is an artist among artists.

Thanks to my agents, Angela Miller and Sharon Bowers, for taking the concept of Calorie Countdown out into the marketplace and making it a reality.

Thanks to Tammi Hancock for the nutritional data.

Thank you also to the folks who created Dragonspeak voice recognition software. Without your product a dyslexic like me would never have been able to write a book.

A special thanks goes out to Michelle Van Kempen of Film Garden, who originally took the concept of *Calorie Commando* to the Food Network. And a heartfelt thanks to Tara Sandler and Jennifer Davidson of Pie Town Productions for believing in me enough to have me host *Weighing In*.

To Bob Tuschman at the Food Network, who saw the potential of *Calorie Commando*. Before I met you, people told me you were a mensch. Now I know what they meant.

A special thanks goes to my producers, Mark Dissin and Margaret Hussey. I am indebted to you both for your encouragement and for your hard work at getting the best out of me.

There are so many others at the Food Network that I would like to thank that I know I will forget someone, so I'll just say thank you to all for the wonderful work you do.

Lastly I would like to acknowledge the dieter who has tried and failed and tried and failed but has decided to try once more. It takes guts and determination. You will have good days and you will have bad days. Don't ever let anyone tell you that what you're doing isn't worth the effort. It is to you that I raise my glass. You are worth every bit of effort you put into this!

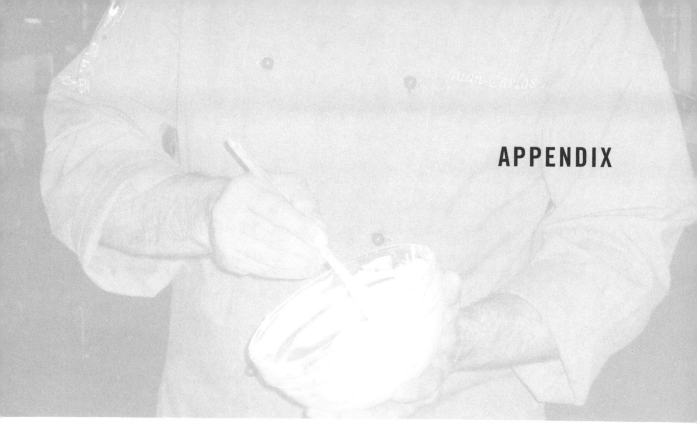

APPENDIX

Here are some of my favorite resources on the Web. Some are a little offbeat, but they're useful.

For calorie counts:

- **http://www.calorieking.com/** For a quick guide for calorie counts, calorie king.com is hard to beat. They also publish a very handy pocket guide.

- **http://www.thecaloriecounter.com/**

- **http://www.dietfacts.com/fastfood.asp** This lists a number of restaurants with nutritional information. If I can't find the information I want from a particular restaurant online, I check out this Web page.

For weight charts and body mass index charts:

- **http://www.halls.md/body-mass-index/bmi.htm**

- **http://nhlbisupport.com/bmi/**

- **http://www.cdc.gov/nccdphp/dnpa/bmi/calc-bmi.htm**

- **http://www.consumer.gov/weightloss/bmi.htm**

- **http://www.healthchecksystems.com**

There are tons of Web pages that will calculate your body mass index. I like the first one because the values are a little more forgiving. But remember, they're only guidelines. If you take them too literally they'll make you crazy. To further illustrate what I mean, check out the National Heart, Lung, and Blood Institute and the Centers for Disease Control Web pages (second on the list). Healthchecksystems.com also sells equipment for measuring body fat.

For calculating your daily caloric needs (prepare to have your jaw drop when you see how little it takes to keep the human body running):

- **http://www.cancer.org/docroot/PED/content/PED_6_1x_Calorie_Calculator.asp** This is the American Cancer Society Web site.

- **http://www.weightlossforall.com/calorie-requirements-daily.htm** If you want to see how to do it by hand, go to this Web page. Bless their heart for posting it. I just don't have the patience myself.

- **http://www.bcm.edu/cnrc/caloriesneed.htm** This is one of my favorites because it calculates your BMI and your caloric needs at the same time. It's put out by Baylor University.

For general information about healthy eating and managing your weight, including keeping food logs, controlling portion size, figuring out your caloric needs, and more:

- **http://weightloss.about.com/**

- **http://mypyramid.gov/mypyramid/index.aspx** This is put out by the Department of Agriculture.

I think my favorite offbeat Web page is mypetfat.com. Yes, you read that right; it's kind of gross but I highly recommend having your own pet fat. Just go check it out.

- **http://www.mypetfat.com/thetools.asp**

And of course, there's my own Web page, **www.caloriecountdown.net**. There you can also find a revolving page of links for some of my favorite products that

I've recommended throughout this book, like Kashi cereals, Molly McButter, spray oils, spices and flavor blends, and nonstick cookware. If you find something cool, go to my page and e-mail it to me. You could spend hours checking out other pages on the Internet, but then you wouldn't be following my advice to get moving. So rather than getting caught up in what I call the paralysis of analysis, take my guidelines and start going forward with the Calorie Countdown. It's an adventure that can be tough at times, but that doesn't mean it can't also be entertaining. I'll see you on the other side.

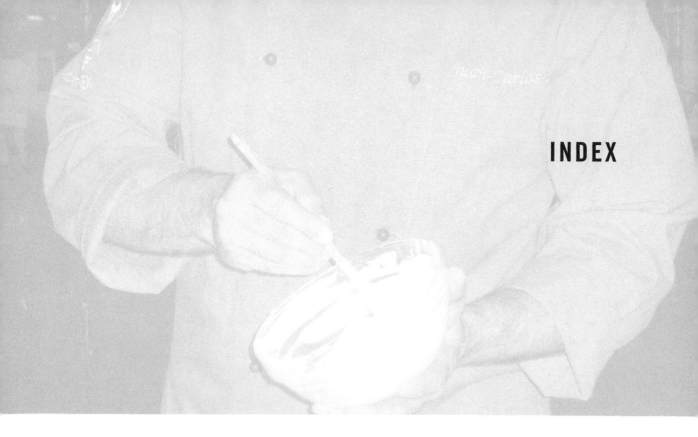

INDEX

E

F

graham crackers, 16, 48

grains, 33, 37

granola
   and carbohydrates, 37
   Crunchy Peanut Granola, 273

grapes, 17

gravy, 204–5

green beans, 266

Green Chile Black Beans, 164

grill, 20

grilled foods, 40, 42

grocery shopping, 20

gyms
   benefits of, 59–61
   choosing a gym, 25, 32, 60–61
   in-home gym equipment, 58
   variety in, 62

H

half-and-half, 40

halibut, 226

ham, 148

hand blenders, 19, 141

Hard Rock Cafe, 43

health and fitness. *See* exercise and
   fitness

healthy foods, 15

Herbed Zucchini Noodles, 258

Herb-Roasted Turkey Breast, 199

Herb Turkey Wraps, 149

hoisin sauce, 22

honey, 33

horseradish
   Garlic-Roasted Tenderloin with Horseradish
     Cream, 198
   Mashed Potatoes with Horseradish,
     261

hot dogs
   Open-Faced Chili Dogs, 150
   Pigs in a Blanket, 160

hunger, 28, 42

hydration, 39, 154

hydrogenated or partially hydrogenated fats, 21,
   37

I

ice cream, 16, 37, 46

ingredient lists, 21, 45

Internet surfing, 48

Italian Dressing, Creamy, 180

J

Jamba Juice, 17, 46

jerk seasoning, 21

jicama
   Creamy Coleslaw, 176
   Light Beef Taco Wraps, 211

journaling food intake
   establishing, 7–13, 23
   reviewing, 17
   utilizing, 18

juice
   juice bars, 16, 48
   sugar in, 49

K

Kalamata Halibut, 226

Kashi
   cereal, 16, 34
   product list, 35
   waffles, 17, 28, 32

kidneys, 39

kitchen equipment and staples
   cleaning out the pantry, 25, 26–28
   essential kitchen equipment, 19–22, 39
   essential kitchen staples, 21

R

S

Spaghetti Squash with Roasted Garlic Pesto, 241

Zucchini Latkes, 268

staples for the kitchen, 21

Starbucks, 44, 69

steak

Ensalada with Charbroiled Steak and Salsa, 46

Pita Steak Sandwich with Dill Sauce, 151

Spicy Korean Rice with Flank Steak, 208

steak fries, 41

stew, 263

stir-fry

Broccoli-Halibut Stir-Fry, 220

Stir-Fried Asparagus and Peppers, 264

storage containers and bags, 20, 33

strategies for eating, xv

strawberries

Chocolate Angel Food Cake with Strawberries, 282

as snack, 17

Strawberry-Toasted Pecan Chicken Salad, 174

strength training, 58, 60

stress, 7, 27, 51

string cheese

Quick String Cheese Quesadillas, 152

as snack, 16, 29

Subway, 33, 44, 69

sugar

in juice, 49

in oatmeal, 35

and simple carbohydrates, 37

substitutions for, 33, 142 (*see also* Splenda)

Sunset Fish Skewers, 230

Sunset Fruit Skewers, 265

Super Size Me, 8, 43

sweet potatoes

Cheese Fries, 256

Roast Beef with Root Veggie Gravy, 204–5

Sweet Potato Casserole with Caramelized Bananas, 269

Sweet Potato Shepherd's Pie, 209–10

T

Taco Bell, 43, 44, 46

tacos

Breakfast Taco, 144

Light Beef Taco Wraps, 211

Turkey Tacos Fiesta, 218

Tea-Smoked Chicken, 212

television, 48

Tequila Chicken Fajitas, 213

teriyaki sauce, 22

Tiramisu, 302

Toasted Almond Green Beans, 266

toaster ovens, 20, 216

tofu, 286

Tofutti Cuties, 16

to-go boxes, 29, 41, 42

tomatoes

Arugula and Tomato Salad, 170

Seared Tuna on Heirloom Tomatoes, 157

tortilla chips, 33, 41

tortillas

Herb Turkey Wraps, 149

My Mom's Tortilla Casserole, 214–15

trainers, 19, 32, 55, 61

treadmills, 60

trigger foods and substitutions

week 1, 26

week 2, 33

week 3, 40

week 4, 46

week 5, 51

triglycerides, 15

tuna

as kitchen staple, 22

Seared Tuna on Heirloom Tomatoes, 157

Tuna Noodle Casserole, 245

Tuna Salad, 178

turkey

Cali Cheesesteak, 147

in Calorie Countdown, 38

Chilaquiles, 191

starting weight, 23, *24*

    target weight, 4–6, 17, 23, *24*

weight training, 58, 60

Weight Watchers, 6, 69

Wendy's, 44, 69

Wheat Thins, 16

white beans, 148

whole grains, 33, 37

whole-wheat crackers, 48

Whole-Wheat Pizza with Assorted Toppings,
    246–47

Wild Mushroom Manicotti, 248

Wilted Garlic Spinach, 267

wine

    substitutions for, 51

    Zinfandel-Poached Pears, 303

women and healthy body fat, 4

wooden kitchen utensils, 19

wraps

    Herb Turkey Wraps, 149

    Light Beef Taco Wraps, 211

Y

yoga, 61–62

yogurts

    Almonds and Yogurt Snack, 276

    carbohydrates in, 37

    and cereal, 34

    Chocolate-Banana Milkshake, 283

    as kitchen staple, 21

    Raspberry Frozen Yogurt, 299

    as snack, 16, 29, 48

    yogurt cheese, 215

Z

Zinfandel-Poached Pears, 303

zucchini

    Air-Fried Zucchini Sticks, 253

    Zucchini Latkes, 268